To our sons,
Mateo and Miles

Copyright © 2024 Diana Licalzi and Ashley Reaver
Published by Blue Star Press
PO Box 8835, Bend, OR 97708
contact@bluestarpress.com
www.bluestarpress.com

All rights reserved. No part of this publication may be reproduced or transmitted in any form or by any means, electronic or mechanical, including photocopy, recording, or any information storage and retrieval system, without permission in writing from the publisher. Trademarks of third parties are used for purposes of identification and information only, and no endorsement is claimed or suggested.

Photography by Roberto Alvarez unless otherwise noted. Stephanie Clark Burman (5th & Market Photography): page iv, Татьяна Ивашкова / Adobe Stock: page vi

Illustrations by Arctic Fever

Cover and interior design by Bryce de Flamand

ISBN: 9781958803967

Printed in Colombia

10 9 8 7 6 5 4 3 2 1

DISCLAIMER: This book is for informational and educational purposes. This book is not intended to be a substitute for the medical advice of a licensed physician. The reader should consult with their doctor in any matters relating to their health.

The information in this book is not intended to treat, diagnose, cure, or prevent disease. This book is not sponsored or endorsed by any organization or company. The information in this book is based on experience and research done by the authors. Neither the publisher nor the authors accept any liability of any kind for any damages caused, directly or indirectly, from the use of the information in this book.

The Postpartum Nutrition Cookbook

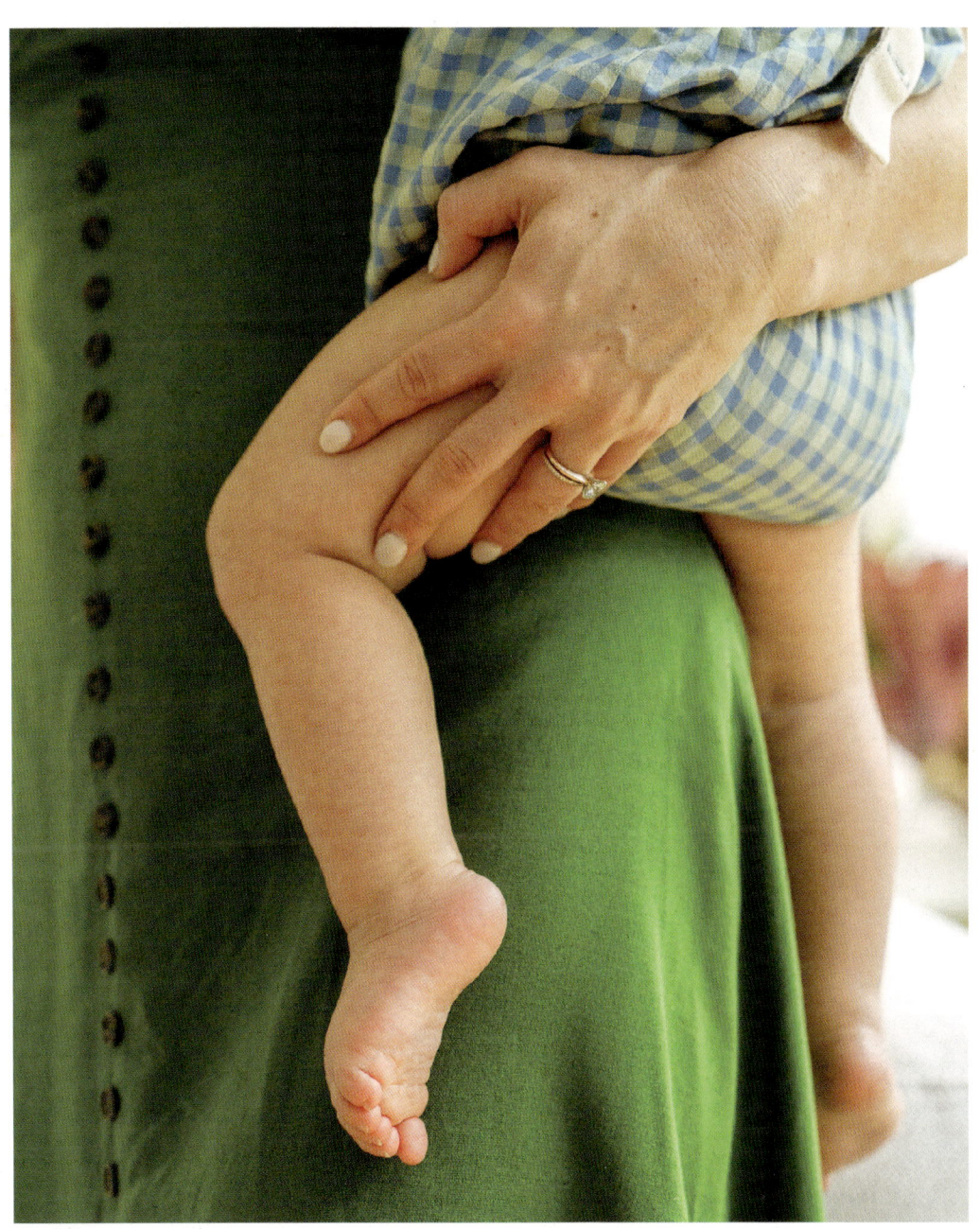

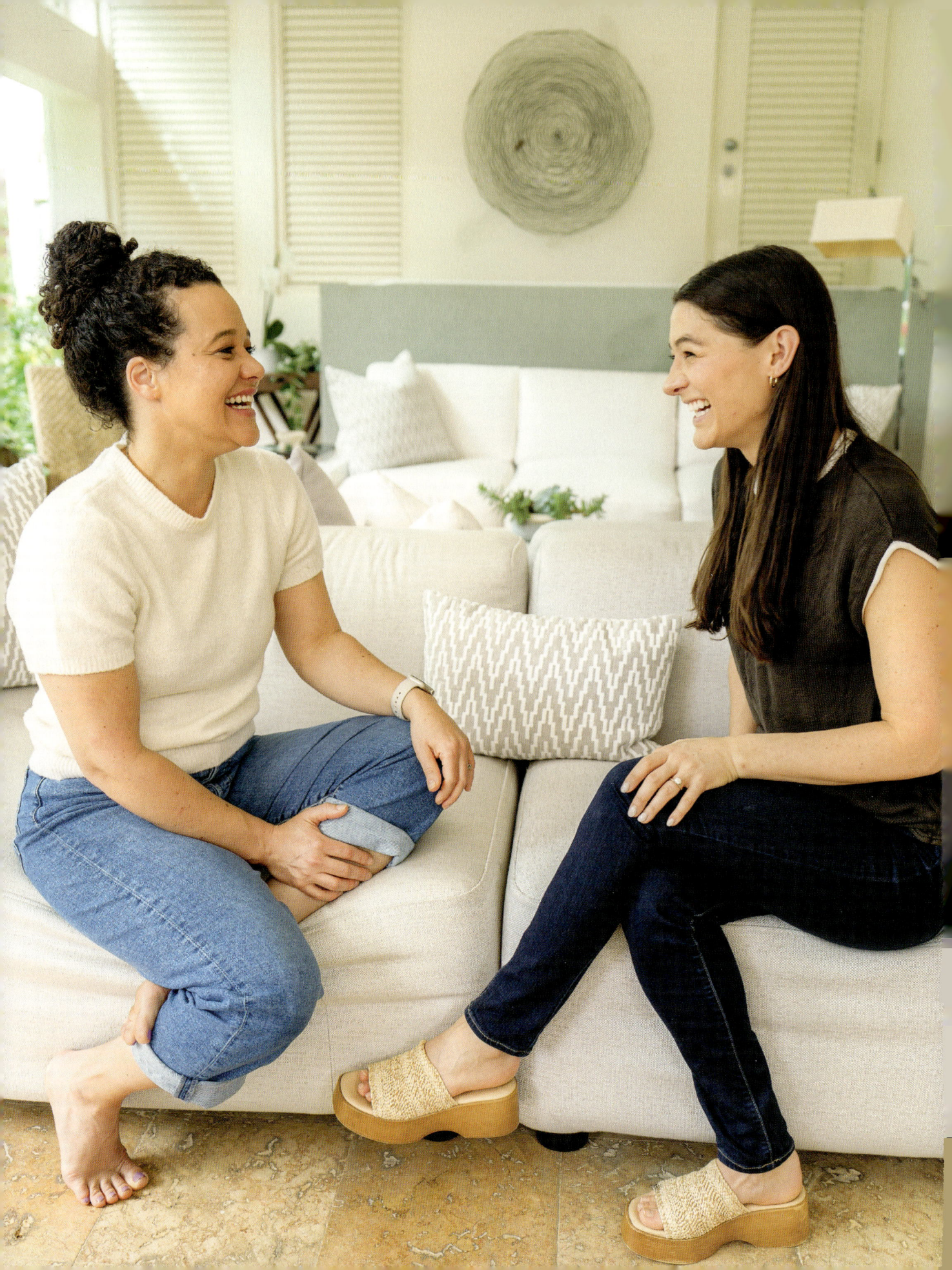

THE Postpartum Nutrition Cookbook

100+ Nourishing Recipes for New Moms

Registered dietitian nutritionists and mothers to little ones
DIANA LICALZI & ASHLEY REAVER

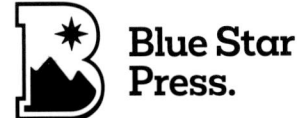
Blue Star Press.

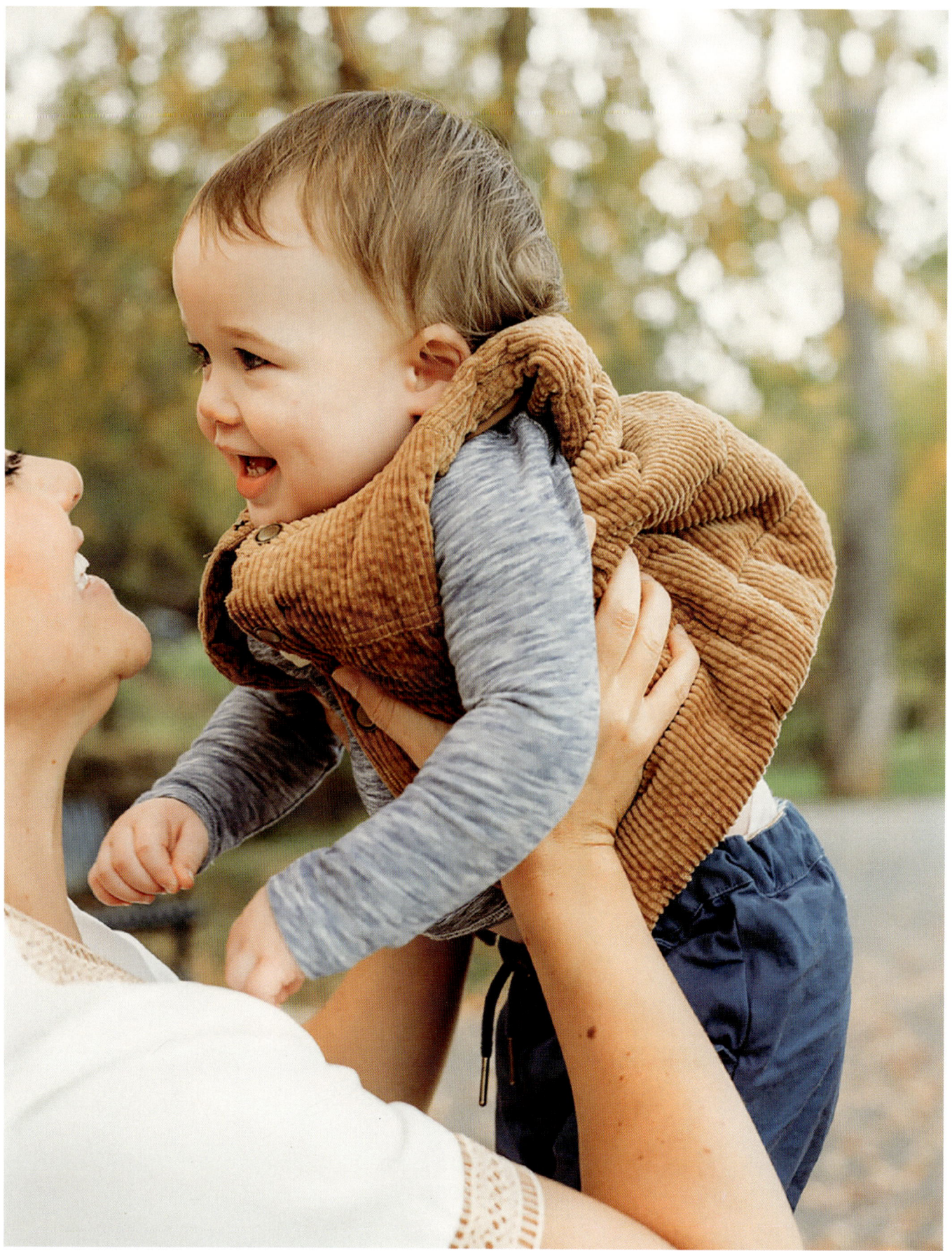

Contents

VII FOREWORD

IX INTRODUCTION

1 PART 1: NUTRITION FOR POSTPARTUM RECOVERY

3 CHAPTER 1: FROM PREGNANCY TO RECOVERY AND LACTATION

13 CHAPTER 2: NUTRITION THAT SUPPORTS POSTPARTUM RECOVERY AND BREASTFEEDING

39 PART 2: HOW TO GET STARTED

41 CHAPTER 3: HELPFUL TOOLS AND PANTRY STAPLES

45 CHAPTER 4: MEAL PLANNING AND PREPPING

55 PART 3: THE RECIPES

59 FREEZER MEALS

91 MAKE-AHEAD BREAKFASTS

117 ONE-HANDED LUNCHES

139 SET-IT-AND-FORGET-IT DINNERS

167 PANTRY MEALS

193 SNACKS AND DESSERTS

213 SMOOTHIES

225 MOCKTAILS AND MORE

246 APPENDIX I: PREPPING YOUR POSTPARTUM FREEZER

260 APPENDIX II: FIRST-WEEK-HOME MEAL PLAN

265 APPENDIX III: SAMPLE WEEKLY MEAL PLAN

270 INDEX

277 ACKNOWLEDGMENTS

278 ABOUT THE AUTHORS

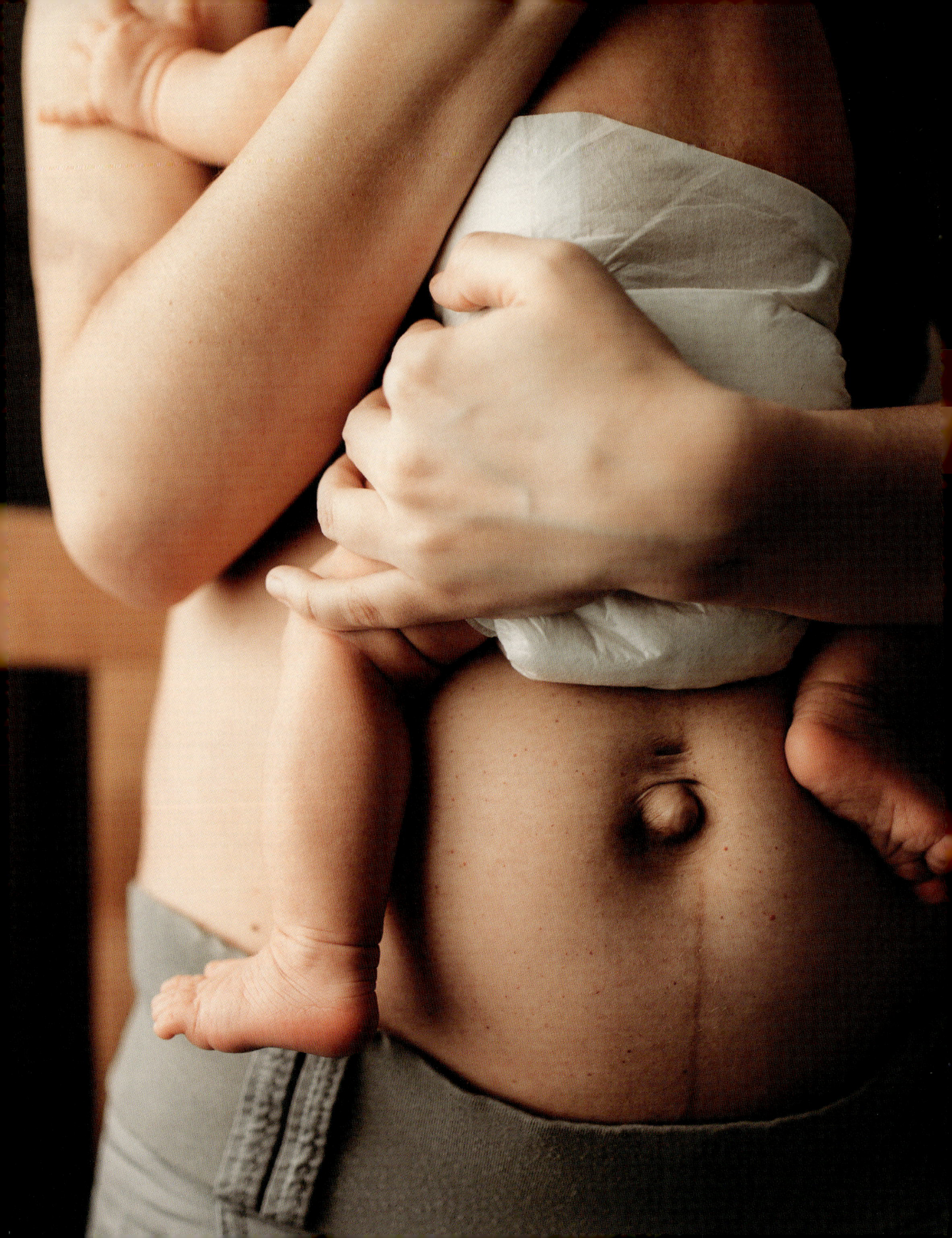

Foreword

As an OB/GYN, I am very excited to introduce this cookbook dedicated to postpartum nutrition. The postpartum period is a truly transformative time in a woman's life. It is marked by moments of overwhelming joy and unique challenges. Amidst the whirlwind of adjusting to life with a newborn, your body is also recovering from the remarkable feats of pregnancy, labor, and delivery. It is crucial not to overlook the importance of nourishing yourself while taking care of the new beautiful life that you created.

Many women feel that they are well-equipped to care for their baby's needs when leaving the hospital but ill-equipped to care for their own. Unlike their newborns, who have several doctor's appointments within the first few months following birth, new mothers typically only have one appointment six weeks after delivery. This appointment focuses primarily on your physical healing following labor and delivery, but there are many other important topics that may not be covered. I know that it is difficult to address every concern a new mother may have during this one postpartum visit.

Postpartum nutrition is an area that is often overlooked yet plays a critical role in supporting your physical recovery, mental well-being, and the demands of breastfeeding. With so many new responsibilities at home, it is easy to forget that your body also requires care. Many women focus on "bouncing back" to their pre-pregnancy bodies as quickly as possible, but the emphasis should be on providing your postpartum body with the right nutrients and hydration to support the recovery process.

This is why I am so excited about the *Postpartum Nutrition Cookbook*. It is a valuable resource for women as they prioritize their health and well-being following birth. Within these pages, you will find not only easy and delicious recipes but a guide for supporting your healing and breastfeeding journey. The detailed explanations of the body's changes during pregnancy, the labor and delivery process, and milk production help to highlight why nutrition is so critical for your postpartum journey.

The recipes are not only realistic for new moms to create but also provide the key nutrients that your body needs as it heals and adapts to the requirements of motherhood. I cannot overstate the importance of your self-care and proper nutrition during this time and hope this book serves as a reference as you embark on this incredible journey of motherhood.

Dr. Mary Margaret McGue
OB/GYN and mom of three

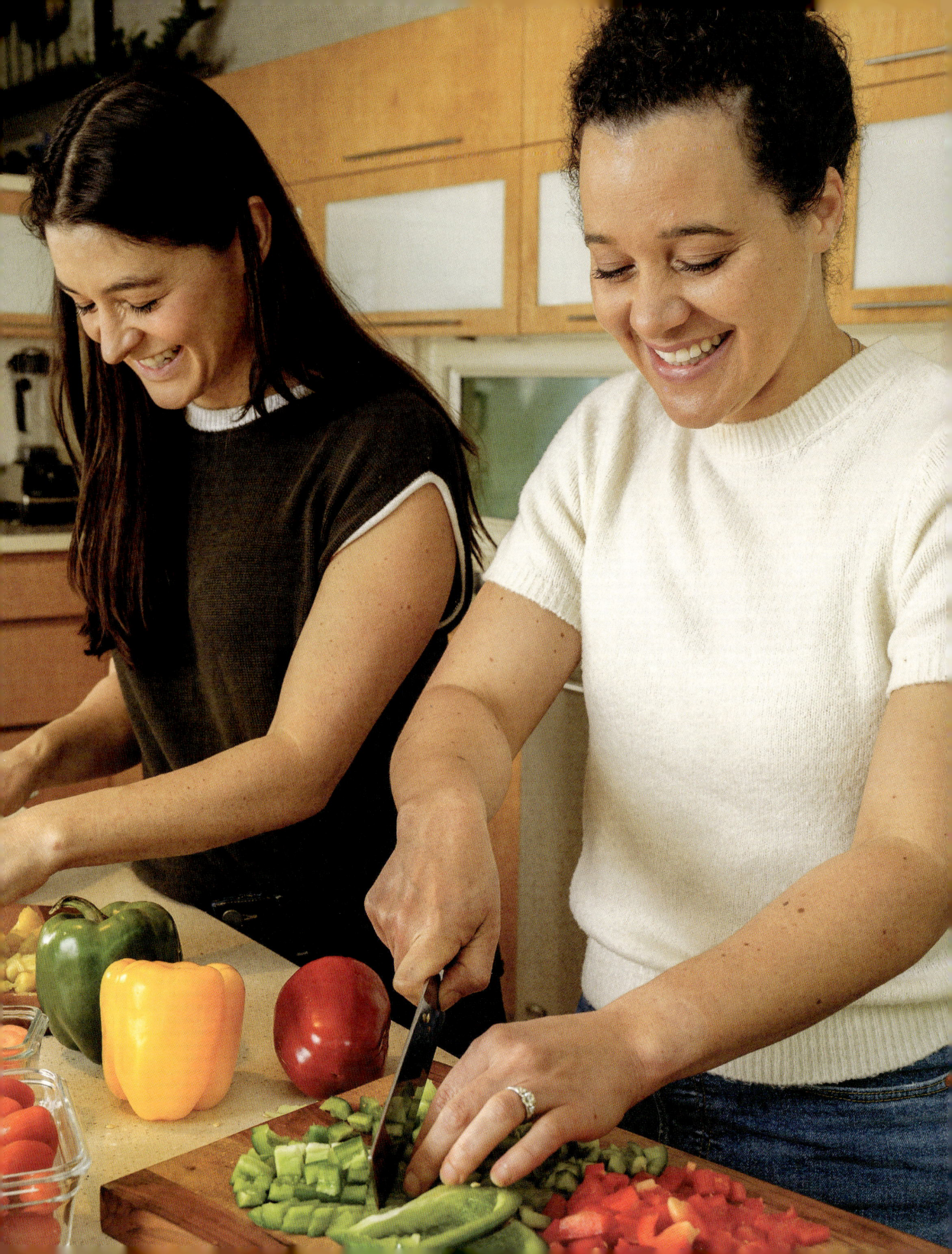

Introduction

Congratulations! If you've picked up this cookbook, you're likely preparing for the arrival of your baby, or perhaps you've recently welcomed your little one into the world. What a remarkable accomplishment. Your body has completed some miraculous feats to get you to this point, and while your baby rightly deserves all of your attention when they arrive, we also want to ensure that you, the extraordinary mama, are well taken care of.

We're Diana and Ashley—registered dietitians and moms to two beautiful baby boys, Mateo and Miles, respectively. We both earned our master's degrees in nutrition science and policy from Tufts University Friedman School of Nutrition, but our paths crossed in 2015 while working for a health analytics company in Boston. We immediately hit it off and have remained close, weathering big moves (Diana moved to Colorado and Ashley to California!), marriages, job changes, and all of life's ups and downs together. We even became moms around the same time, sharing the incredible journey of pregnancy and the postpartum period.

On our paths to become registered dietitians, we learned a lot of general nutrition information for pregnancy, but we couldn't recall much about postpartum nutrition. So, like many new moms, we found ourselves scrolling through Google for answers during our 2:00 a.m. feedings, only to be bombarded with questionable information—from detox plans to parasite cleanses to "hormone-balancing" diets. It left us both shocked and appalled at the scarcity of evidence-based guidance for new moms.

The void of information compelled us to create a comprehensive resource addressing the crucial role that nutrition plays in supporting your breastfeeding journey and the postpartum recovery process—whether you've given birth vaginally or via C-section. We created the resource that we so desperately wished we'd had during those initial postpartum months.

Of course, just knowing the information isn't always enough. Finding the time and energy to nourish yourself with a newborn to care for is no small feat. So, in crafting this resource, we included meal-prepping guidance, meal plans, grocery lists, advice on pantry staples, and over 120 recipes that support postpartum recovery and breastfeeding. Taking care of yourself should be as uncomplicated and achievable as possible during this incredible, yet challenging, time.

During pregnancy, so much focus is on preparation for labor and delivery, which is a relatively small amount of time (although it can feel like forever); on the other hand, the postpartum period often gets overlooked, even though it can last up to eighteen months. By diving into this book, you're taking a proactive step toward optimal recovery, successful breastfeeding, and flourishing as a new mom!

PART 1

Nutrition for Postpartum Recovery

In the first two chapters, we explore the incredible journey of growing, delivering, and breastfeeding a baby. In chapter 1, we'll touch on the transformational changes your body goes through during pregnancy, the exceptionally demanding feat of labor and delivery, the lengthy recovery process, and the efforts of milk production.

All of this sets the stage for chapter 2, where we explore the nutrients that are important for postpartum recovery and breastfeeding. At the end of the section, you'll find a comprehensive chart where you can quickly reference any nutrient to see its recommended daily amount and primary food sources. We also dispel many nutrition myths along the way!

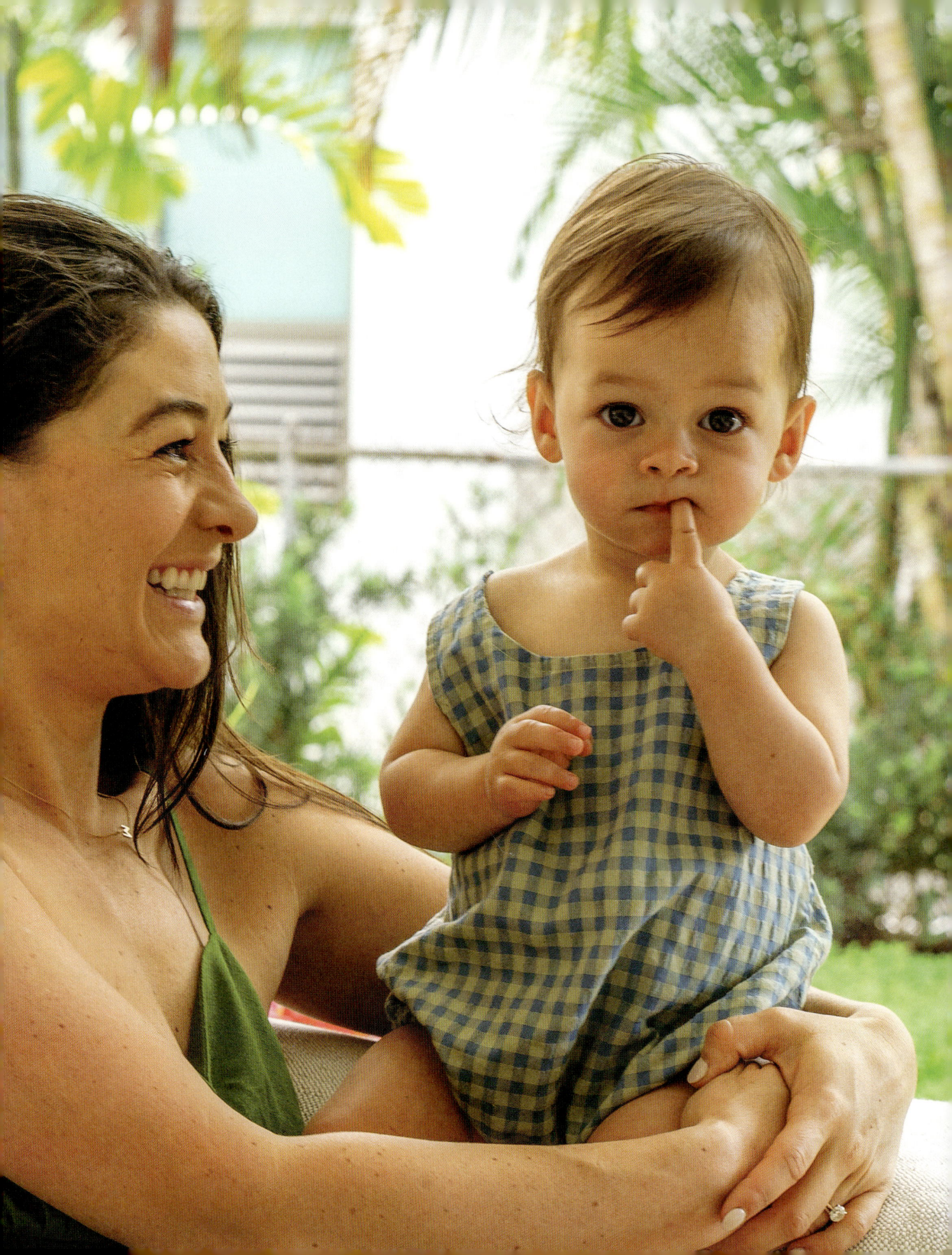

CHAPTER 1

From Pregnancy to Recovery and Lactation

In this chapter, we detail all the processes your body is going through, from pregnancy to recovery and lactation, so that you'll understand why your body's nutritional needs have changed and why they are too important to neglect during the postpartum phase.

Pregnancy

First, let's start with the nine-and-a-half-month journey during which your body provided all the building blocks to grow a human being. Stop for a moment and think about that—virtually everything (except for a teeny sperm carrying DNA) came from your body! Every facet of your baby's being, from the tips of their tiny toes to the crown of their head, was crafted from the nutrients within you. It's no wonder many nutrient requirements, including protein, folate, and iron, increase significantly during this time. Even the water within your baby's body originated from yours! It's truly a remarkable realization. And if you choose to breastfeed, this incredible connection will continue.

Throughout pregnancy, the body undergoes a multitude of physical changes to support the growth of a new human. It's a period where you grow an entirely new organ—the placenta—an incredible feat that occurs at no other stage of life. These extensive changes start from conception and impact various systems within your body, and many of them directly influence your nutritional requirements during pregnancy and the postpartum recovery period.

CARDIOVASCULAR SYSTEM

The cardiovascular system is an intricate network that circulates blood throughout your body. Its primary role is to supply your cells with the essential nutrients and oxygen they require while efficiently removing waste products. During pregnancy, we add an additional demand to the cardiovascular system: transporting nutrients and oxygen to a new organ (the placenta) and to your developing baby.

To accommodate these extra responsibilities, your blood volume significantly increases as your body works harder to nourish the growing baby. By the end of pregnancy, your blood volume can increase by up to 60%, resulting in three to four pounds of additional blood circulating through your body. To keep pace with the expanding blood volume, your body ramps up the production of new red blood cells—a key reason why your iron needs essentially double during pregnancy. Iron is crucial to making hemoglobin, a protein in red blood cells that carries oxygen to all the parts of the body.

Because your body requires more iron during this time, it naturally enhances its ability to absorb iron from the foods you consume. But these measures aren't enough—your iron intake must increase too. Iron requirements increase from 18 milligrams per day for premenopausal women to 27 milligrams per day during pregnancy. Toward the end of their nine-month development, your baby also stockpiles iron to meet the needs of their first six months of life.

With this increase in blood volume, your heart rate also increases to facilitate its circulation. More blood vessels develop, and you might notice variations in blood pressure or the effort your heart uses to move that blood. Furthermore, the physical size of your heart can also increase to more efficiently circulate blood.

RESPIRATORY SYSTEM
During pregnancy, the respiratory system provides the increased oxygen needed to sustain your growing baby and the developing placenta. Oxygen consumption increases by roughly 30%. Hemoglobin, the protein found in red blood cells that contains iron, transports the oxygen throughout the body, contributing to your drastically increased iron needs. You may notice you are breathing more rapidly and find yourself out of breath more often as your body strives to meet these enhanced oxygen demands, while your lungs and rib cage begin battling for space against your growing uterus.

DIGESTIVE SYSTEM
Your digestive system changes during pregnancy, reconfiguring itself to make room for the baby growing within your abdomen. This often leads to discomfort such as indigestion, constipation, and heartburn, which can influence your food choices and the frequency with which you eat. Fortunately, these usually subside shortly after delivery. The digestive tract also becomes more efficient at absorbing specific nutrients during pregnancy, such as calcium and iron, to meet your heightened needs.

BREAST TISSUE
During pregnancy, your breast tissue undergoes the last stage of maturation, gearing up for its vital role in milk production. You likely noticed these breast changes early in pregnancy, but the final weeks of pregnancy officially usher in the phase of providing milk to your baby, driven by shifts in your hormone levels. Breast tissue accounts for one to two of the additional pounds you've gained throughout pregnancy, and this extra breast tissue lingers until you are no longer breastfeeding. Your increased nutrition needs during pregnancy provide the building blocks for these tissue changes and will remain elevated during breastfeeding to support lactation.

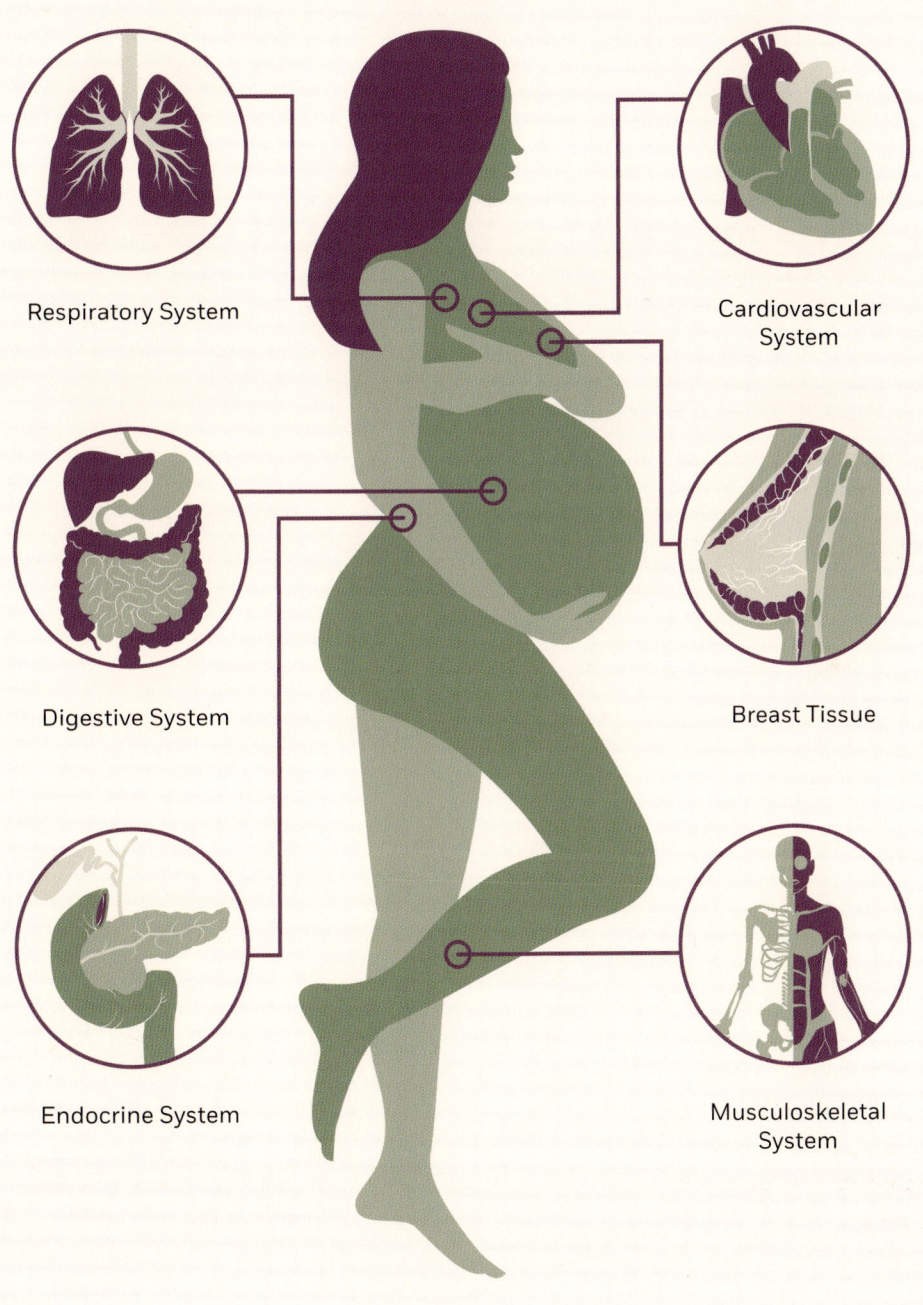

ENDOCRINE SYSTEM

Your endocrine system creates and regulates hormones, the body's chemical messengers that send signals through the bloodstream to tissues. The placenta, while just a temporary organ, acts as an endocrine gland, secreting large amounts of estrogen and progesterone. You may also have noticed transformations in your hair and nails—changes in hormones can make them grow faster and become stronger. Following childbirth, hormones fluctuate due to the delivery of the placenta, production of breast milk, and initiation of bonding with the baby, among other things. This can elicit a wide range of emotions for new moms, making the postpartum period a time that's often emotionally charged, to say the least.

MUSCULOSKELETAL SYSTEM

The tissues in your abdomen expand as the baby steadily progresses up toward your rib cage. Simultaneously, your bones shift in position to accommodate the growing baby and to prepare for the moment of birth. You may also lose bone mass in the final months of pregnancy, since your baby's calcium needs are highest during this time. Your digestive tract more than doubles the absorption of calcium from foods to help meet this demand, but the reservoir of calcium in your own bones can be used when diet is not enough. Any calcium lost from your bones can typically be regained during the postpartum period.

Muscles across your body, particularly those in the pubic region, adapt to the demands of pregnancy, while your skin is also stretched to its limits. The protein in your diet provides the essential components for collagen, the primary type of protein found in your body's connective tissues, such as skin and muscle.

After nine and a half incredible yet challenging months, it's time for the baby to arrive, marking the beginning of labor and delivery.

Labor and Delivery

The process of giving birth is so physically demanding that it is widely acknowledged as one of the most challenging ordeals a female will undergo in her lifetime. Whether you have a vaginal birth or a C-section, your tissues have a lot of repairing to do, and nutrition can help support this process. Let's take a moment to review the physical demands of labor and delivery to fully understand and appreciate the recovery process.

The average labor lasts twelve to twenty-four hours for a first baby, whereas subsequent births typically take eight to ten hours. During the first stage of labor, the body endures intense and frequent contractions of the uterine muscles to push the baby through the birth canal. The second stage is often referred to as the "pushing" stage, where the woman becomes actively involved in pushing the baby through the birth canal to the outside world. Pushing can last for hours and can be an intensely laborious and demanding undertaking. Lastly, the final stage of labor is the delivery of the placenta, which involves the passage of the placenta out of the uterus through the vagina.

The placenta leaves behind a roughly ten-inch wound (around the size of a dinner plate) inside of your uterus, which contributes to postpartum bleeding, known as lochia, and takes up to six weeks to heal.

In vaginal labor, the perineum, the area between the vagina and anus, may stretch, tear, or require an episiotomy (a surgical cut made at the opening of the vagina). This area often requires stitches and may remain sore during the several weeks it takes to heal. In contrast, a C-section involves major abdominal surgery to deliver the baby. During this procedure, an incision is made through seven layers of tissue, including the mother's abdominal wall and uterus, allowing direct access to the baby. The surgical incision and the manipulation of organs can cause major discomfort and pain, and the recovery period typically involves a longer hospital stay and more postoperative care.

Women usually lose about half a quart (500 mL) of blood during vaginal birth or about one quart (1,000 mL) after a C-section. Postpartum bleeding can span several weeks before gradually tapering off. Additionally, the pelvic floor muscles and the uterus, which stretch during pregnancy and contract during labor, need time to heal and regain their strength.

Both vaginal and C-section deliveries can result in physical exhaustion, dehydration, discomfort, and pain. However, it's crucial to recognize that the physical demands of childbirth often coincide with emotional and psychological challenges, too. These dual burdens highlight the remarkable resilience of the female body in adapting to these demands.

Recovery

After learning about the process of pregnancy, labor, and delivery, are you at all surprised that the American College of Obstetrics and Gynecology recommends waiting up to eighteen months between pregnancies? It takes significant time for the body to fully recuperate and prepare for another pregnancy. It's crucial to approach the postpartum recovery process with the seriousness that it deserves, especially when it spans nearly two years.

ACUTE RECOVERY (BIRTH TO SIX WEEKS)

Imagine this scenario. You've just completed an ultramarathon, undergone major abdominal surgery, or perhaps both. In the immediate aftermath of such an event, you'd likely prioritize rest, hydration, and nourishing food to support your recovery. However, after the unbelievable feat of delivering a baby, mothers generally experience sleep deprivation, heavy bleeding, dehydration, and poor nutrition. Emotionally, this phase can be demanding as well, as new mothers navigate fatigue, hormonal changes, and the trials and rigors of breastfeeding. In the United States, we don't treat the first few weeks after childbirth with the same reverence that we treat recovery from any other major physical trauma or surgical procedure, yet the body's needs are similar.

The postpartum period, particularly the first two weeks following delivery, mirrors the recovery process after surgery. Whether you've experienced a vaginal birth, with or without tearing, or a C-section, your body's tissues require significant repair and recuperation. Plus, after pregnancy, the separation of the placenta from the uterine wall leaves an internal wound, and eventual scab, that's roughly the size of a dinner plate, and the subsequent bleeding can last for weeks following delivery.

Wound healing has four distinct phases: hemostasis, inflammation, proliferation, and remodeling. During hemostasis, blood vessels in the wound area constrict to reduce blood flow and stop bleeding. Once blood loss has stopped, the inflammatory phase can start. During this phase, which lasts for several days, white blood cells and other inflammatory cells access the wound to clean it, clear away bacteria, and prepare it for new tissue growth. The nutrients that support the healing process—vitamin C, beta-carotene, and zinc—play a critical role during this inflammatory phase.

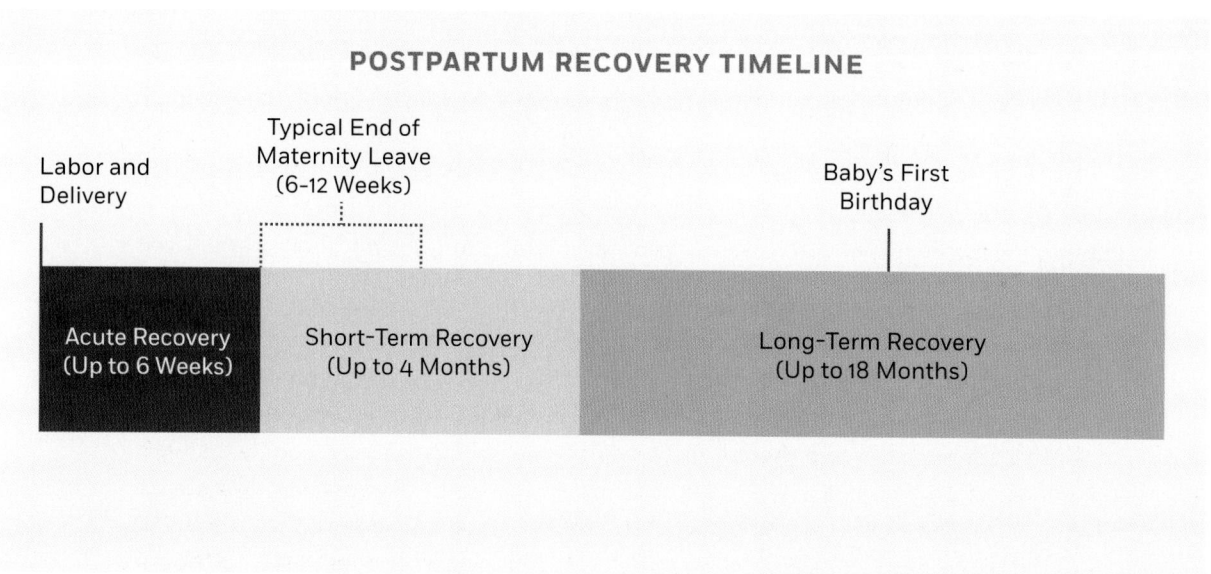

Over the next week, the wound starts the process of proliferation, where protein and calories are particularly important, along with vitamin C and zinc. In a process called angiogenesis, new blood vessels are created to replace those that were damaged. The body begins to produce collagen, making the scaffolding that will ultimately fill in to close the wound and return the tissue to normal function. The final remodeling phase can occur over months or years, depending on the severity of the wound. During this phase, collagen production continues to build the strength and elasticity of the tissue and skin.

The acute recovery postpartum period generally encompasses the first three phases of wound healing, as well as the initiation of the final remodeling phase (depending on the circumstances of birth). Acute recovery can last up to six weeks, which is why most women will schedule their first postnatal appointment around the six-week mark to monitor the progress of their healing. The intensity and duration of healing may be longer following a C-section, but the nutrition principles remain the same.

SHORT-TERM RECOVERY (FOURTH TRIMESTER)

The short-term recovery period, or the three-month period following birth, is commonly referred to as the fourth trimester. During this time, your uterus returns to its normal size, allowing your organs to return to their usual position. You may find yourself feeling less physical discomfort toward the end of this period.

Around this time, the focus also tends to shift from the healing associated with birth to regaining muscle mass and function, the demands of breastfeeding or pumping, hormonal fluctuations, and coping with exhaustion from frequent nighttime feedings and a disrupted sleep schedule. Hair typically starts to fall out around this time, and while it's hormone-driven, proper nutrition can help lessen the severity of hair loss. The fourth trimester is also when your body can start to replenish the nutrients that may have been depleted during the heightened demands of pregnancy.

After the fourth trimester, the general consensus in US culture is that you are "recovered," as maternity leave comes to an end. But while your bodily tissues may be returning to normal, the postpartum recovery is far from over. You might feel well enough to walk or do gentle exercise, especially if you're looking to rebuild the muscle mass and core strength that was lost during pregnancy and recovery. Remember, though, your body dedicated nine and a half months to growing a baby, and it will likely take that long, or longer, to feel completely like yourself again.

While your physical health is important, so is your mental health. Approximately 12% of women will experience postpartum depression (PPD), which typically starts one to three weeks after delivery and can last for several months. No single cause of PPD has been identified, but the increased risk of nutritional deficiencies caused by the high demands of pregnancy may play a role in the development of depressive symptoms. In particular, low levels of vitamin D and omega-3s, as well as overall poor diet quality, may be associated with PPD development. Research also suggests that at-home confinement increases the risk of PPD, which should encourage you to take walks as soon as you're cleared by your provider. Walking can not only help with your mental health, it can also help to regain your muscle mass.

LONG-TERM RECOVERY (UP TO EIGHTEEN MONTHS)
While we often think of postpartum recovery as the time immediately following childbirth, the long-term recovery period may last up to eighteen months. It's the longest, and perhaps the most difficult, stage in recovery to see or feel. The long-term recovery process, often referred to as the interpregnancy period, focuses on continuing to replenish the nutrients that your body provided to your growing baby and the gradual rebuilding of muscle mass. This period should optimize a woman's health between her pregnancies and for the remainder of her lifespan. During this phase, you may be engaging in more recreational activity, breastfeeding, addressing any lingering health issues from pregnancy, and (maybe!) even contemplating the possibility of another pregnancy.

Lactation

Because breastfeeding further increases many of our nutrient requirements, it's important to review the process of lactation. Throughout pregnancy, your body has been gearing up to become the sole food source for your new baby. The changes in breast tissue that we discussed earlier are now complete, and your breasts are ready to debut their new talent of milk making.

During the last weeks of pregnancy and the first few days after delivery, your body produces colostrum, a nutrient-dense milk that also provides antibodies to support your baby's immune system. Often called liquid gold, this is the first milk your baby will have when they start breastfeeding. Your body slowly transitions to produce mature milk over the next two weeks and will continue to provide mature milk throughout breastfeeding.

Breast milk is a complex and dynamic substance that provides all the necessary nutrients and components for a baby's growth and development up to six months of age. It changes based on your baby's needs. As your baby requires more energy and nutrients, you'll provide them through your milk. These nutrients are derived from your body's fat stores and from the foods you consume.

Milk production begins as nutrients enter into the cells of the breast's mammary glands. Inside the cells, amino acids are used to create proteins that are specific to milk and easily digested by your baby. Fatty acids are used to create triglycerides, the primary type of fat found in breast milk. Lastly, glucose is used to create galactose, which then binds with other glucose molecules to form lactose—the carbohydrate found only in milk. Protein, triglycerides, and lactose are excreted from the cells with other vitamins and minerals. They combine with water in what is called the milk space and, eventually, the fluid is expressed as milk.

Along with calories, protein, fat, and carbohydrates, breast milk also contains many other components required for growth and development, such as micronutrients, immune factors, hormones, digestive enzymes, and bioactive factors to support the baby's gastrointestinal health. All of these come from your body!

The female body goes through some impressive changes to support the growth and delivery of your little one. It's no wonder many nutrient requirements skyrocket during pregnancy, and they don't stop there. If you choose to breastfeed, many of your nutritional needs increase even more for the first year. Nutrition plays an important role during the acute recovery period, the six weeks immediately following birth, as well as the long-term process that can take up to eighteen months. We'll dive into all of your specific nutritional needs in the next chapter.

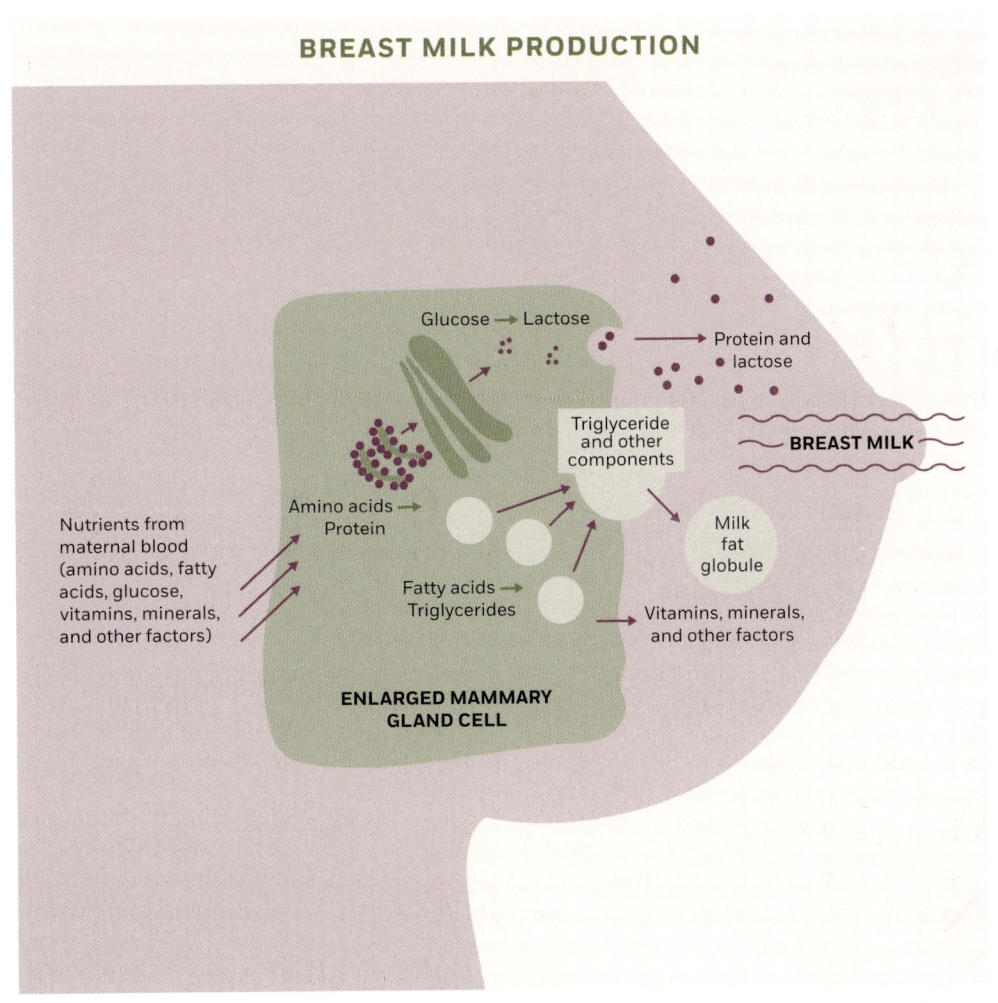

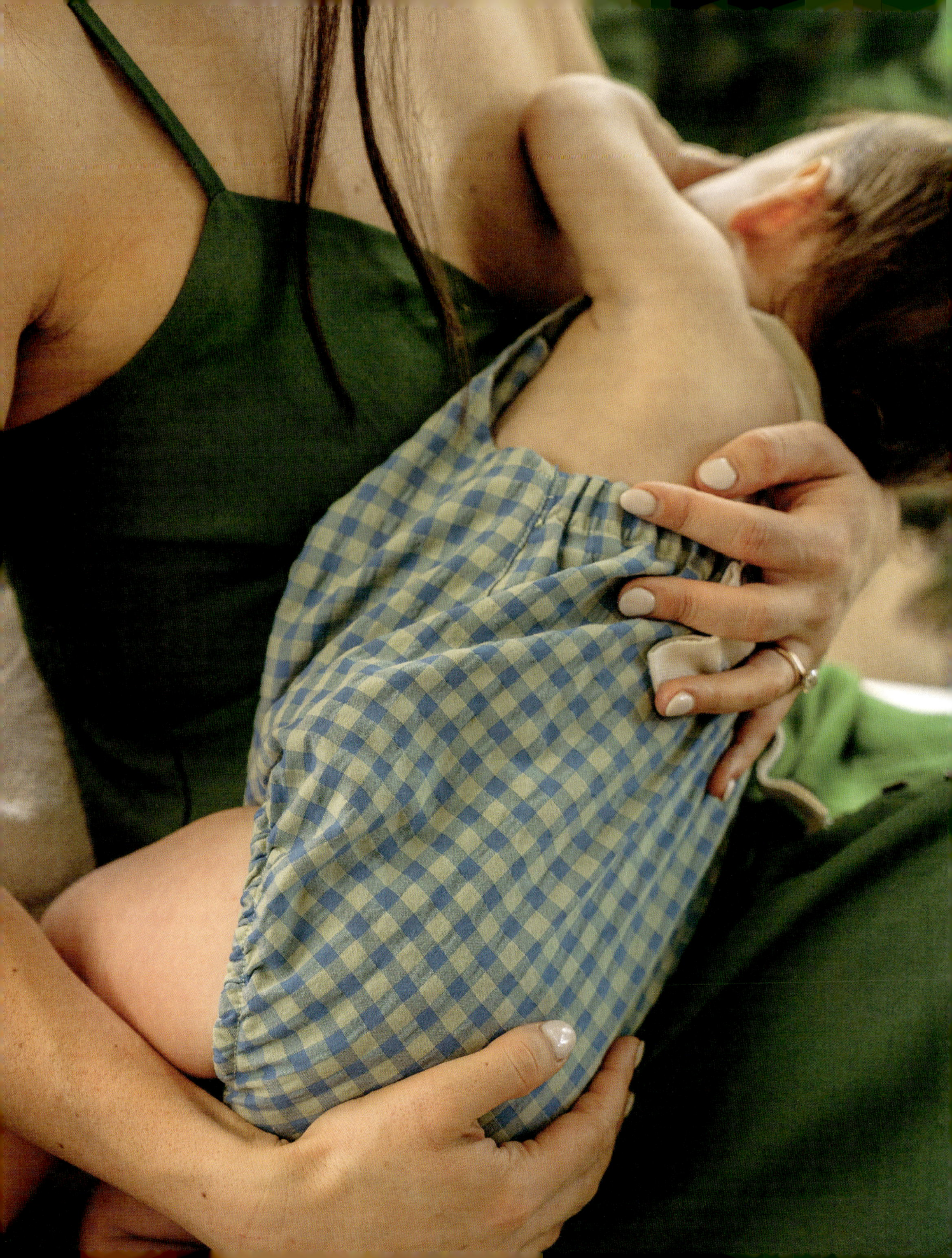

CHAPTER 2

Nutrition That Supports Postpartum Recovery and Breastfeeding

We were inspired to write this book because we couldn't find a comprehensive resource on nutrition for postpartum recovery and breastfeeding while we were navigating this time. There are no official guidelines for acute postpartum recovery. Our recommendations are based on nutrition guidelines for recovery from other major surgeries or injuries. So we are very excited to present what we think is the most comprehensive guide on this topic!

Throughout pregnancy and the first year of breastfeeding, your nutritional needs increase, putting you at a higher risk of not meeting them. Fortunately, a balanced diet with the help of supplements (such as prenatal vitamins) can help to meet this increased demand. This chapter explores the vital nutrients that contribute to postpartum recovery and healthy breastfeeding. If you feel overwhelmed, don't worry—we've included a high-level summary of the most important nutrients that many women fall short on. You can also find the full version at the end of the chapter, where you can reference any nutrient to find its recommended amount and primary food sources.

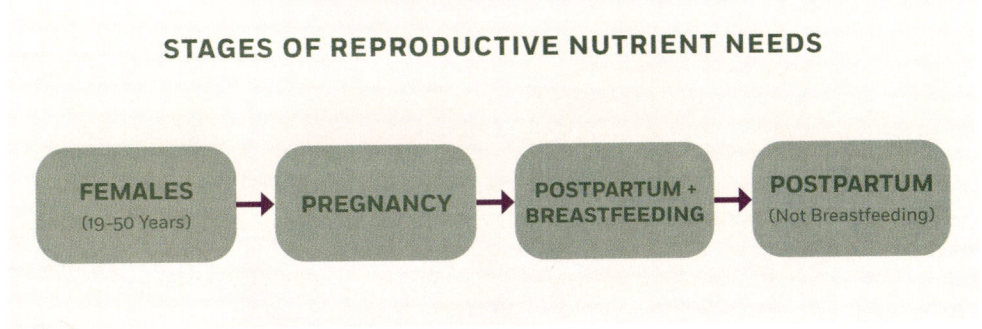

NUTRIENT NEEDS FOR POSTPARTUM RECOVERY

NUTRIENTS	POSTPARTUM + BREASTFEEDING	POSTPARTUM (NOT BREASTFEEDING)
CALORIES*	Acute: 30–35 kcal/kg + an additional 330 per day Long-term: 25–30 kcal/kg + an additional 330–400 per day	Acute: 30–35 kcal/kg Long-term: 25–30 kcal/kg
CARBOHYDRATES	At least 210 g/day + additional based on activity	Acute: at least 175 g/day Long-term: at least 130 g/day + additional based on activity
PROTEIN**	1.3–1.5 g/kg	Acute: 1.3–1.5 g/kg Long-term: 1.0–1.5 g/kg to encourage continued regain of muscle mass
OMEGA-3S	1.3 g/day	1.1 g/day
VITAMIN A	1,300 mcg RAE/day	Acute: 1,300 mcg RAE/day Long-term: 700 mcg RAE/day
VITAMIN C	Acute: 250 mg/day Long-term: 120 mg/day	Acute: 250 mg/day Long-term: 75 mg/day
CHOLINE	550 mg/day	425 mg/day
IODINE	290 mcg/day	150 mcg/day
IRON	Acute: 18 mg/day or recommended level from doctor based on hemoglobin level Long-term: 9 mg/day until menstrual cycle resumes, then increase to 18 mg/day	Acute: 18 mg/day or recommended level from doctor based on hemoglobin level
ZINC	12 mg/day	8 mg/day

Acute = first six weeks, Long-term = up to eighteen months

*These are rudimentary and easy formulas to calculate your calorie needs. If you are active, multiply this number by:
    1.375 if you are lightly active, 1.55 if you are moderately active, 1.725 if you are very active

Note: To calculate your weight in kilograms divide your body weight in pounds by 2.2.

** If you are very active, your protein needs may be as high as 1.7 g/kg.

Calories and Carbohydrates

ROLE IN THE BODY

Calories provide the energy needed by every cell in the body. Without calories, the body wouldn't be able to carry out the basic processes needed to live. Calories come from three main components (or macronutrients) of food: carbohydrates, protein, and fat. Alcohol also contributes calories. Carbohydrates should make up the largest portion of the diet, as they provide the body with glucose, the preferred energy source of the brain and every cell in the body. It's incredibly difficult to meet our energy needs without consuming adequate carbohydrates.

IMPORTANCE DURING POSTPARTUM RECOVERY

During the postpartum period, the body requires additional energy to rebuild the tissue needed to heal wounds from childbirth. Guidelines recommend consuming 30 to 35 calories per kilogram of body weight during the acute recovery phase to meet these heightened energy needs. An inadequate calorie and carbohydrate intake can slow wound healing and lead to muscle breakdown. One of the primary roles of carbohydrates is to prevent protein, particularly from our muscles, from being used as an energy source, especially during this time of healing. In addition, consuming carbohydrates stimulates the release of insulin, an anabolic hormone that is integral in many processes required for tissue growth and repair.

> To calculate your body's caloric needs, first convert your body weight to kilograms. To do this, simply divide by 2.2.
> Ex: 150 lb / 2.2 = 68 kg

> Next, multiply your weight in kilograms by 30–35.
> Ex: 68 kg × 30–35 = 2,040–2,380 calories

> So, a 150-pound woman needs 2,040 to 2,380 calories per day during acute recovery.

Calorie needs outside of the acute recovery period decrease back to normal levels for healthy adults. The recommendation is to consume 25 to 30 calories per kilogram of body weight. This number is the minimum baseline for those with a healthy body weight and increases with any physical activity. But remember, there's no one-size-fits-all answer, and your needs will vary based on many factors, so please adjust as needed.

IMPORTANCE DURING BREASTFEEDING

Breastfeeding is a remarkable and demanding journey that utilizes a significant amount of energy and calories. It's common to experience increased hunger, particularly during nighttime feedings. Most breastfeeding moms need an extra 500 calories a day to support the energy needs required for milk production. However, not all of those calories need to come from food.

In the first six months postpartum, the Dietary Guidelines for Americans suggests adding an additional 330 calories per day from food. The remaining 170 calories will come from body fat stores developed during pregnancy and will help you return to prepregnancy body weight. After six months, your calorie needs increase to an additional 400 calories per day as the baby requires more calories from both breast milk and food.

SOURCES

Most foods contain calories, and many foods are good sources of carbohydrates, including grains, legumes, fruit, vegetables, and some dairy products. We encourage you to consume the majority of your calories from foods that are also dense in the nutrients listed throughout this chapter.

Fiber

ROLE IN THE BODY

Fiber is a type of carbohydrate naturally found in plant foods that the body can't digest. It has a wide range of health-supporting roles, including regulating blood sugar and cholesterol levels and aiding in healthy bowel movements. Fiber also increases satiety after meals and supports a healthy body weight. What's more, fiber serves as a food source for the healthy bacteria in our gut. Eating enough fiber helps to maintain a healthy environment in our digestive tract.

IMPORTANCE DURING POSTPARTUM RECOVERY

In the initial weeks postpartum, constipation is quite common. Adequate intake of fiber, coupled with proper hydration, lubricates the gut and promotes natural elimination. It also reduces the downward pressure required for elimination, which is especially helpful while the pelvic floor and abdominal muscles recover.

IMPORTANCE DURING BREASTFEEDING

Fiber is not an essential nutrient specifically for breastfeeding; however, all women should consume 25 to 36 grams of fiber or more per day for overall health.

SOURCES

Good sources of fiber include whole grains, legumes, fruit, vegetables, nuts, and seeds.

PROBIOTICS AND GUT HEALTH

Pre- and probiotics have risen in popularity over the last few years; however, research does not conclusively demonstrate the health benefits of such supplements (outside of very specific clinical diagnoses). This is why the American Gastroenterological Association does not recommend the widespread use of probiotics. Consuming enough fiber is one of the best ways to support good gut health.

Protein

ROLE IN THE BODY

Most people are familiar with protein's role in muscle, but few know that it's also needed to strengthen bones and connective tissue. In addition, protein is required for the transportation of compounds in the body, the formation of hormones, the production of antibodies in our immune system, fluid regulation, and the production of enzymes.

IMPORTANCE DURING POSTPARTUM RECOVERY

Vaginal tears, episiotomies, C-sections, placenta wounds, and other aspects of pregnancy and childbirth all require healing during the postpartum period. Protein is so essential to wound healing that the requirements increase to 1.3 to 1.5 grams of protein per kilogram of body weight during acute recovery.

Protein needs remain elevated to between 1.0 and 1.5 grams per kilogram as the body continues to heal and muscle mass is regained throughout the long-term recovery phase. Light to moderate resistance training is also essential to regain muscle mass. Your protein needs may go up to 1.7 grams per kilogram if you are very active.

> To calculate your protein needs, first convert your body weight to kilograms. To do this, simply divide by 2.2.
> Ex: 150 lb / 2.2 = 68 kg
>
> Next, multiply your weight in kilograms by 1.3–1.5.
> Ex: 68 kg × 1.3–1.5 = 88–102 g
>
> So, a 150-pound woman needs roughly 88 to 102 grams of protein per day.

Collagen—a structural protein found in the body's connective tissues, such as skin, tendons, cartilage, and bone—provides strength and elasticity to these tissues. In the proliferative phase of wound healing, collagen serves as the scaffolding for the growth of new tissue and facilitates the formation of blood vessels. As the healing progresses into the remodeling phase, collagen continues to strengthen the healed tissue, improving its structure and contributing to the formation of scars and the overall integrity of the tissue. This phase typically starts around two weeks post-injury and can extend for a year. Remodeling requires sufficient protein, calories, vitamin C, and zinc intake to facilitate collagen production, tissue recovery, and regaining full function.

IMPORTANCE DURING BREASTFEEDING

Protein needs also increase during breastfeeding, primarily to support the baby's growth and development. Breast milk is rich in protein, which is crucial for an infant's

Collagen Supplements: Fact or Fiction?

The body produces collagen from amino acids—the building blocks of protein—along with vitamin C and zinc. While collagen supplements are popular, there is not much scientific evidence to show they speed up wound healing. Collagen supplements, like any other protein, cannot be directly absorbed into our bodies. The collagen must be broken down into amino acids that are then absorbed within the digestive tract. Once absorbed, our body uses these amino acids to create various proteins (not necessarily collagen). A diet rich in protein, vitamin C, and zinc is the best way to ensure natural collagen production.

---

rapid growth, brain development, and overall health. To meet the increased protein demands, the body requires additional dietary protein to ensure it doesn't utilize its own protein stores.

Breastfeeding women need roughly 1.3 grams of protein per kilogram of body weight per day. However, some studies suggest that consuming at least 1.5 grams of protein per kilogram of body weight per day is a more optimal intake, especially if you are regularly exercising.

SOURCES
Animal-based sources of protein include beef, poultry, fish, shellfish, eggs, yogurt, and cottage cheese, while plant-based protein sources include lentils, beans, and soy products (tofu, soy milk, edamame, tempeh). Nuts, seeds, and whole grains also provide smaller amounts of protein.

Fat and Omega-3s

ROLE IN THE BODY
Fat is a significant energy source in the diet and the most efficient way to store energy (which is one reason we gain six to eight pounds of fat during pregnancy). Beyond providing energy, fat insulates our body from the cold and protects our internal organs. It's also required for the absorption of four essential fat-soluble vitamins: A, D, E, and K. Additionally, dietary fats provide essential fatty acids such as omega-3 and omega-6, integral components of every cell in our body. There are three main omega-3 fatty acids: alpha-linolenic acid (ALA), eicosapentaenoic acid (EPA), and docosahexaenoic acid (DHA). Notably, DHA plays a remarkably vital role in the developmental processes of the baby's brain, retina, and nervous system during pregnancy and infancy.

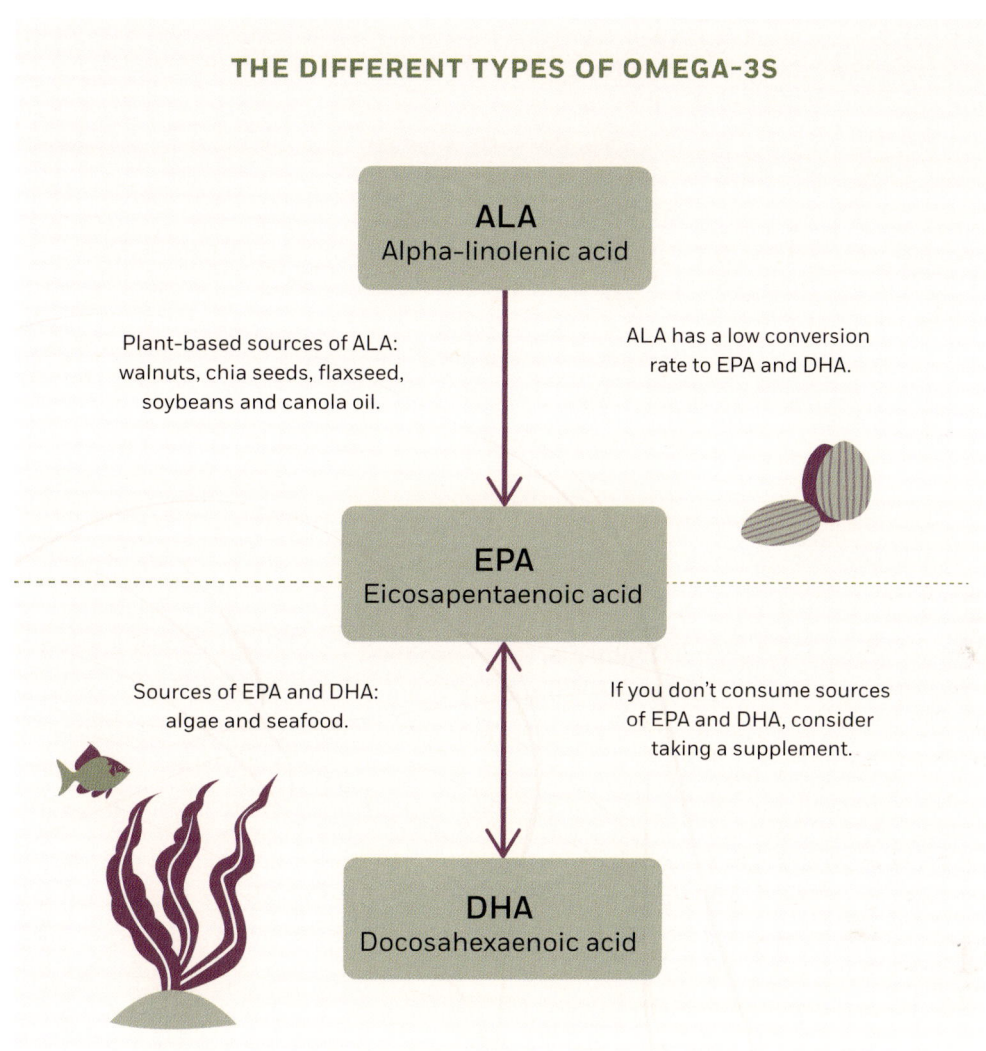

IMPORTANCE DURING POSTPARTUM RECOVERY

During the postpartum period, fat provides a concentrated source of energy for the body to use while recovering from pregnancy and childbirth and adjusting to the demands of caring for a newborn. Adequate fat intake also prevents protein, particularly from our muscles, from being used as an energy source. Failing to eat enough fat can contribute to low energy availability and slow wound healing. Notably, omega-3 fatty acids may also help to reduce the incidence, severity, and duration of postpartum depression.

IMPORTANCE DURING BREASTFEEDING

Similar to its role in postpartum recovery, fat also provides energy for breastfeeding. What's more, omega-3 fatty acids are transferred to the baby through breast milk. Ensuring an adequate intake of omega-3 fatty acids, especially DHA, is essential for promoting optimal development in infants.

SOURCES
Sources of healthy fats include fatty fish, avocados, nuts, seeds, and olive oils. EPA and DHA are found in fatty fish, including salmon, tuna, mackerel, and trout. ALA is found in plant oils, such as chia, flaxseed, soybean, and canola oils; chia seeds; hemp seeds; flaxseed; and walnuts. While ALA can be converted into EPA and then to DHA, the conversion is quite poor. For individuals on a vegan diet or those who don't eat fish, opting for an algae-based DHA supplement may be necessary.

MERCURY IN FISH
You can avoid potential mercury or contaminant exposure from fish by limiting varieties with higher mercury levels, such as pike, marlin, mackerel, tilefish, and swordfish.

Vitamin A

ROLE IN THE BODY
Vitamin A exists in two main forms: preformed vitamin A retinoids, such as retinol, which are found in animal products, and provitamin A carotenoids, such as beta-carotene, found in plant-based foods. Preformed vitamin A is readily usable by the body, while carotenoids need to be converted into the active form of vitamin A. A diverse diet will ensure that vitamin A needs are met, as deficiencies are quite rare in the United States.

Vitamin A has many functions in the body, including developing and maintaining tissues and vision, and it also supports the immune system. It is crucial for fetal development, turning generic stem cells into specialized tissues such as cardiovascular tissue, digestive tissue, and skin. As a fat-soluble nutrient, it also requires fat for absorption.

IMPORTANCE DURING POSTPARTUM RECOVERY
Vitamin A contributes to the body's natural wound-healing processes by supporting tissue repair and regeneration. It also maintains the health of the skin and mucous membranes. Notably, the form of vitamin A found in plants, beta-carotene, assumes a critical role in the body's antioxidant defense network, helping to support the inflammatory phase of wound healing.

IMPORTANCE DURING BREASTFEEDING
The demand for vitamin A nearly doubles during breastfeeding, as infants rely on their mothers for this essential nutrient during their initial six months of life. Ensuring an adequate intake of vitamin A is crucial for breastfeeding mothers and infants.

SOURCES
Preformed vitamin A is highest in liver, fish, eggs, and dairy products. Provitamin A forms, meanwhile, are found in leafy greens and red, orange, and yellow fruit and vegetables such as mangoes, cantaloupe, apricots, sweet potatoes, carrots, butternut squash, and pumpkin.

HOW MUCH IS TOO MUCH?
Overconsumption of preformed vitamin A in food and supplemental form may be toxic. Never exceed a level of 3,000 mcg or 10,000 IU per day.

B Vitamins

ROLE IN THE BODY
B vitamins are a category of eight vitamins involved in energy metabolism—the conversion of energy from food into a form of energy that our cells can use. They all have other specific functions as well, ranging from red blood cell formation and neurotransmitter production to DNA synthesis. You may have heard of many of them: thiamin (B1), riboflavin (B2), niacin (B3), pantothenic acid (B5), vitamin B6, biotin (B7), folate (B9), and vitamin B12.

IMPORTANCE DURING POSTPARTUM RECOVERY
Although all B vitamins play crucial roles in postpartum recovery, B6 and B12 contribute significantly to replenishing blood loss from labor and after delivery. Vitamin B6 facilitates the synthesis of hemoglobin (a protein in red blood cells), while vitamin B12 supports the proper formation of red blood cells.

Biotin Supplements: Fact or Fiction?

Popular hair, skin, and nail supplements are often recommended to counteract postpartum hair loss. Our take: save your money! During pregnancy, increased levels of estrogen prolong the growth phase of hair, leading to thicker and fuller hair. After giving birth, hormone levels drop significantly, and the hair shifts into the shedding phase, with noticeable hair loss typically starting a few months after childbirth. No supplement, biotin-containing or not, will stop postpartum hair loss. While a biotin deficiency can lead to hair loss, such deficiencies are incredibly rare given how little biotin we need and how abundant it is in food. Focusing on a proper diet with adequate calories and protein is a more effective way of lessening the severity of postpartum hair loss.

IMPORTANCE DURING BREASTFEEDING

During lactation, your body needs more of all the B vitamins, with the exceptions of thiamin, niacin, and folate. Folate needs are elevated in pregnancy due to the development of the baby's neural tube that eventually becomes the brain and spinal cord.

SOURCES

Most plant and animal-based foods contain high amounts of B vitamins, except for B12, which is exclusively found in animal products. Optimal sources are whole foods, as B vitamins may degrade with high levels of processing. Fortified foods, especially grain-based products, can also serve as good sources of B vitamins.

PLANT-BASED DIETS AND B12

Mothers following strict vegetarian or vegan diets should take B12 supplements. Consult with your healthcare provider.

Vitamin C

ROLE IN THE BODY

Fun fact: Did you know that most animals can produce their own vitamin C and therefore don't need to consume it? Humans and fruit bats are two of the only animals that rely on their diet for this essential nutrient. Hence the name "fruit" bats—they get their vitamin C from fruit! Vitamin C acts as an antioxidant, supports the immune system, aids in iron absorption, and contributes to collagen synthesis for skin, bones, and connective tissues.

IMPORTANCE DURING POSTPARTUM RECOVERY

Along with adequate protein and zinc, vitamin C is needed to create collagen for wound healing following a vaginal or C-section delivery. Collagen production remains particularly important through the first year of postpartum as tissues continue to recover. What's more, during the recovery process, vitamin C also acts as an antioxidant, helping to support the inflammatory phase of wound healing.

IMPORTANCE DURING BREASTFEEDING

Vitamin C needs increase by almost 50% during breastfeeding, as this essential nutrient is vital to the baby's immune system and the formation of healthy skin, bones, and blood vessels.

SOURCES

Fruits and vegetables are the best sources of vitamin C. Vitamin C-rich foods include citrus fruits, kiwis, strawberries, and certain vegetables such as red and green bell peppers, broccoli, Brussels sprouts, and cabbage. It is important to incorporate raw or very minimally cooked fruits and vegetables into your diet, as vitamin C degrades with extended heat exposure. If you plan to rely heavily on freezer meals during postpartum, be sure to add fresh sources of vitamin C. (We've included suggestions with all of our freezer meals.)

Vitamin E

ROLE IN THE BODY
Like vitamin A, vitamin E is a fat-soluble nutrient that requires fat for absorption. Vitamin E's primary role in the body is as part of the antioxidant defense network, specifically protecting the outer layer of our cells from damage caused by oxidative stress. It works with the support of vitamin C to stop the production of free radicals (unstable molecules that can cause cellular damage). Vitamin E also supports immune function, plays a role in preventing platelet aggregation, and dilates blood vessels.

IMPORTANCE DURING POSTPARTUM RECOVERY
The requirements for vitamin E remain the same as for non-pregnant women throughout pregnancy and postpartum recovery.

IMPORTANCE DURING BREASTFEEDING
Vitamin E needs increase by 25% during lactation. As with many other vitamins, this increased requirement is to compensate for the amounts secreted into breast milk.

SOURCES
Vitamin E is found in many plant foods, especially those that contain fat. Wheat germ, sunflower oil, and safflower oil are among the best sources. Sunflower seeds, almonds, hazelnuts, and peanuts are also good sources.

Vitamin D

ROLE IN THE BODY
Vitamin D helps the body absorb calcium from the digestive tract. When calcium levels in the blood are low, the inactive form of vitamin D that is stored in the body is converted to the active form and signals the digestive tract to absorb more calcium from foods. Therefore, a deficiency in vitamin D can lead to a lower absorption of calcium and subsequent lower calcium availability in the body. During pregnancy and breastfeeding, adequate vitamin D and calcium are incredibly important for growing your baby's bones and teeth. As a fat-soluble nutrient, vitamin D requires fat for absorption.

IMPORTANCE DURING POSTPARTUM RECOVERY
Vitamin D remains important in the postpartum period, as it ensures that your body will absorb sufficient calcium to maintain bone mineral density. Adequate levels of vitamin D postpartum have also been linked to a decreased incidence of, and faster recovery from, postpartum depression.

IMPORTANCE DURING BREASTFEEDING
Breast milk alone does not provide infants with sufficient vitamin D, which becomes crucial shortly after birth. To prevent a deficiency, the Dietary Guidelines for Americans and the American Academy of Pediatrics suggest supplementing breastfed or partially breastfed infants with 400 IU of vitamin D daily, starting within the first few days of life. Breastfeeding mothers may also supplement with vitamin D in order to provide an adequate amount through breast milk. Studies suggest that substantial doses of 6,000 IU or more are needed. Prolonged exclusive breastfeeding without vitamin D supplementation can cause rickets in infants.

SOURCES
Vitamin D is naturally found in only a handful of foods. Fatty fish, including trout, salmon, tuna, and mackerel, as well as fish liver oils, are notable sources. Fortified foods, including orange juice, milk, and some cereals, may also be good sources. Additionally, exposing the skin to sunlight triggers the body's production of vitamin D. However, factors such as age, limited sun exposure, sunscreen use, and geographic location can hinder the body's ability to generate an adequate amount.

Calcium

ROLE IN THE BODY
Bone mineralization and maintenance is perhaps the most well-known function of calcium, but it is also involved in blood clotting, the transmission of nerve impulses, and voluntary and involuntary muscle contractions. During pregnancy, calcium is used to form the baby's bones and teeth. Did you know that babies have all of their baby teeth when they are born? It just takes them a few months to pop through the gums.

IMPORTANCE DURING POSTPARTUM RECOVERY
During postpartum healing, any calcium lost from your bones can be regained by eating enough to meet your needs.

IMPORTANCE DURING BREASTFEEDING
Interestingly, dietary calcium needs do not increase during pregnancy and lactation. Instead, the body increases its absorption of calcium from the foods we eat and taps into its stores (primarily from bones), if needed, to meet the baby's calcium needs.

Research indicates that women experience a 3 to 7% reduction in bone mass during breastfeeding. Once you are done breastfeeding, it's important to restore the calcium that was used for milk production by consuming the recommended daily amounts. The good news is that this bone loss is typically recovered within six months once you stop breastfeeding.

SOURCES
Dairy products such as milk, cheese, and yogurt are good sources of calcium, but they are not the only sources. Plant-based milks, such as almond or soy, which are fortified with calcium, often contain more calcium per serving than dairy products. Vegetables such as broccoli, kale, and cabbage are good sources, too. Lastly, canned sardines and salmon contain soft bones that also contribute calcium.

CALCIUM AND PREECLAMPSIA
Supplementation with calcium may help to reduce the risk of preeclampsia in those with a low calcium intake. This should be discussed with your healthcare provider.

Choline

ROLE IN THE BODY
Choline is a component of the outer structure of every cell in the body. It is also needed to produce acetylcholine, a neurotransmitter essential for the development of a child's brain and nervous system during pregnancy and infancy.

IMPORTANCE DURING POSTPARTUM RECOVERY
Choline doesn't directly influence recovery during the postpartum period. However, all women require adequate choline for optimal health.

IMPORTANCE DURING BREASTFEEDING
Shockingly, 90 to 95% of pregnant and nursing women fall short of the recommended daily intake of choline, as many prenatal supplements lack this nutrient. Lactating mothers should prioritize adequate choline intake through diet or supplementation for both their well-being and that of the baby.

SOURCES
Animal-based products, especially eggs and liver, are particularly rich in choline. Other dietary sources include soybeans, tofu, cruciferous vegetables, kidney beans, nuts, seeds, and whole grains.

SUPPLEMENTS
If you are pregnant or breastfeeding, be sure to take a prenatal vitamin or multivitamin that contains choline.

Galactagogues: Fact or Fiction?

Galactagogues are substances that are often used to boost milk supply. They can include herbal supplements, prescription drugs, and even certain foods. Experts have explored numerous supplements, such as fenugreek seed and milk thistle, for their potential impact on lactation. However, the research on them is mixed. There isn't a solid and consistent body of evidence to conclusively prove that supplements effectively boost milk supply. While some studies have shown positive results such as increased milk volume and higher infant weight, others have demonstrated a negative impact on lactation. If you are considering herbal supplements, always consult with a healthcare provider knowledgeable in lactation medicine to weigh the potential benefits against any risks.

Oats, flaxseed, and Brewer's yeast are popular foods thought to boost milk supply. However, as with supplements, the research is mixed. While these foods may not directly improve milk supply, they will not negatively impact it either, and they provide other nutritional benefits such as fiber, B vitamins, omega-3s, and protein. Overall, adequate calorie intake and hydration are the two best ways to ensure adequate milk supply.

Iodine

ROLE IN THE BODY
Iodine is required for the production of thyroid hormones, as well as the proper development of the skeletal and nervous systems in utero and during infancy. Thyroid hormones influence many biochemical reactions and play a role in determining metabolic requirements.

IMPORTANCE DURING POSTPARTUM RECOVERY
Iodine doesn't directly influence recovery during the postpartum period. However, all women require adequate iodine for proper thyroid function.

IMPORTANCE DURING BREASTFEEDING
Iodine requirements notably increase while breastfeeding to support the cognitive development of the baby, and a significant number of pregnant and lactating women in the United States do not meet the necessary iodine requirements. While breast milk contains iodine, its concentration varies depending on maternal iodine levels. Exclusively breastfed infants rely on maternal iodine for their development.

SOURCES

Iodized salt, or table salt, is fortified with iodine. Seaweed, including kelp, nori, kombu, and wakame, are among the richest food sources of iodine since iodine comes from the sea. Fish and seafood such as cod and oysters are also good iodine sources, as are eggs. Dairy products generally contain iodine, but the content will vary based on whether the cows received iodine feed supplements and whether iodophor-sanitizing agents were utilized in cleaning the cows and milk-processing equipment.

One simple way to ensure adequate iodine intake is to use iodized salt. Sea salt, Himalayan salt, Kosher salt, and other specialty salts are not fortified with iodine and are, therefore, not good sources.

Iron

ROLE IN THE BODY

Iron plays diverse roles in the body, including metabolizing energy, producing neurotransmitters, maintaining immune function, and metabolizing alcohol and drugs. Most notably, though, iron is a key component of hemoglobin and myoglobin, the compounds in red blood cells and muscle cells, respectively, that are responsible for transporting oxygen in the bloodstream.

IMPORTANCE DURING POSTPARTUM RECOVERY

Women usually lose about two cups of blood during vaginal birth or about four cups after a C-section! Plus, after pregnancy, the separation of the placenta from the uterine wall leaves an internal wound roughly the size of a dinner plate, which causes bleeding, called lochia, that can last for weeks following delivery. While there are no formal recommendations to increase iron intake after delivery, iron needs are likely higher during the acute recovery phase to help replenish red blood cells lost during labor and after delivery. Iron supplements may be recommended by your healthcare provider. Low or deficient levels of iron can cause shortness of breath, fatigue, rapid heartbeat, and lightheadedness.

After lochia has stopped and your hemoglobin level is within the normal range, your iron needs decrease significantly. Until your period resumes, your iron needs are similar to the requirements of men and postmenopausal women. Once your period resumes, it is important to increase your iron intake to replenish the red blood cells lost in your monthly cycle.

IMPORTANCE DURING BREASTFEEDING

Babies are born with significant iron stores that fulfill their needs for roughly six months. Breast milk provides highly bioavailable iron, but in insufficient quantities to meet the baby's iron needs after six months. This is why foods, in particular iron-rich foods, should be introduced at around six months.

Placentophagia: Fact or Fiction?

Placentophagia, or the ingestion of the placenta, is a common behavior among many animals and, more recently, among women. A growing number of women are consuming their placenta in different forms, including raw, cooked, dehydrated, processed, or encapsulated. The placenta plays a very important role during pregnancy—transporting vital nutrients to the growing fetus—and because of this, contains a variety of vitamins and minerals. It also houses different hormones, including oxytocin (the "happy hormone"). Proponents of consuming the placenta believe it provides a range of benefits, including higher energy levels, improved mood, increased milk production, increased newborn weight gain, and decreased postpartum depression. But is there any scientific evidence to support these claims?

Unfortunately, research has not shown any benefits of consuming your placenta, even in controlled studies using encapsulated placenta. Although likely rare, some researchers cite a potential health risk from bacterial or viral infections as reason enough to not consume the placenta.

The placenta is an organ that, like other animal organs, provides nutrients, namely B vitamins, iron, and protein. The amount of these nutrients present in the placenta can easily be consumed from common foods. While each woman's placenta is a different size, on average a placenta contains roughly 50 grams of protein, the equivalent of 7 ounces of animal protein, and 45 milligrams of iron, which is the standard dose in a prenatal supplement. The non-nutritional benefits attributed to consuming hormones present in the placenta have not demonstrated any impact on maternal health, likely because these hormones are destroyed in the processing of the placenta.

Lastly, it is often said that animals instinctively eat their placenta and that these instincts in humans may have been lost due to modern birthing practices. However, veterinarians note that some animals may just enjoy the taste of placenta, or they may consume it to protect their young by preventing the smell of blood from attracting predators. In summary, there likely aren't any benefits. However, if placentophagia is important to you, then ensure proper preparation to avoid any potential health hazards.

SOURCES

Iron from food comes in two forms: heme and nonheme. Heme iron is more easily absorbed than nonheme iron, although nonheme iron can still be utilized to meet iron needs. Dietary sources rich in heme iron include red meat such as beef, bison, and lamb, and seafood such as clams, oysters, mussels, octopus, and whelk. Nonheme iron, on the other hand, is found in plants such as hemp seeds, pumpkin seeds, beans, lentils, peas, and fortified grain products.

IRON AND VITAMIN C

The absorption of nonheme iron can be enhanced by pairing it with vitamin C–rich foods, such as citrus fruits.

Zinc

ROLE IN THE BODY

Zinc is a heavily utilized mineral in the body and participates in nearly every chemical reaction. Some of its critical roles include DNA synthesis, the formation of hemoglobin to carry oxygen throughout the body, bone and collagen formation, and immune function, as well as supporting reproduction, growth, and development.

IMPORTANCE DURING POSTPARTUM RECOVERY

Zinc is important in all stages of wound healing. It is required for protein synthesis, which includes creating new collagen used in connective tissues in the skin and muscle. It also participates in cell proliferation, contributing to the formation of new cells necessary for tissue repair and resumed blood flow. Despite its necessity, research does not support supplementation with zinc. Meeting your dietary requirements during postpartum should be sufficient to support wound healing.

IMPORTANCE DURING BREASTFEEDING

The need for zinc increases by 4 milligrams per day during lactation compared to prepregnancy. Zinc concentrations in breast milk are at their highest in the first month after birth, then drop by 75% by the ninth month. Due to this significant decrease, human breast milk is insufficient to meet an infant's zinc requirement after the age of six months, and therefore, it must be sourced from food.

SOURCES

The top sources of zinc are meat, shellfish (oysters are the best source), legumes, nuts, and seeds. Additionally, fortified breakfast cereals, oats, and pumpkin seeds are other good sources of zinc.

Water and Hydration

ROLE IN THE BODY

Approximately 60% of the human body is water, so as you might expect, hydration is key to the proper functioning of many bodily systems. A few of its most important roles include:

- maintaining blood volume, which allows oxygen and nutrients to be transported throughout the body
- forming special fluids such as tears and amniotic fluid
- keeping exposed tissues in the eyes, mouth, nose, and skin moist
- lubricating joints
- regulating body temperature
- removing waste from the body via urine

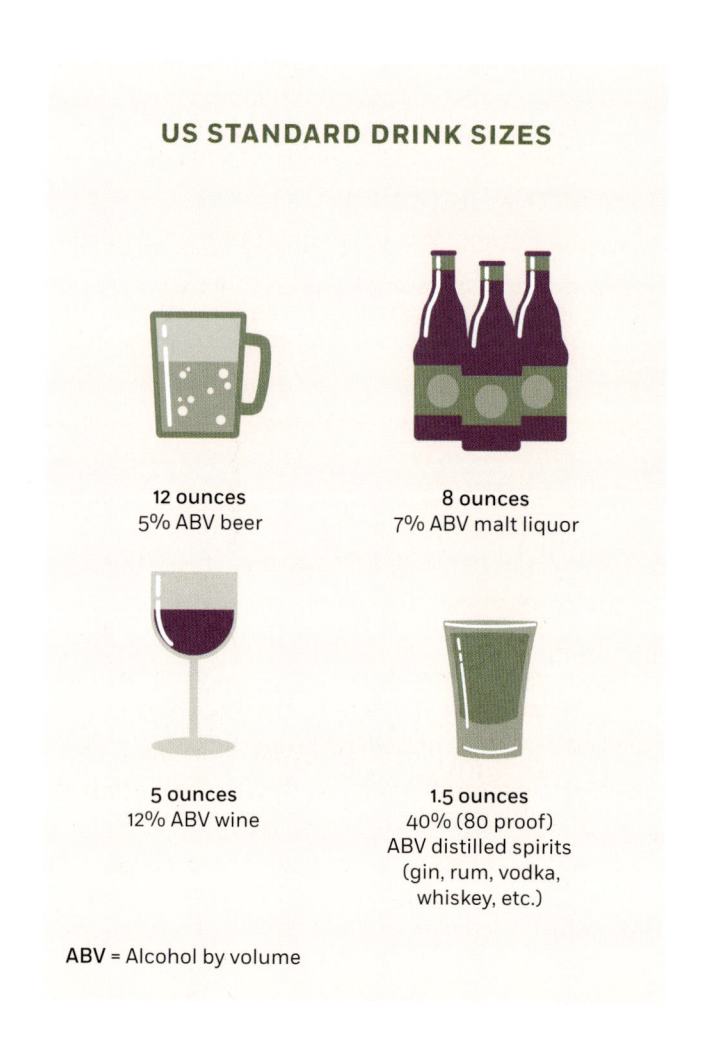

US STANDARD DRINK SIZES

12 ounces
5% ABV beer

8 ounces
7% ABV malt liquor

5 ounces
12% ABV wine

1.5 ounces
40% (80 proof) ABV distilled spirits (gin, rum, vodka, whiskey, etc.)

ABV = Alcohol by volume

IMPORTANCE DURING POSTPARTUM RECOVERY

Adequate hydration is crucial during the postpartum period as the body undergoes various physical adjustments and continues to recover from the demands of pregnancy and childbirth. Proper hydration aids in tissue repair by providing adequate oxygen and nutrients to tissues and replenishing fluids lost during labor and delivery. It also prevents constipation, a common postpartum issue. A general goal for fluids during the acute recovery period is 1 milliliter of fluid per calorie consumed or 30 to 35 milliliters per kilogram of body weight.

> To calculate how much fluid you need each day, first convert your body weight to kilograms. To do this, simply divide by 2.2.
> Ex: 150 lb / 2.2 = 68 kg

> Next, multiply your weight in kilograms by 30–35.
> Ex: 68 kg × 30–35 = 2,040–2,380 mL

> So, a 150-pound woman needs 2,040 to 2,380 mL, or 8 ½ to 10 cups, of liquid per day.

IMPORTANCE DURING BREASTFEEDING

Staying well hydrated is key for successful breastfeeding and ensuring a healthy milk supply. As a breastfeeding mom, aim for about 16 cups of fluids each day from both food and drink.

Research has shown that overloading fluids will not boost your milk supply. So there's no need to go overboard with water consumption—just focus on staying adequately hydrated.

SOURCES

Aside from water, other good sources of hydration include herbal teas, green or black tea, coffee, seltzer water, and cow- or plant-based milk. Foods with a high water content include melons, strawberries, pineapples, oranges, tomatoes, cucumbers, bell peppers, celery, and lettuce.

A NOTE ON ELECTROLYTES

Electrolytes are minerals such as sodium, potassium, calcium, and magnesium that help regulate bodily functions, including balancing the amount of water in the body, moving nutrients into our cells and waste out of our cells, balancing the body's pH level, and supporting muscle and nerve function. In general, proper hydration and a well-balanced diet will provide an adequate amount of electrolytes naturally. However, in certain situations where you're experiencing excessive sweating, prolonged physical activity, or illness that causes dehydration, electrolyte-rich beverages may be beneficial. A few signs that may indicate an electrolyte imbalance include muscle cramping, a persistent headache, or transparent urine.

Caffeine and Alcohol: Fact or Fiction?

It is generally safe to drink caffeine while you are breastfeeding your baby. However, experts recommend limiting your intake to 300 milligrams of caffeine per day (about three 8-ounce cups of coffee) while nursing, as small amounts can transfer to the breast milk and affect some babies.

What about alcohol? The claim that alcohol increases milk supply is an old wives' tale. Research has not only debunked this but has shown the opposite to be true. Not only does alcohol not build your supply, it can actually decrease it and inhibit milk letdown. While frequent, excessive drinking is strongly discouraged, alcohol does not need to be avoided completely while nursing, if you choose to drink. However, the timing is important when it comes to drinking.

Alcohol levels are usually highest in breast milk thirty to sixty minutes after consuming a standard drink and can be detected in it for two to three hours. If you choose to drink, the American College of Obstetricians and Gynecologists recommends waiting at least two hours after a standard drink before breastfeeding. However, the more alcohol you consume, the longer you should wait (i.e., if you consume two drinks, you should wait four hours; after three drinks, wait six hours; etc.). It is important to note that "pumping and dumping" doesn't speed up the time needed to eliminate alcohol from your body or breast milk.

Postpartum Health Conditions That May Be Impacted by Nutrition

Gestational diabetes, high cholesterol, and high blood pressure are all conditions that may occur during pregnancy and may impact your nutritional requirements in the postpartum period.

Gestational diabetes mellitus (GDM) is a type of diabetes that may impact as many as 10% of pregnancies in the United States. GDM occurs when the body can't make enough insulin to meet the heightened demands during pregnancy. Insulin, a hormone made by the pancreas, helps funnel blood sugar (glucose) into the cells of the body. As a result, with GDM, the glucose level in the blood is higher than normal. Additionally, during pregnancy the body increases its hormone production, which can affect how the body uses insulin. In some people, this can lead to some degree of insulin resistance, where the body can't effectively use insulin. GDM tends to resolve after pregnancy; however, as many as 60% of women with GDM will go on to develop type 2 diabetes over the following ten to twenty years. Prioritizing fiber-rich foods and minimizing refined carbs, added sugars, and saturated fats are all important in managing type 2 diabetes.

Cholesterol levels, especially triglyceride levels, increase during pregnancy and stay elevated during breastfeeding in order to support the growth and development of the baby. While producing breast milk, your body mobilizes your fat stores, which are primarily triglycerides. These triglycerides move through the blood to the mammary glands and are incorporated into your breast milk. This elevation is normal. If your levels remain high after you stop breastfeeding, though, you should consult your doctor and work with a dietitian to lower them. Fiber, in particular soluble fiber, and saturated fat are the two primary nutrients to focus on when lowering cholesterol.

High blood pressure, or preeclampsia, is diagnosed after the twentieth week of pregnancy as a blood pressure of higher than 140/90 mmHg and the presence of protein in the urine. Preeclampsia typically resolves on its own following delivery. Postpartum preeclampsia, or post-eclampsia, is elevated blood pressure and protein in the urine after delivery. It is a rare but serious condition that should be treated by your doctor immediately. Returning to a healthy body weight between pregnancies can help to reduce the risk of preeclampsia in subsequent pregnancies.

If any of these conditions persist during the postpartum period, it's important to consult with a doctor and work with a registered dietitian.

We hope this chapter makes you more aware of your increased needs during the postpartum period. You don't need to track or measure your food to perfectly hit these numbers. Simply incorporating some of the food sources listed can make a big difference in your postpartum and breastfeeding journey—and we're going to show you how! In the following chapter, we'll go over some pantry staples, essential tools, and meal-planning strategies to make nourishing yourself through the postpartum phase more realistic.

Avoid Cold Foods: Fact or Fiction?

Is your body capable of recovering while eating cold foods? Some cultures believe that cold or raw foods should be avoided for four to six weeks after delivery to aid in postpartum recovery. It is thought that consuming cold foods 1) decreases blood flow to the recovering uterus and 2) requires a substantial amount of energy to digest compared to room-temperature or hot foods, thereby decreasing the energy (or calories) available for recovery.

While Western medicine is not always perfect, as nutrition scientists we rely on data-driven outcomes from scientific research to inform our recommendations. Based on our research, we did not find any evidence that consuming cold foods negatively impacts postpartum recovery.

During the process of digestion, blood flow is diverted from other areas of the body to support the oxygen requirements needed for this demanding task, but this diversion happens regardless of the temperature of the food consumed. Exposure to cold temperatures does constrict blood vessels, which is why ice is often used as a treatment for swelling. However, the ingestion of cold foods (in usual amounts) does not decrease blood flow to the reproductive organs.

While it is true that consuming cold water requires more energy for digestion compared to room temperature or hot beverages, it is not a significant difference. Energy is used to heat the water in the stomach to body temperature in a process called thermogenesis. The amount of energy required to heat one cup of cold water is about 10 calories, which is the equivalent of one strawberry. This small amount of energy used to digest cold foods is not enough to create a drastic energy deficit that would negatively impact your healing.

There are a lot of traditional beliefs about the postpartum period. Many of these traditions are passed on with love from family members. If it is important to you and your family to follow these customs, please employ them as you'd like. However, if avoidance of certain foods or food preparation techniques prevents you from meeting your heightened nutrient needs, we hope you will be more lenient with these beliefs. If you choose to stick with hot foods, you'll find many soup, stew, and sipping recipes in the book to enjoy.

Most cultures have food traditions specific to the postpartum period, and while writing this book, we learned about many incredible postpartum recipes from around the world. We wanted to celebrate these wonderful recipes with their own spotlight in the book, so we spent time researching cultural ingredients and interviewing friends from different countries about their postpartum practices. We encourage you to talk about your postpartum experience with friends from different cultures to learn about their traditional practices.

Nana's Aynar Spiced Tea, page 242

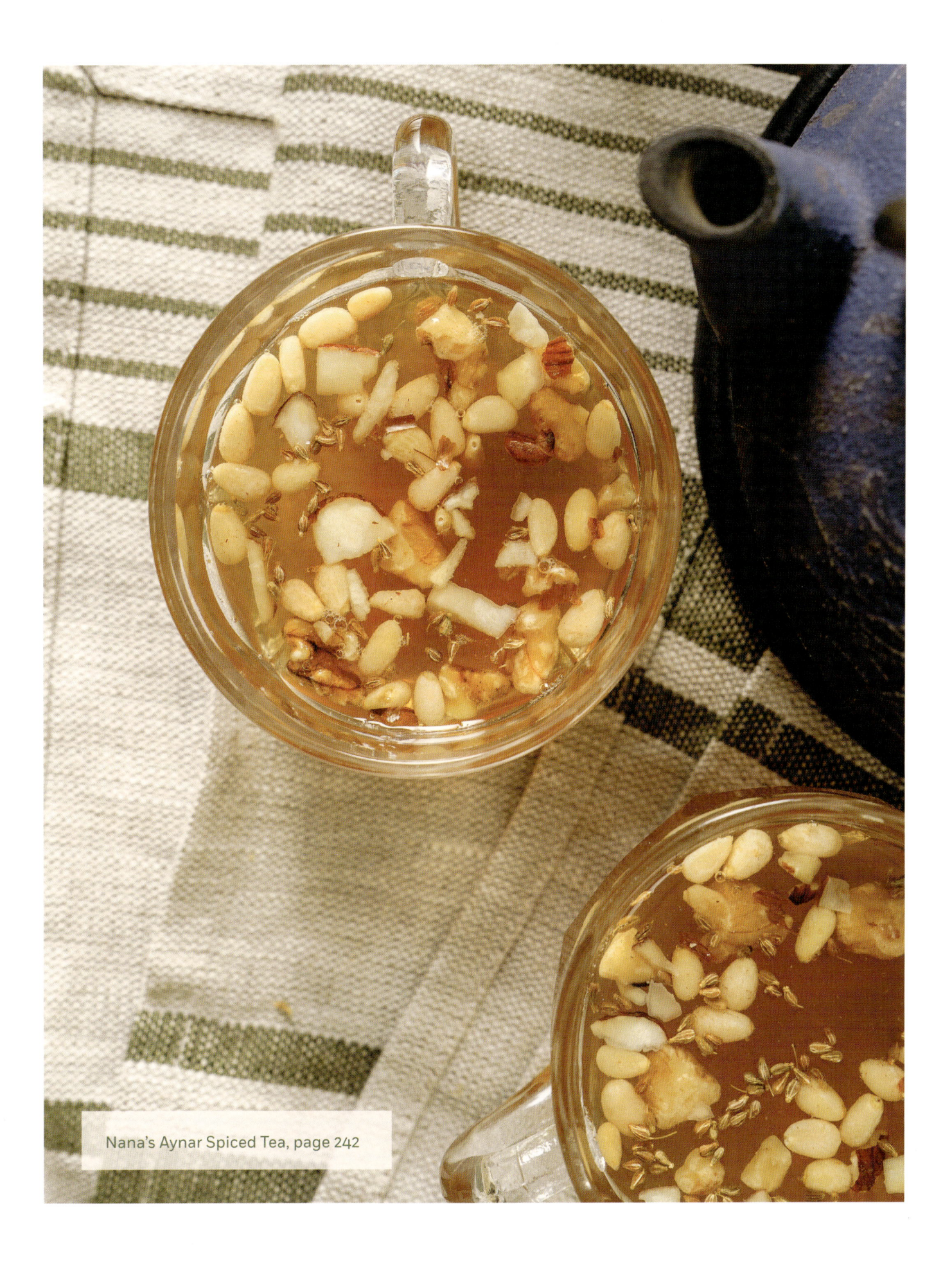

NUTRIENT NEEDS FOR POSTPARTUM RECOVERY

NUTRIENT	FEMALES (19–50 YEARS)	PREGNANCY	POSTPARTUM + BREASTFEEDING
CALORIES*	25–30 kcal/kg	1st trimester: no increase 2nd trimester: additional 340 kcal/day 3rd trimester: additional 450 kcal/day	Acute: 30–35 kcal/kg + an additional 330 per day Long-term: 25–30 kcal/kg* + an additional 330–400 per day
CARBOHYDRATES	At least 130 g/day + additional based on activity	At least 175 g/day + additional based on activity	At least 210 g/day + additional based on activity
FIBER	25 g/day	25–36 g/day	31–34 g/day
PROTEIN**	At least 0.8 g/kg	1st trimester: no increase 2nd & 3rd trimester: at least 1.1 g/kg	1.3–1.5 g/kg
OMEGA-3S	1.1 g/day	1.4 g/day	1.3 g/day
VITAMIN A	700 mcg RAE/day	770 mcg RAE/day	1,300 mcg RAE/day
VITAMIN B2 (RIBOFLAVIN)	1.1 mg/day	1.4 mg/day	1.6 mg/day
VITAMIN B5 (PANTOTHENIC ACID)	5 mg/day	6 mg/day	7 mg/day
VITAMIN B6	1.3 mg/day	1.9 mg/day	2.0 mg/day
VITAMIN B7 (BIOTIN)	30 mcg/day	30 mcg/day	35 mcg/day
VITAMIN B9 (FOLATE)	400 mcg/day	600 mcg/day	500 mcg/day
VITAMIN B12	2.4 mcg/day	2.6 mcg/day	2.8 mcg/day
VITAMIN C	75 mg/day	85 mg/day	Acute: 250 mg/day Long-term: 120 mg/day
VITAMIN E	15 mg/day	15 mg/day	19 mg/day
VITAMIN D	600 IU/day	600 IU/day	600 IU/day
CALCIUM	1,000 mg/day	1,000 mg/day	1,000 mg/day
CHOLINE	425 mg/day	450 mg/day	550 mg/day
IODINE	150 mcg/day	220 mcg/day	290 mcg/day
IRON	18 mg/day	27 mg/day	Acute: 18 mg/day or recommended level from doctor based on hemoglobin level Long-term: 9 mg/day until menstrual cycle resumes, then increase to 18 mg/day
ZINC	8 mg/day	11 mg/day	12 mg/day
MAGNESIUM	310–320 mg/day	350–360 mg/day	310–320 mg/day

POSTPARTUM (NOT BREASTFEEDING)	FOOD SOURCES
Acute: 30–35 kcal/kg Long-term: 25–30 kcal/kg	All foods containing carbohydrates, protein, and fat contribute calories
Acute: at least 175 g/day Long-term: at least 130 g/day + additional based on activity	Fruit, vegetables, legumes, grains, some dairy products
Acute: 28 g/day Long-term: 25 g/day	Legumes, vegetables, whole grains, nuts, seeds
Acute: 1.3–1.5 g/kg Long-term: 1.0–1.5 g/kg to encourage continued regaining of muscle mass	Animal sources: beef, poultry, dairy products, eggs, pork, seafood Plant sources: beans, lentils, soy; whole grains, nuts, and seeds contribute smaller amounts
1.1 g/day	Fatty fish, walnuts, flaxseed, chia seeds, hemp seeds, algae
Acute: 1,300 mcg RAE/day Long-term: 700 mcg/day 700 mcg RAE/day	Apricots, broccoli, carrots, fortified milk, eggs, kale, sweet potatoes
1.0 mg/day	Dairy products, eggs, meat, fortified cereals, almonds, spinach
5 mg/day	Shiitake mushrooms, salmon, avocados, chicken, beef, sunflower seeds, whole milk
1.3 mg/day	Fish, meat, poultry, whole grains
30 mcg/day	Eggs, meat, fish, seeds, nuts
400 mcg/day	Beans, dark green vegetables, fortified foods such as cereals and juices
2.4 mcg/day	Dairy products, eggs, meat, poultry, seafood, fortified products such as cereals and plant-based milks
Acute: 250 mg/day Long-term: 75 mg/day	Citrus fruits, kiwi, strawberries, vegetables (including red and green bell peppers, broccoli, Brussels sprouts, and cabbage)
15 mg/day	Wheat germ oil, sunflower seeds, almonds, hazelnuts, pine nuts, peanuts
600 IU/day	Fatty fish, eggs, fortified foods such as orange juice and milk
1,000 mg/day	Dairy products, green leafy vegetables (including broccoli, kale, and cabbage)
425 mg/day	Beef, chicken, eggs, soy, salmon, wheat germ, mushrooms
150 mcg/day	Dairy products, seafood, iodized salt, seaweed, fortified products such as cereals and plant-based milks
18 mg/day or recommended level from doctor based on hemoglobin level	Animal-based (heme) sources: clams, oysters, mussels, meat, poultry Plant-based (nonheme) sources: fortified cereals, lentils, beans, hemp seeds, chia seeds, pumpkin seeds
8 mg/day	Red meat, oysters, crab, hemp seeds, pumpkin seeds, cashews, lentils, chickpeas
310–320 mg/day	Legumes, spinach, almonds, pumpkin seeds, cashews, wheat, oats, barley, quinoa

Acute = first six weeks,
Long-term = up to eighteen months

These are based on nutrition guidelines for recovery from other major surgeries or injuries.

*These are rudimentary and easy formulas to calculate your calorie needs. If you are active, multiply this number by: 1.375 if you are lightly active, 1.55 if you are moderately active, and 1.725 if you are very active.

Note: To calculate your weight in kilograms divide your body weight in pounds by 2.2.

**If you are very active, your protein needs may be as high as 1.7 g/kg.

PART 2

How to Get Started

Eating healthily often takes a back seat, especially with a little one on the way. However, planning your meals and nutrition should be a key part of getting ready for your baby's arrival. Now that you've learned about the importance of postpartum nutrition, it's time to create a plan so you feel confident and prepared for this exciting journey.

Meeting your nutrient needs won't just happen, especially right after a life-altering addition to your household. Once your baby comes, your time and mental capacity for any type of self-care, including feeding yourself, becomes limited. So over the next two chapters, we'll discuss ways to help set you up for success during this exciting but nutrient-demanding time!

Lactation Cookies (3 Ways), page 208

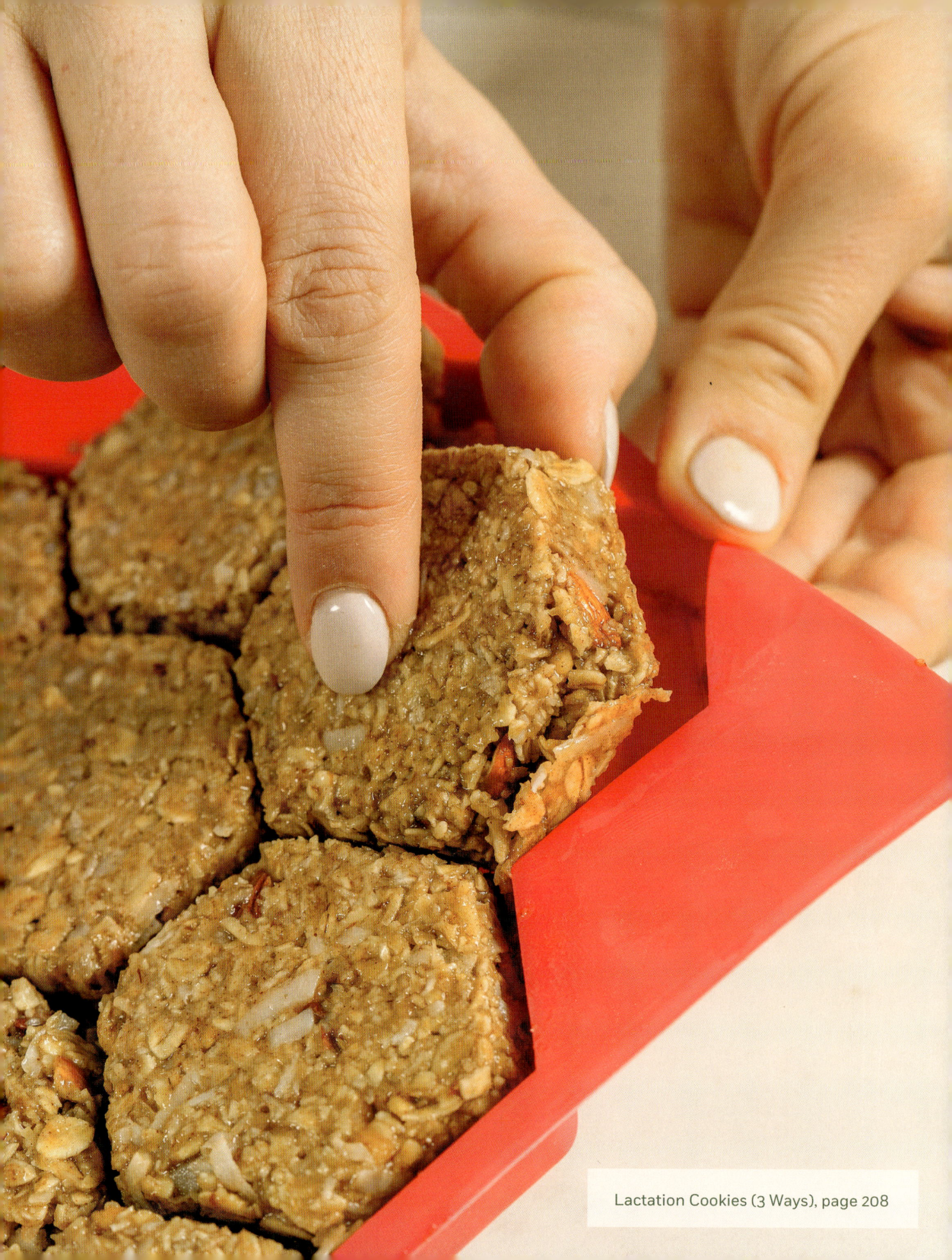

CHAPTER 3

Helpful Tools and Pantry Staples

In this chapter, we list the kitchen tools and appliances that will make cooking easier and your time in the kitchen more efficient. They'll also come in handy for many of the recipes in this book. If you don't have any of these tools or appliances, you can always put them on your registry! A well-nourished mom is the ultimate necessity for the postpartum period. We also include a list of pantry staples to make meal planning easier. Scan the QR code on page 42 for a list of our recommended products.

Kitchen Tools and Appliances

FOOD STORAGE

- **Glass or plastic containers:** various sizes; great for leftovers and meal prepping
- **Mason jars (or recycled jars):** use different sizes for overnight oats, salads, soups, smoothies, and other foods
- **Silicone cube trays:** for freezing individual portions of broth, soup, or stews
- **Reusable ziplock bags:** save money on traditional plastic storage bags; great for taking snacks on the go; use different sizes to freeze foods
- **Aluminum pans:** some freezer meals can be made right in the pan and frozen once cooled

APPLIANCES

- **High-powered blender:** great for blending larger batches of food such as sauces, soups, dressings, smoothies, and ice cream
- **Food processor:** helps with food prep by chopping, mincing, mixing, and blending
- **Instant Pot or other electric multi-cooker:** allows you to quickly make grains, beans, and other foods and acts as a slow cooker
- **Air fryer:** a great tool to quickly cook and crisp up foods
- **A separate freezer:** we know this is extra and not an option for everyone, but if you have the space and resources, you will not be disappointed in the extra freezer space for food and breast milk

KITCHEN TOOLS

- **Measuring spoons and cups**
- **Sharp chef's knives**
- **Silicone baking mat**
- **Veggie chopper:** not essential, but helps save time chopping vegetables
- **Large baking sheets**
- **Muffin tin**
- **9 x 5-inch loaf pan**
- **8 x 8-inch and/or 9 x 13-inch baking dish**

Pantry Essentials

Since you won't always have time to get to the grocery store, we've included a list of fridge, freezer, and pantry staples to make meal planning easier. There's also a whole chapter with recipes you can make from these essential pantry items. Stocking your house with these ingredients will make meal preparation and cooking much easier.

TO KEEP IN YOUR PANTRY

LONG-LASTING VEGETABLES

Carrots

Celery

Garlic

Onions, including white, yellow, and red

Potatoes, white and sweet

NUTS AND SEEDS

Almond or sunflower seed butter

Nuts, such as almonds, walnuts, pistachios, and cashews

Chia seeds

Flaxseed

Hemp seeds

Peanut butter

Tahini

BEANS, LEGUMES, AND CANNED/BOTTLED GOODS

Capers

Canned clams

Canned artichoke hearts

Canned chickpeas

Canned black beans

Canned butter, cannellini, or Great Northern beans

Chicken or vegetable broth

Diced tomatoes

Dried lentils

Marinara sauce

Salsa

Tomato paste

GRAINS AND PASTAS

Bean-based pasta

Bread

Brown rice

Brown-rice ramen noodles

Oats

Quinoa

Long pasta, such as linguini or angel hair

Macaroni and cheese

Tortillas

White or wheat flour

DRIED HERBS AND SPICES

Ground cinnamon

Dried parsley

Dried thyme

Garlic powder

Italian seasoning

Onion powder

Pepper

Red pepper flakes

Salt

Taco seasoning

CONDIMENTS

BBQ sauce

Fish sauce

Mayonnaise

Mustard

Nonstick cooking spray

Olive oil

Sesame oil

Soy sauce or soy sauce alternative

Sriracha

Teriyaki sauce

Worcestershire sauce

OTHER

Cocoa powder

Chocolate chips

Protein powder

Vanilla extract

SCAN FOR MORE INFORMATION AND RESOURCES

TO KEEP IN YOUR FRIDGE

Bottled lemon juice and/or lime juice	Cottage cheese	Eggs
Butter or vegan butter	Cheese, such as cheddar and Parmesan	Tofu
		Yogurt

TO KEEP IN YOUR FREEZER

Broccoli	Fruit, such as bananas, berries, mango, pineapple	Pepper-onion mix
Brown rice		Pizza
Chicken sausage	Green beans	Salmon
Edamame	Peas and carrots mix	Shrimp
		Spinach

Next up, we'll discuss how to combine these pantry staples with fresh ingredients to maximize your nutrition while minimizing the time and effort spent in the kitchen!

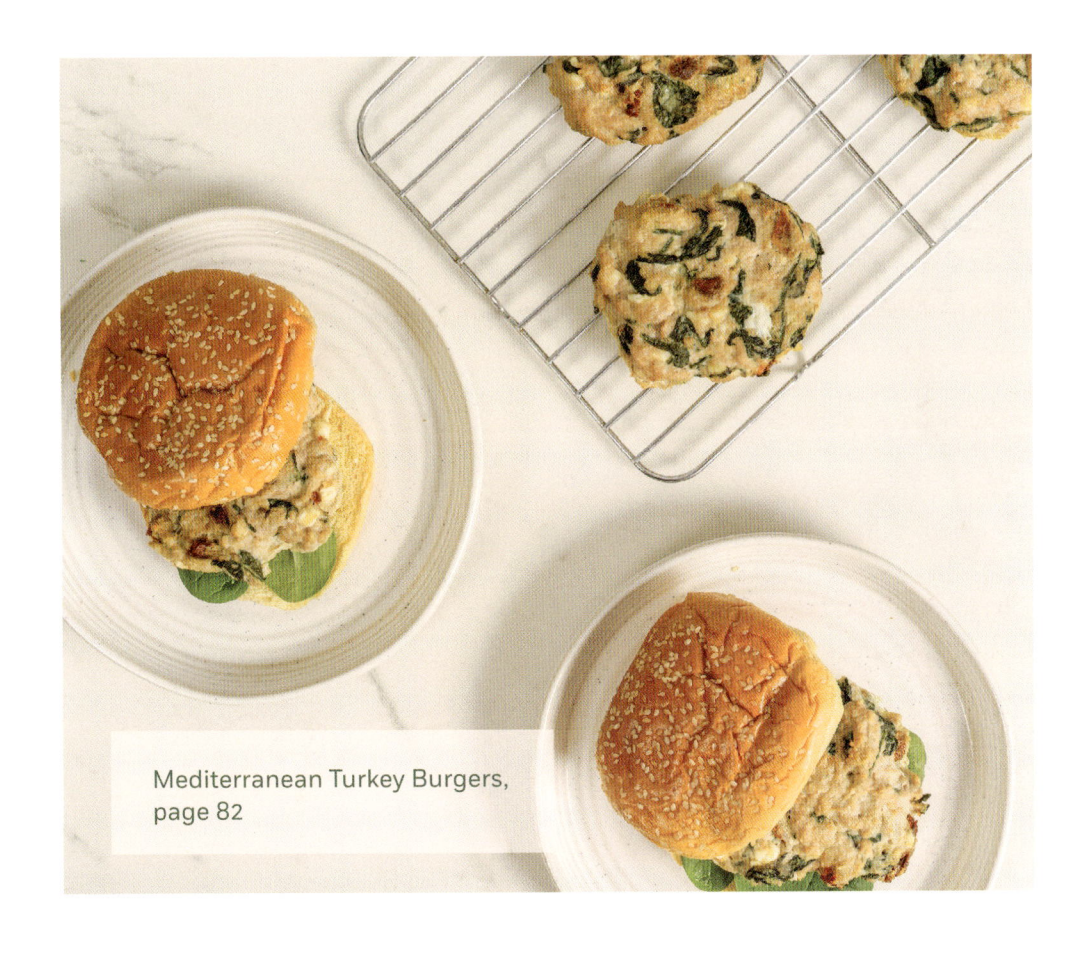

Mediterranean Turkey Burgers, page 82

Egg Breakfast Burritos,
page 84

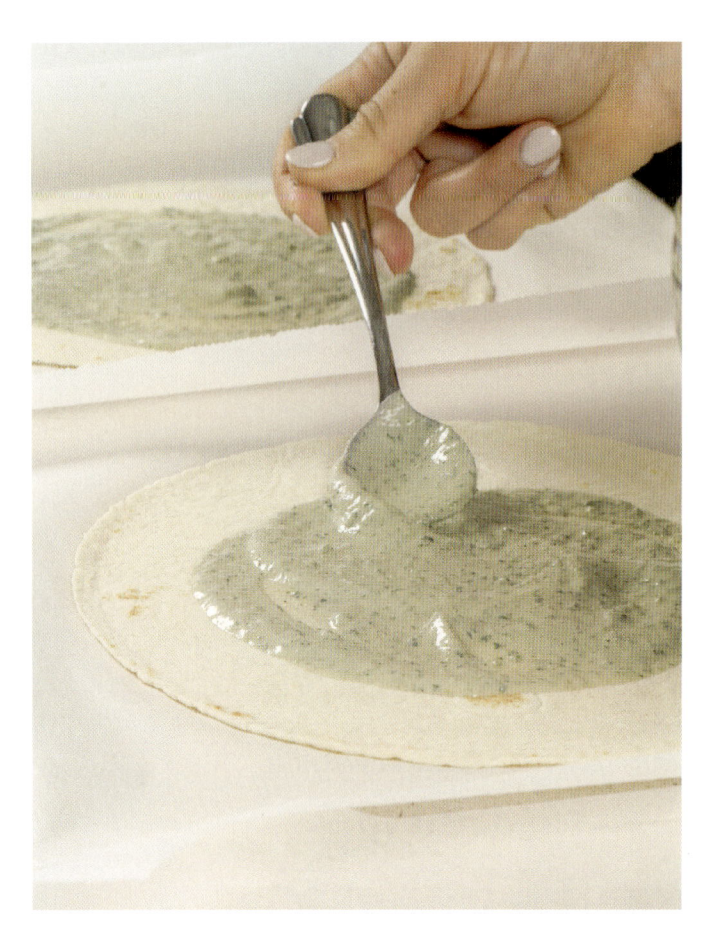

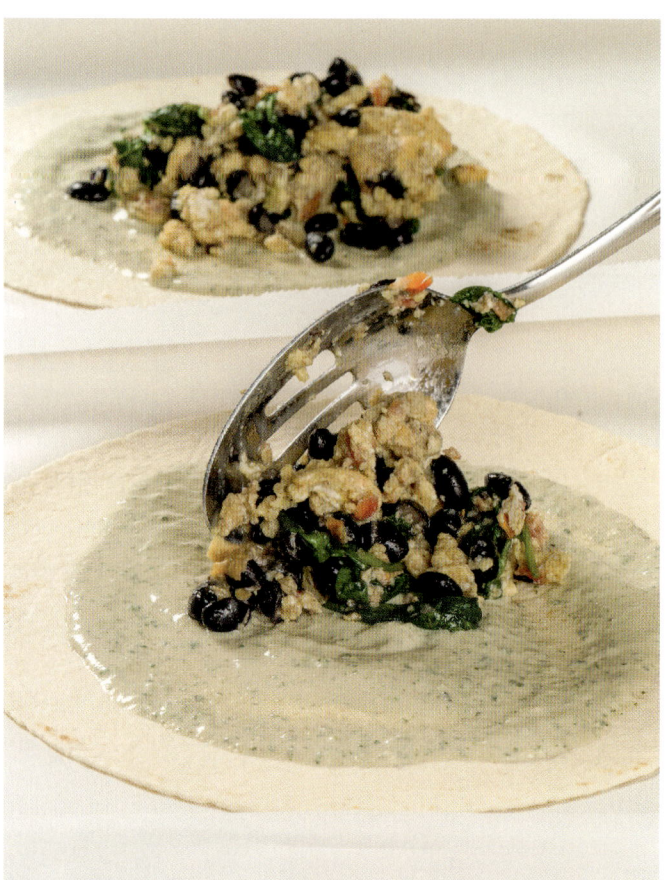

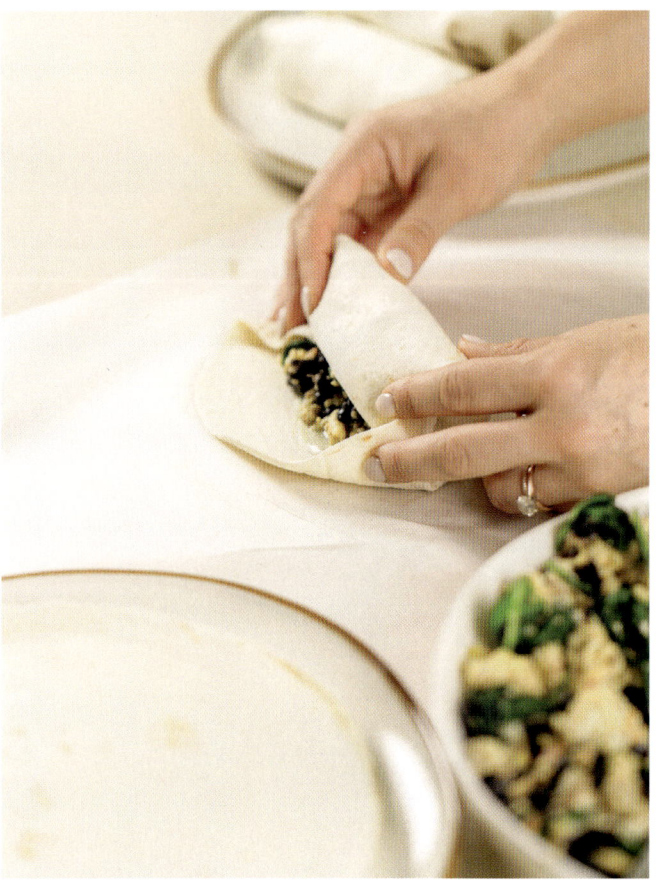

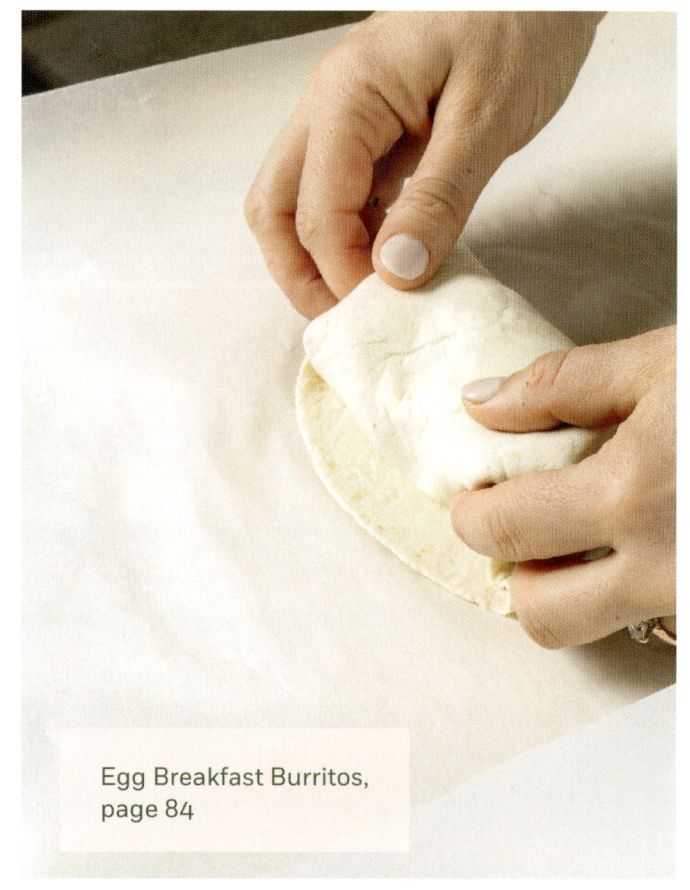

CHAPTER 4

Meal Planning and Prepping

Meal planning doesn't have to be time- or labor-intensive. Investing just one hour in the kitchen each week can save you time and mental energy on deciding what to eat every day. Don't know where to even begin in meal planning? Don't worry, in this chapter, we'll teach you how to:

- Stock your freezer before delivery
- Maximize your freezer meals post-baby by pairing them with fresh ingredients
- Approach meal planning in a realistic way
- Meal plan for the whole family
- Enlist help from your community to make your nutrition a priority

Stock Your Freezer Before Delivery

Maintaining a supply of frozen foods is a lifesaver during the postpartum period. Eventually, the meal train will end, family will leave, and your maternity support will dwindle. But your freezer supply will be there waiting for you! Having some meals, or meal components, that you can easily incorporate into your weekly meal plan (or prepare in just a few minutes) lessens the burden of planning and preparing over twenty-one meals, plus snacks, every week. As you start to nest and get ready for the baby, don't forget about getting yourself ready, too. Beyond stockpiling diapers and heavy-duty pads for postpartum recovery, ensure your freezer is well stocked with convenient and nourishing options for you and your family.

If you don't already have some of the tools that we mentioned in chapter 3, then add them to a baby registry. The tools we outlined will save you time in the kitchen and increase your likelihood of eating nutritious meals, which, in turn, will help you feel your best during the postpartum period. Appliances such as the Instant Pot and reusable containers for freezing foods will make food preparation easier, not only during the postpartum period but for years to come, especially if you have your sights set on expanding your family or making baby food, too.

Chapter 5: Freezer Meals is dedicated to meals to store in your freezer. In addition to complete meals, such as breakfast burritos and lasagna, we've also included a range of meal components, such as shredded beef and pork meatballs, that can easily be added to any dish, as well as breads and muffins that are perfect for a quick snack or on-the-go breakfast. If you don't have a lot of freezer space, pick the ones that you are most likely to eat. But if you have space to store all of the freezer meal recipes before the baby comes, go for it! Consider asking your friends and family to help

One of the easiest ways to boost your vitamin C intake is with bottled lemon or lime juice. They mix well with water and can be refrigerated for a long time.

During your first week home, you will likely be relying on your freezer stock the most. This is also when your vitamin C needs are the highest, because you are in the acute recovery phase of wound healing. Appendix II includes a meal plan for that first week at home. It uses mostly freezer meals paired with recipes high in vitamin C or with "Vitamin C Boost" suggestions.

You'll be able to draw on your freezer meals for weeks or months to come—and we encourage you to restock the freezer when supplies get low. Even with a freezer full of meals, though, it's important to put a bit of thought into how you are going to feed yourself each week. Next, we've laid out a strategy for meal planning that is approachable and requires minimal time.

Make a Realistic Meal Plan

Finding time to nourish yourself postpartum becomes challenging, but dedicating a small amount of time each week to planning and preparing your meals can lead to a big payoff. What follows are some tips for keeping nutrition practical and achievable in the midst of the new demands of caring for your baby.

NORMALIZE MONOTONY AND MANAGE EXPECTATIONS

Some days are going to be easier than others, and normalizing monotony with your food choices can be a helpful strategy as you navigate the challenges of caring for a newborn. It's perfectly acceptable to embrace a repetitive routine, such as having the same breakfast or lunch daily for a couple of weeks. By limiting food choices and sticking to a few reliable meals, you can alleviate the decision-making burden that often accompanies postpartum life. This not only streamlines meal planning but also helps prevent you from feeling overwhelmed, allowing you to prioritize you and your baby's well-being without the added stress of varied and elaborate meal preparations. And remember, not every meal must be perfectly balanced.

BATCH COOK

Batch cooking is a time-saving, cost-effective, and health-conscious approach to meal preparation. You will spend less time in the kitchen, you will save money by buying meal ingredients in bulk, and you can properly size the portions you store for later consumption.

MEAL PLAN AND PREP EACH WEEK

Sit down for a few minutes over the weekend to plan out meals for the following week. Follow our guide to make your week as simple as possible, combining a variety of freezer and make-ahead meals with a few simple freshly made or pantry-based meals.

Sample menu:
For the full menu and grocery list, check out Appendix III.

	MON	TUES	WED	THURS	FRI	SAT	SUN
BREAKFAST	Apple Cider Oatmeal Bread **and** Green Eggs and Ham Cups or Eggless "Egg" Cups	Banana Bread Baked Pancakes	Apple Cider Oatmeal Bread **and** Green Eggs and Ham Cups or Eggless "Egg" Cups	Banana Bread Baked Pancakes	Apple Cider Oatmeal Bread **and** Green Eggs and Ham Cups or Eggless "Egg" Cups	Banana Bread Baked Pancakes	Apple Cider Oatmeal Bread **and** Green Eggs and Ham Cups or Eggless "Egg" Cups
LUNCH	Thai Peanut Chicken Salad	Creamy Enchilada Casserole	Sheet-Pan Steak Fajitas	Creamy Enchilada Casserole	Thai Peanut Chicken Salad	Creamy Enchilada Casserole	Takeout
DINNER	BeaBea's Lasagna	Sheet-Pan Steak Fajitas	Thai Peanut Chicken Salad	BeaBea's Lasagna	Grandma's Tomato Soup and Grilled Cheese	Takeout	Fancified Frozen Pizza

Once you've chosen your meals, decide when to transfer your freezer meals into your fridge to let them defrost. Next, write out a list of ingredients you'll need for the rest of your meals. Hopefully, your pantry will already be stocked with these items, saving you a trip to the grocery store. Depending on your situation, have your partner or a loved one head to the grocery store, or head there yourself, as it could be a good excuse to get out of the house. If going to the grocery store is too daunting, you can always use a grocery delivery service if that's available to you. Then spend an hour or two preparing for three to four meals.

Each week, choose:
- One breakfast freezer meal
- One to two make-ahead breakfasts
- Two lunch/dinner freezer meals
- Two pantry meals
- Two freshly made recipes
- Two takeout meals

Meal Plan for the Whole Family

It's important to acknowledge that you may not be the only person eating in your household! Whether it be a partner or other kids, dealing with different food preferences can add to mealtime stress. Here are a few strategies that can help to make this easier, especially if you are usually the grocery shopper and meal preparer in the home.

INVOLVE THE WHOLE FAMILY IN MEAL PLANNING

On top of everything else you are dealing with postpartum, grouchy grumbles about what's for dinner are not helpful for your sanity. In an effort to minimize complaints, involve the whole family in meal planning. Let each person pick one dinner option for the week (or breakfast, lunch, or snack depending on your family size). For younger kids, you can provide two to three options for them to pick from—bonus points if they are your freezer meals! When it's time for their meal during the week, celebrate that it's their dinner choice to help them feel more excited about the meal.

If a child (or even a partner) isn't excited about what's offered, you can gently remind them that it's their sibling's night to pick dinner. Just as they have chosen a meal for the whole family to enjoy, now it's someone else's turn. Not every meal needs to be their favorite, and it's important that everyone gets to choose a meal one night. Remind them that they will pick again soon.

REMEMBER YOU ARE NOT A SHORT-ORDER COOK

Feeling the pull to make everyone happy at mealtimes is a big drain on energy and time. It also sets the precedent that every single meal has to be a child's favorite food. In the world outside of the home, kids won't always have their favorite foods as options. We also know that we get a variety of nutrients from an assortment of foods. Children may not like every food they try, but a wide range of nutrient-rich foods will help them grow big and strong.

With this in mind, try to resist the urge to make separate meals for everyone in the house to keep the peace. Having a few favorite items in the fridge or ready to go in the freezer to supplement what is being served for dinner can make at least part of each meal palatable to everyone. Most research suggests that children, especially after age two, need to be introduced to a new food around fifteen times before they are comfortable eating it. Don't lose hope after one failed attempt. Keep trying!

DON'T BE AFRAID TO ADD WHAT YOU NEED TO MEALS

If little mouths are requesting chicken nuggets every night for dinner, it might make sense to have a few options that you can add to your plate of chicken nuggets to help meet the heightened needs of your postpartum body. In particular, protein and vitamin C are two key nutrients to help with your recovery. Fiber is also an important component to add to meals to keep you feeling your best. Having fiber-rich options, such as bagged salads, in the refrigerator to add to any meal can help you boost your fiber intake while still allowing you to participate in family mealtime. Easy protein sources such as shredded chicken thighs from the freezer or tofu in the fridge can also ensure you get in that important protein for your healing. Your littles will benefit from vitamin C, too, and can share your morning smoothie or water with lemon.

These tips are general rules of thumb and won't always be appropriate to apply, but they can help to lessen the stress of feeding your family and ensure that you're giving your body what it needs to recover optimally. And all of these should be done without guilt, because a mom who is feeling well will benefit the entire family.

Enlist Help from Your Community

During the postpartum period, our number one tip is: *Don't hesitate to ask for and accept help.* Enlisting support from your community and using convenient options will help make your nutrition a priority. Involve friends and family in food prep—have them make freezer meals, or better yet, consider hosting a freezer-stocking day where everyone comes together to prepare and store meals for you. Bookmark different recipes that sound appealing, and share them with your friends and family. Create a standard grocery shopping list, and have someone restock these ingredients every so often. If your mother-in-law comes to visit, show her this chapter!

A fun idea to get your loved ones involved is having a nesting party, where you invite friends and family to help you "nest" and prepare for the postpartum period. They can help you wash bottles and pumps, get the nursery ready, organize and fold baby clothes, make padsicles, stock your pantry, and prepare freezer meals.

Have a loved one organize a meal train using platforms such as Meal Train, Take Them A Meal, or CareCalendar, which allows friends and family to coordinate meal contributions. Don't be ashamed to utilize meal delivery services such as Uber Eats or DoorDash for convenient options. Make grocery shopping seamless with delivery services offered by your local grocer or Instacart. Explore meal-kit subscriptions such as Dinnerly, Sunbasket, Home Chef, or Blue Apron for simplified cooking. Additionally, consider the support of a postpartum doula or, as previously mentioned, involve friends and family in food prep to ensure that nourishing yourself remains a shared priority during this transformative time.

Need more step-by-step guidance and examples? At the end of this book, you can find three appendices with meal plans and grocery lists to guide your postpartum nutrition plan:

- **Appendix I: Prepping Your Postpartum Freezer.** A three-day cooking plan to make all eighteen recipes from the Freezer Meals chapter, complete with a grocery list, cooking timeline, and step-by-step instructions.

- **Appendix II: First-Week-Home Meal Plan.** A survival guide on what to eat during your first week home, pulling from your freezer meals and incorporating a few fresh ingredients to support your healing. This grocery list can even be ordered on your way home from the hospital!

- **Appendix III: Sample Week Meal Plan.** Daily menus feature a mixture of recipes from all of our chapters, including both frozen meals and freshly prepared recipes.

We hope you're feeling inspired to fuel your postpartum recovery! You can't control or plan for your baby's sleep, tummy troubles, diaper rashes, or illnesses, but hopefully, with the help of the *Postpartum Nutrition Cookbook*, you'll feel more in control of your postpartum nutrition needs for healing and breastfeeding.

One-Pan Shrimp Boil, page 145

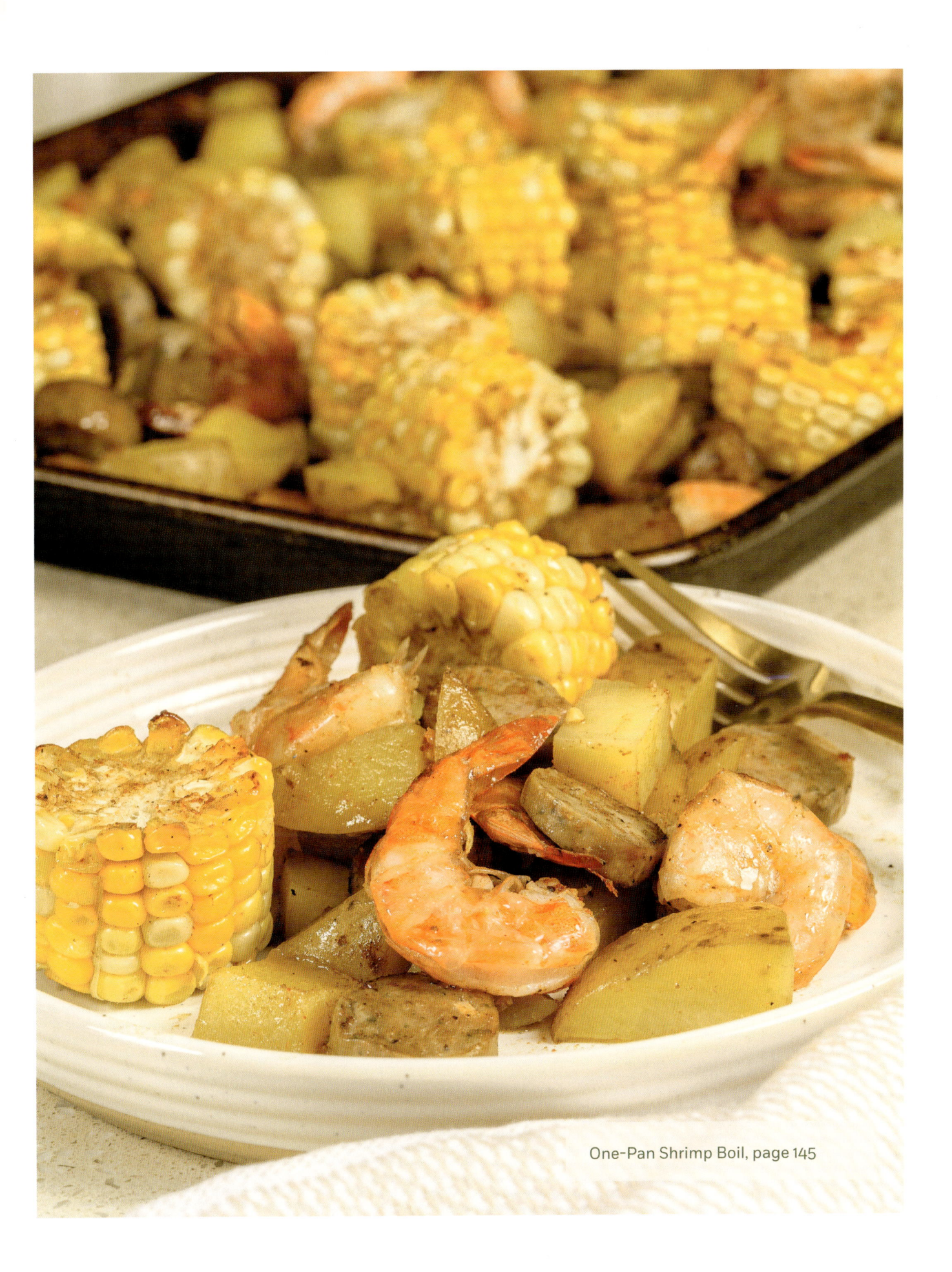

Creamy Chicken Quinoa Bake, page 142

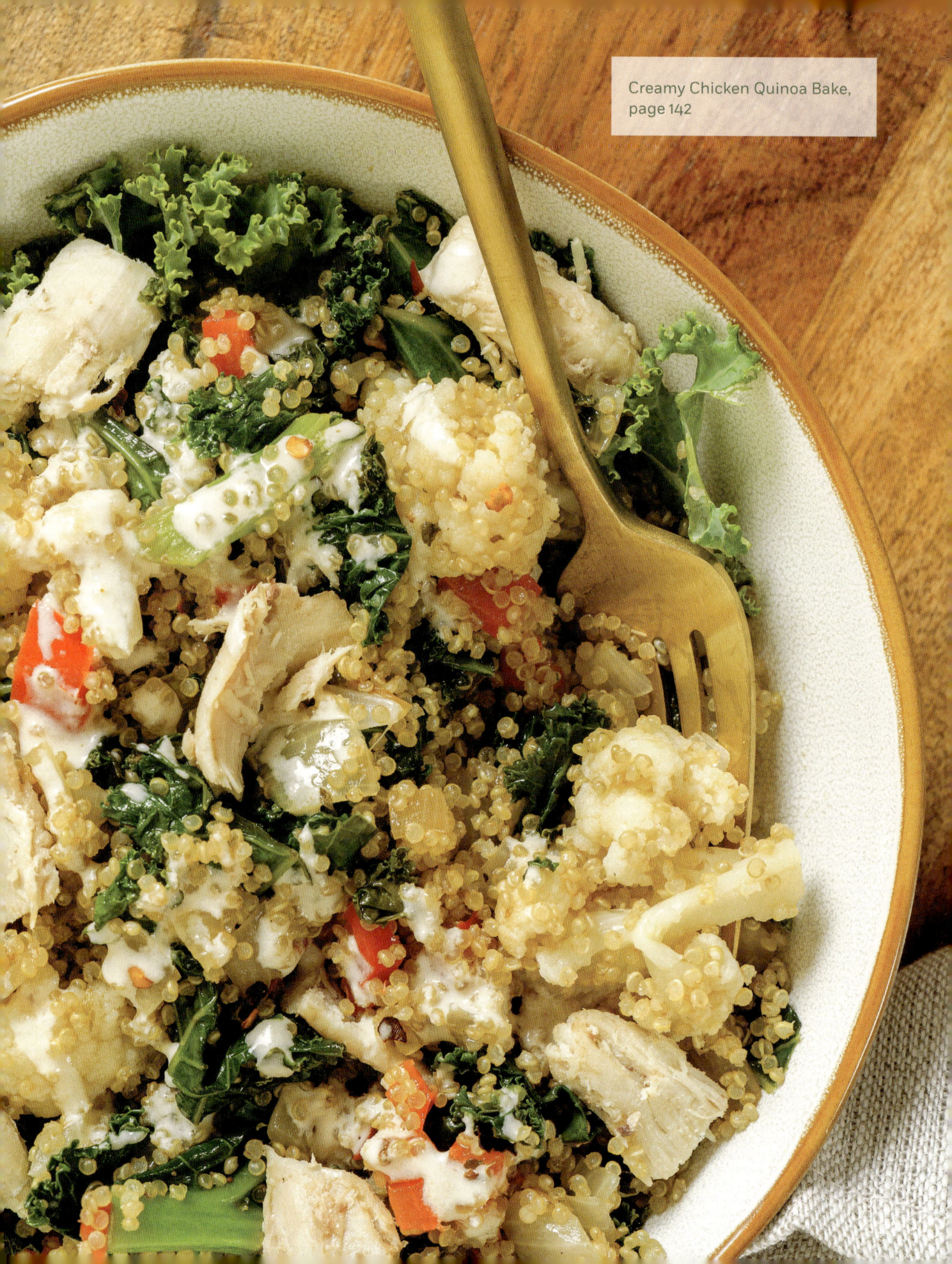

PART 3

The Recipes

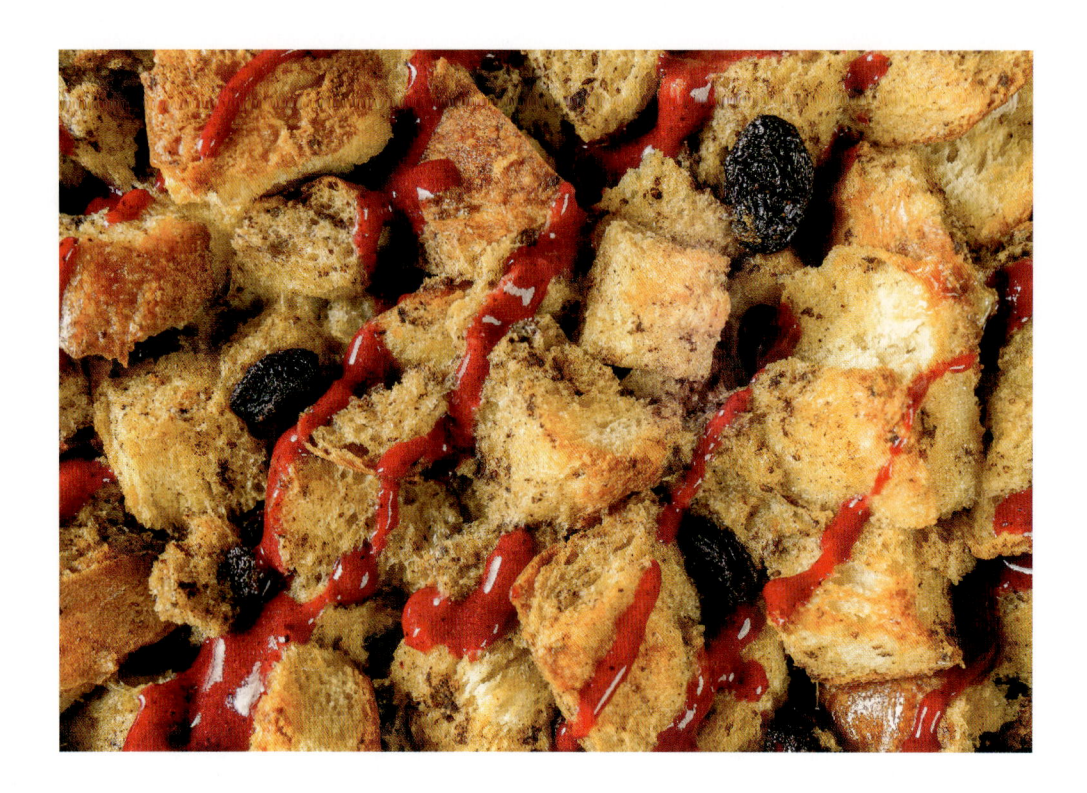

How to Navigate the Recipes

Welcome to the recipes! With every recipe, you'll find helpful tips and ways to modify and/or enhance each dish. To find these at a glance, look for the following notes throughout the recipe chapters:

● **MAKE IT PLANT-BASED:** Many recipes are already naturally plant-based; however, for many that aren't, we've included suggestions on how to make a plant-based version.

● **VITAMIN C BOOST:** Vitamin C is a critical antioxidant during the recovery phase. We've included a vitamin C boost with each of our freezer recipes since vitamin C gets degraded in the cooking process.

● **PROTEIN ADD:** Because protein needs are elevated during the postpartum period, we included a protein add for recipes with less than 20 grams of protein. We've offered both plant-based and animal-based options to help you boost the protein per serving.

● **MAKE IT GLUTEN-FREE:** For any recipe that contains gluten, we've included a gluten-free option. If a recipe includes oats, substitute with gluten-free oats.

● **MAKE IT NUT-FREE:** Because nuts are a top allergen, we've included nut-free options for any recipe including nuts.

You'll see that we call for "milk of choice" throughout our recipes. We generally recommend fortified soy or cow's milk over other varieties, as these are protein- and calcium-rich and provide more of a creamy consistency in recipes. Therefore, we used soy milk in our calculations for the nutritional information for recipes containing milk. However, feel free to use your favorite non-dairy milk, such as almond, oat, coconut, or any other variety. Most milks can be used interchangeably in these recipes, but we recommend always buying the unsweetened versions. If you choose to use plant-based yogurts, we suggest an option with over 10 grams of protein and less than 3 grams of saturated fat per serving. We like Kite Hill's Greek-style yogurt.

You'll learn more about the recipes in the recipe introductions, where we include information on specific ingredients and other beneficial aspects of each recipe—for example, whether it is high in certain micronutrients such as vitamin C, vitamin A, iron, or calcium.

Every recipe also includes nutrition information: calories, fat, carbohydrates, fiber, and protein. We did not include these to encourage you to count and track your foods. We do not want you to focus on logging your meals during postpartum recovery. However, we felt it was important for us to share nutrition details to ensure that you are getting enough of certain nutrients, especially calories, protein, and fiber. As discussed in chapter 2, the requirement for many nutrients increases during the postpartum phase. We've chosen to highlight these in our recipes since they tend to be underconsumed, which can have a significant impact on your recovery and on regaining muscle mass and normal digestion.

As dietitians, we also have your long-term health in mind. These recipes are great for the whole family as well as for your health through the many upcoming stages of life. They are high in fiber and moderate in saturated fat, which are two important considerations for preventing many of the chronic diseases that individuals develop later in life.

Lastly, we encourage you to make these recipes your own. Tweak them to your preferences or make changes to accommodate your family's needs. We intentionally included many different cooking techniques and flavors from cultures around the world to highlight the vast possibilities of making meals at home.

Most cultures have food traditions specific to the postpartum period, and while writing this book, we learned about many incredible postpartum recipes. We wanted to celebrate these wonderful recipes, so we sprinkled some throughout! We hope that many of these recipes will become staples at your family's dinner table for years to come.

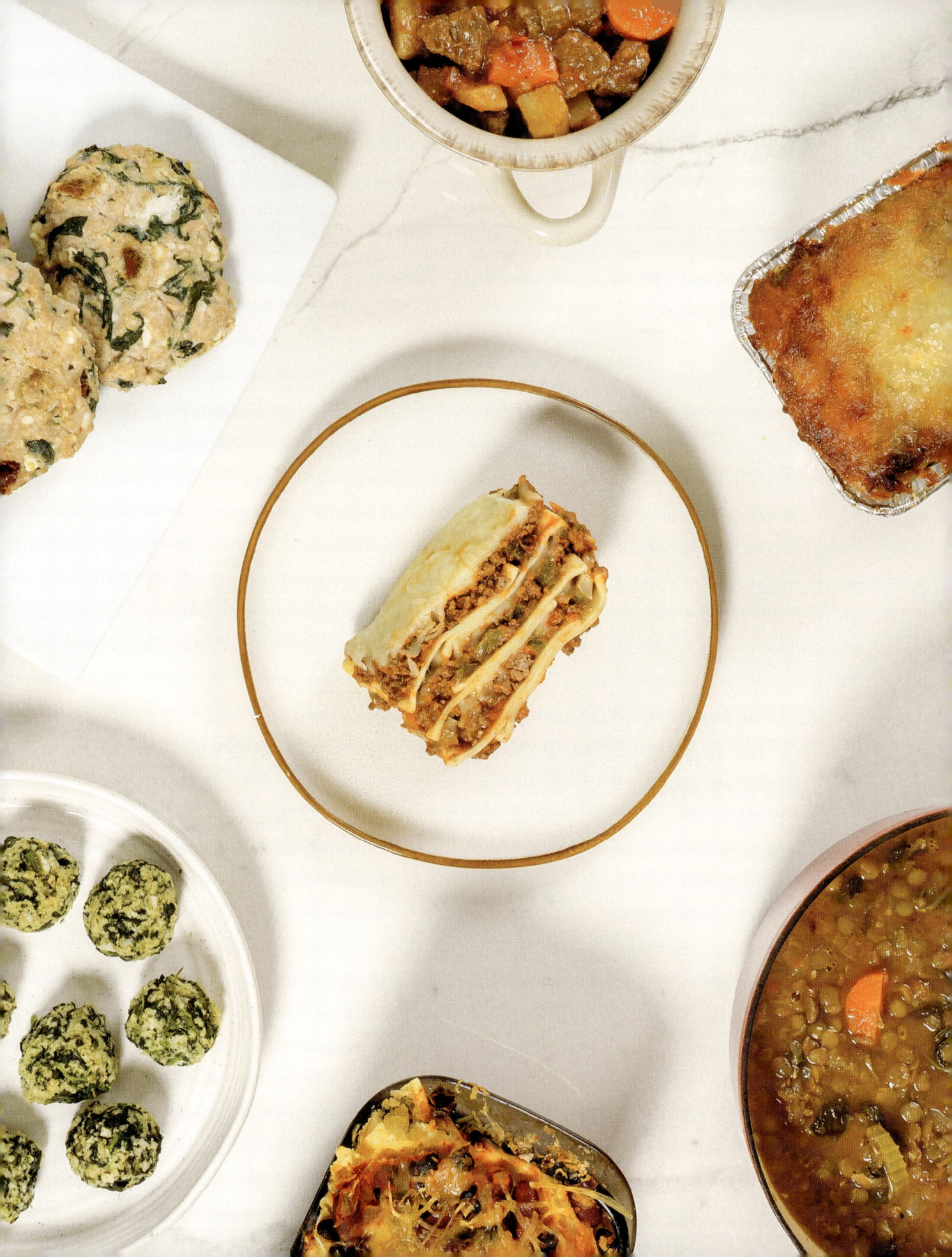

Freezer Meals

Prepare for your baby's arrival by creating a cozy nest for yourself. Dedicate some time to filling your freezer with the delicious meals featured in this chapter. As you transition into the early days at home with your newborn, you'll be focused on nourishing your baby, but who will take care of feeding you? Your freezer will become your best friend, especially during those crucial weeks following delivery. Trust us when we say adding an extra freezer to your registry wasn't a joke!

Although these recipes are designed for the freezer, you can certainly enjoy these meals on the same day you prepare them if you prefer. We've also provided reheating instructions with every recipe.

To ensure your recovery is supported, each recipe comes with a "vitamin C boost." This essential nutrient is crucial during this time, but the vitamin C in fresh ingredients can degrade during cooking. Therefore, we've included strategies to ensure you're getting enough of it. For more details on the importance of vitamin C, refer to chapter 2.

Mom's Spaghetti Sauce

SERVES 8
PREP TIME: 10 MINUTES
COOKING TIME: 35 MINUTES

1 tablespoon olive oil

1 large onion, diced

2 green bell peppers, diced

8 ounces mushrooms, sliced

2 pounds ground beef

4 garlic cloves, chopped

1 (28-ounce) jar marinara sauce

● **VITAMIN C BOOST**

Serve with a side salad with half a red bell pepper (+75mg) and a simple vinaigrette of ¼ cup lemon juice (+25mg), olive oil, and salt.

● **PROTEIN ADD**

Serve with bean pasta (+8g) or whole-wheat pasta (+7g).

● **MAKE IT PLANT-BASED**

Check out our Lentil Spaghetti Sauce recipe on page 61.

Per serving: Calories: 282
Fat: 16g | Carbohydrates: 12g
Fiber: 3g | Protein: 26g

This iron-rich meat sauce will help to replenish iron stores lost during delivery and provide much-needed protein for tissue repair.

1. In a large pot, heat the olive oil over medium heat. Add the onions, bell peppers, and mushrooms and sauté. Once they are soft (5–7 minutes), add in the ground beef and cook until completely browned, mashing it with a fork to get it to crumble. Add the garlic and cook for 1 more minute.

2. Pour in the jarred marinara sauce and simmer for 5–10 minutes. Cool completely and ladle back into the marinara sauce jar. Be sure to leave a bit of space at the top. Ladle the remaining sauce into another jar or freezer-safe container and freeze.

3. To defrost, place the jar in the refrigerator 2 days before you want to serve it, or submerge it in warm water until it's soft enough to scoop out.

NOTE: Use this in our lasagna recipe (page 62), serve over pasta, or mix with rice for stuffed peppers.

Lentil Spaghetti Sauce

SERVES 6
PREP TIME: 10 MINUTES
COOKING TIME: 35 MINUTES

1 large yellow onion, diced

6 garlic cloves, roughly chopped

4 cups vegetable broth, plus more for sautéing

1 ½ cups small diced carrots

2 teaspoons dried oregano

1 ½ teaspoons salt

½ teaspoon black pepper

¼ teaspoon red pepper flakes

¼ teaspoon ground cumin

¼ cup plus 4 teaspoons tomato paste

4 medium tomatoes, diced, with juices reserved

1 ⅓ cups dried red lentils

6 tablespoons hemp seeds

● **VITAMIN C BOOST**

Serve with a side salad with half a red bell pepper (+75mg) and a simple vinaigrette of ¼ cup lemon juice (+25mg), olive oil, and salt.

● **PROTEIN ADD**

Serve with bean pasta (+8g) or whole-wheat pasta (+7g), or add 3 more tablespoons of hemp seeds (+3g).

Per serving: Calories: 287
Fat: 8g | Carbohydrates: 23g
Fiber: 15g | Protein: 18g

Looking for a plant-based version of our spaghetti sauce? Instead of beef, this recipe uses lentils, which are also rich in protein and iron—two essential nutrients for postpartum healing.

1. In a large pot over medium heat, sauté the onion and garlic in a splash of vegetable broth for 2–3 minutes, adding more vegetable broth as needed.

2. Add the carrots, oregano, salt, pepper, red pepper flakes, and cumin. Cook for 7–8 minutes, stirring occasionally, adding more vegetable broth as needed to prevent sticking.

3. Add the tomato paste and tomatoes and their juices and cook for 2–3 minutes.

4. Add the vegetable broth, lentils, and hemp seeds. Bring to a boil, then cover tightly, lower the heat to low, and simmer gently for 20–25 minutes, or until the lentils are tender.

5. Cool completely and ladle into a ziplock bag or jar.

6. To defrost, place the bag or jar in the refrigerator 2 days before you want to serve it, or submerge it in warm water until it's soft enough to scoop out.

NOTE: Use this in our lasagna recipe (page 62), serve over pasta, or mix with rice for stuffed peppers.

BeaBea's Lasagna

MAKES TWO (8 X 3-INCH) LOAF PANS, ABOUT 12 SERVINGS
PREP TIME: 15 MINUTES
COOKING TIME: 50 MINUTES

½ (16-ounce) box lasagna noodles

1 recipe of Mom's Spaghetti Sauce (page 60) or Lentil Spaghetti Sauce (page 61)

2 (6-ounce) bags shredded mozzarella cheese

● **VITAMIN C BOOST**

Serve with our Pomegranate Fizz Mocktail (+26mg) (page 229) or a cup of water with ¼ cup lemon juice (+25mg).

● **MAKE IT PLANT-BASED**

Use Lentil Spaghetti Sauce and plant-based shredded mozzarella cheese.

● **MAKE IT GLUTEN-FREE**

Substitute noodles with gluten-free noodles or thinly sliced zucchini or eggplant.

Per serving: Calories: 393
Fat: 19g | Carbohydrates: 20g
Fiber: 4g | Protein: 30g

Use our Mom's Spaghetti Sauce to create this ultimate freezer meal. Complete with protein, carbs, beta-carotene, and iron, this meal will help your body heal during those first few weeks. It's also incredibly comforting and filling to help satisfy your postpartum hunger.

1. Boil the noodles according to the package instructions.

2. Preheat the oven to 350°F.

3. Place a small amount of sauce on the bottom of each of two 8-inch square aluminum pans. Lay lasagna noodles in a single layer over the sauce until the bottom layer is covered (note: lasagna noodles may need to be cut to completely cover the layer). Add about 1 cup of spaghetti sauce to each pan, then top with about ½ cup of mozzarella cheese. Repeat, adding another layer of noodles, sauce, and cheese. Top each pan with a final layer of noodles and the remaining sauce. Top with the remaining mozzarella.

4. Cover with foil and bake for 45–50 minutes, or until the lasagna is bubbling.

5. Allow to cool completely before wrapping in foil and freezing.

6. To defrost, remove from the freezer 2–3 days before you plan to eat it. To reheat, bake, covered in foil, at 350°F for 45 minutes. Remove the foil and allow the cheese to crisp before removing from the oven. Or for a single serving, microwave a slice for approximately 2 minutes.

NOTE: We recommend baking the lasagna before you freeze it so that you can simply defrost it and reheat a slice in the microwave. However, you can also assemble the lasagna and freeze it unbaked. Just remember to thaw completely before cooking.

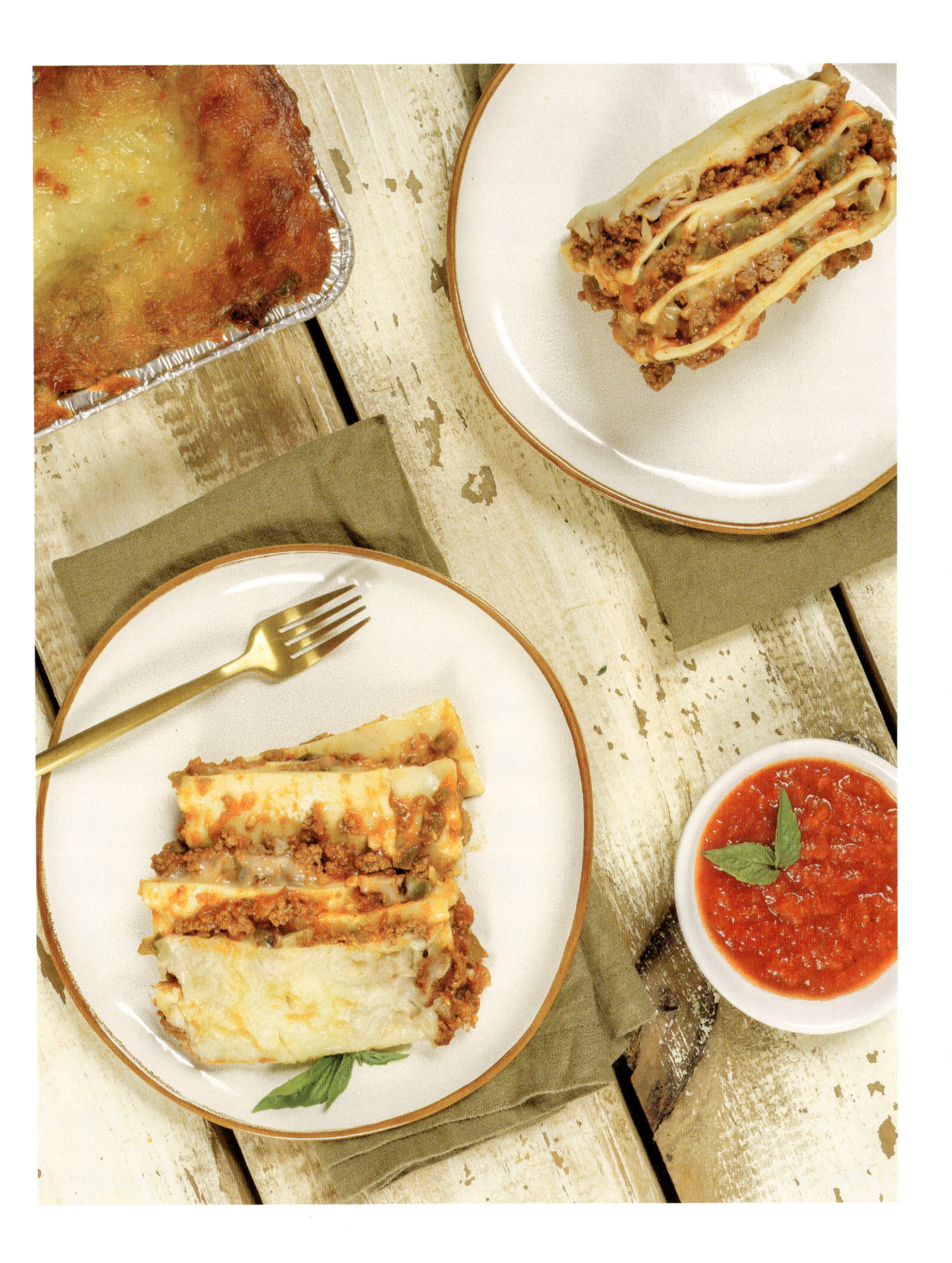

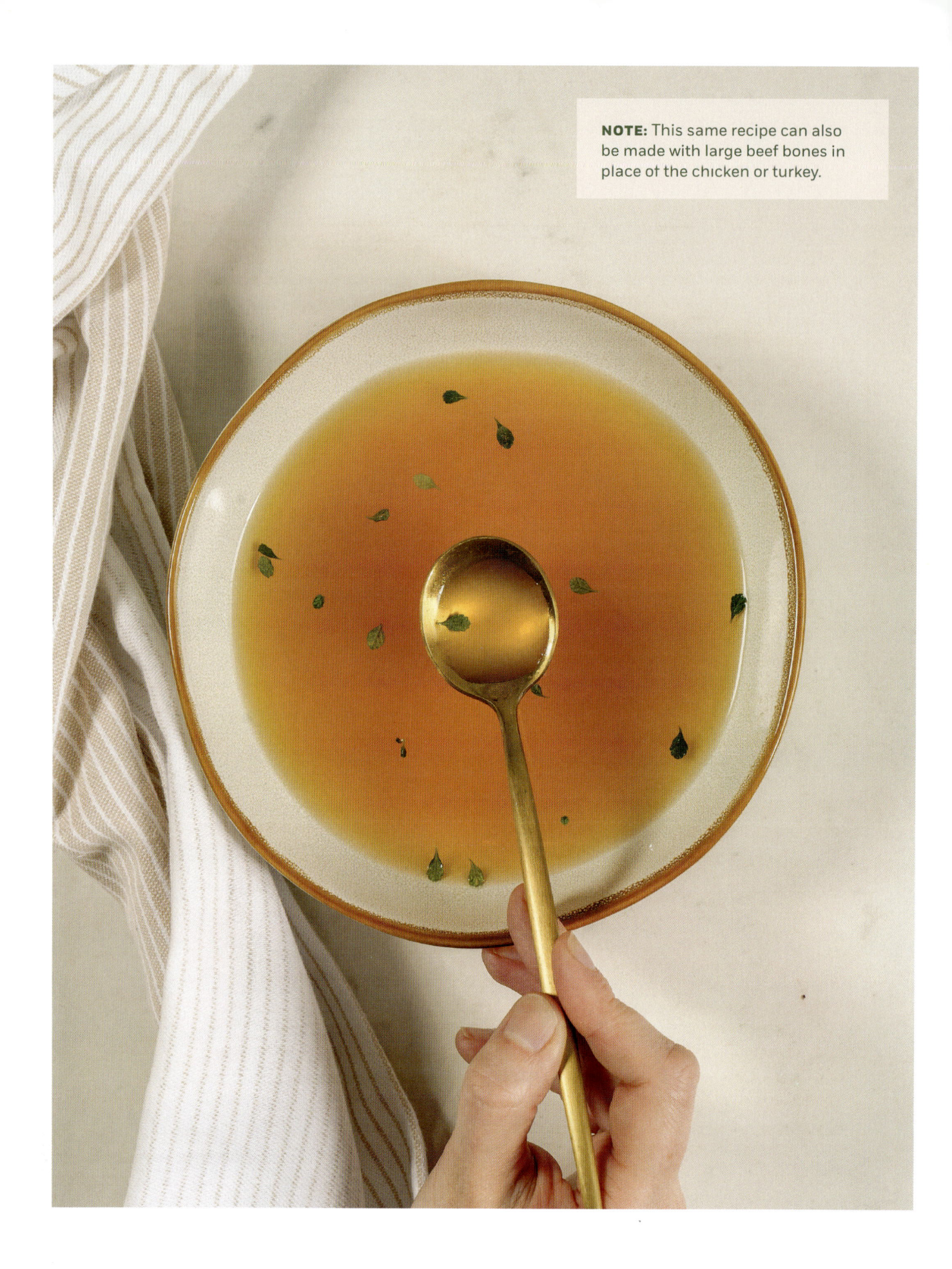

NOTE: This same recipe can also be made with large beef bones in place of the chicken or turkey.

Homemade Chicken Broth

MAKES 4 QUARTS, ABOUT 16 (1-CUP) SERVINGS
PREP TIME: 10 MINUTES
COOKING TIME: 24 HOURS

6 carrots, roughly chopped

4 celery stalks, roughly chopped

2 large onions, roughly chopped

3 garlic cloves, smashed with skin removed

4 chicken backs or 1 turkey back (ask at the meat counter)

3 bay leaves

2 teaspoons salt

1 teaspoon black pepper

1 teaspoon dried thyme

● **VITAMIN C BOOST**

Have a serving of broth with 1 orange (+70mg) or 2 kiwis (+130mg).

● **PROTEIN ADD**

Serve with 3 ounces of shredded protein, such as chicken, beef, or pork (+21g).

● **MAKE IT PLANT-BASED**

Check out our Vegetable Broth recipe on page 66.

Per 1-cup serving: Calories: 52
Fat: 3g | Carbohydrates: 1g
Fiber: 0g | Protein: 5g

Sipping on warm broth immediately after delivery is incredibly soothing. By making your own bone broth, you control the ingredients and can benefit from additional protein from the long cooking process. Mostly water and electrolytes, this broth is also a great option to enhance hydration and can be used in place of boxed chicken broth in any recipe.

1. Combine all the ingredients in an Instant Pot or slow cooker. Add enough water to cover the ingredients, or at least 4 quarts.

2. In Instant Pot, select the slow cooker function and set the time to 20 hours. In a slow cooker, cook on low for 24 hours. You may need to check occasionally and add more water in a slow cooker.

3. When the time has finished, allow it to cool slightly, then place a colander inside a large bowl. Slowly pour the broth through the colander to catch and discard all the solid ingredients.

4. Portion the broth into individual containers (such as quart-size leftover takeout containers or glass jars). Allow the broth to cool completely before freezing.

5. To defrost, remove from the freezer and thaw in the refrigerator for 24 hours. Depending on the shape of the container, you may also be able to run the container under hot water to loosen the broth from the sides and then add the frozen broth directly to your dish.

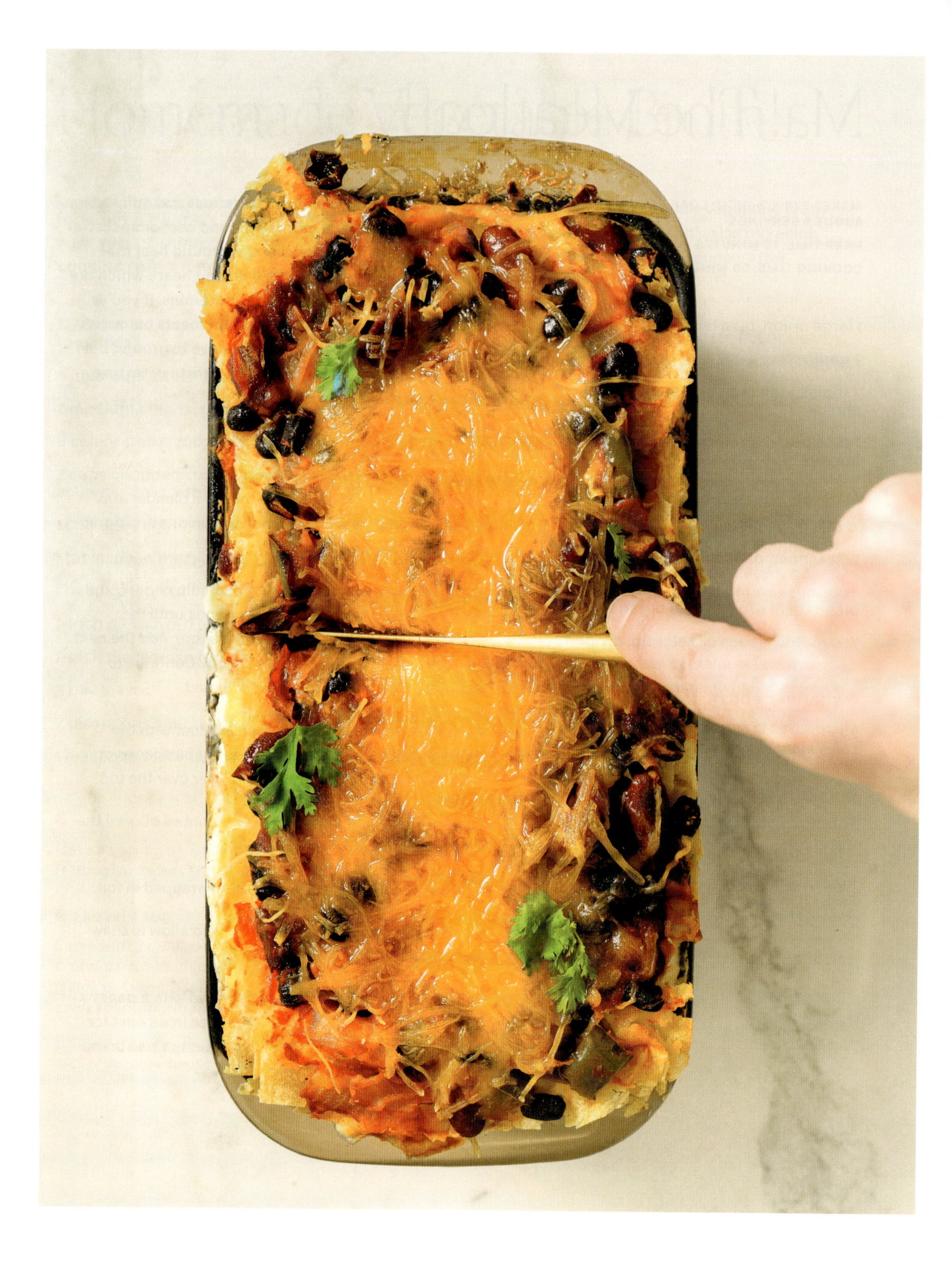

Creamy Enchilada Casserole

SERVES 6
PREP TIME: 20 MINUTES
COOKING TIME: 25 MINUTES

2 tablespoons olive oil

1 red bell pepper, diced

1 onion, diced

4 cups dark leafy greens (spinach, kale, chard)

2 (15.5-ounce) cans pinto, black, or kidney beans, rinsed

1 (15-ounce) jar enchilada sauce

8 (6-inch) corn tortillas, halved

1 ½ cup cottage cheese

¼ cup water

½ cup shredded cheddar or Monterey Jack cheese

Optional toppings: fresh cilantro and lime juice

● **VITAMIN C BOOST**

Serve with our Frozen Strawberry-Lime Mock-a-Rita (page 232, +97 mg).

● **PROTEIN ADD**

Add 3 ounces of shredded meat (+21g) or 3 ounces of baked tofu (+13g).

Per serving: Calories: 340
Fat: 10g | Carbohydrates: 46g
Fiber: 10g | Protein: 17g

Layered like a lasagna, this enchilada casserole comes together quickly and is full of flavor and fiber. The cottage cheese adds protein to make this recipe creamy and filling.

1. Preheat the oven to 375°F.

2. Heat the olive oil in a large skillet over medium heat. Add the bell pepper and onions and sauté until tender (about 4 minutes).

3. Add the greens, beans, and enchilada sauce. Cook until the greens are wilted (about 4 minutes).

4. Spray an 8 x 3-inch aluminum loaf pan with nonstick spray. Place one-quarter of the enchilada filling on the bottom of the pan. Spread evenly to coat. Then arrange 5–6 tortilla halves on top of the sauce, trying to completely cover the layer. Add another quarter of the filling mixture on top of the tortillas. Then top with ¾ cup of the cottage cheese.

5. Repeat this process with another layer of tortillas, another quarter of the filling, and the remaining cottage cheese. Top with a last layer of tortillas, then combine the remaining filling with the water. Pour over the tortillas and top with the shredded cheese.

6. Cover with aluminum foil and bake for 20–25 minutes, or until the cheese is completely melted.

7. To freeze, cool completely before wrapping the entire dish in foil.

8. To defrost, remove from the freezer 1–2 days before you plan to eat. Reheat the entire dish in the oven, covered with foil, at 375°F for 30 minutes. You can also reheat the defrosted casserole in the microwave: remove a slice from the pan and heat for 90 seconds.

9. Serve topped with cilantro and fresh lime juice, if desired.

White Bean Chicken Chili

SERVES 4
PREP TIME: 15 MINUTES
COOKING TIME: 30 MINUTES

2 tablespoons olive oil

1 pound boneless, skinless chicken thighs, cut into 1 x 1-inch pieces

1 large red onion, diced

1 (4-ounce) can green chiles

2 garlic cloves, chopped

1 tablespoon ground cumin

¼ teaspoon salt

¼ teaspoon black pepper

1 (32-ounce) carton chicken or vegetable broth (if using low-sodium broth, add more salt)

2 (15.5-ounce) cans white beans, drained and rinsed

2 cups frozen corn

Optional toppings: fresh cilantro, shredded cheddar cheese

● **VITAMIN C BOOST**

Squeeze the juice of half a lime (+7mg) over the chili and pair with our Summer Shandy (page 235, +16mg).

● **MAKE IT PLANT-BASED**

Replace the chicken with an extra 15.5-ounce can of white beans.

Per serving: Calories: 447
Fat: 12g | Carbohydrates: 55g
Fiber: 12g | Protein: 35g

A winning recipe to store in the freezer, this hearty chili is high in protein and fiber, two nutrients that aid in the postpartum recovery process. Green chiles are very high in vitamin C, but unfortunately much of it is lost in processing and cooking. Not to fear, though, we've added a vitamin C boost that will ensure you are still taking in enough.

1. In a large saucepan, heat the olive oil over medium heat. Add the chicken and onions. Cook, stirring often, until the onions are soft and the chicken is opaque (about 7 minutes). Add the chiles, garlic, cumin, salt, and pepper. Cook for 2 minutes, then add the broth and bring up to a low boil.

2. Add 1 can of white beans to the pan. Thoroughly mash the beans from the other can with a fork and stir into the chili. Bring back up to a low boil for 5 minutes, then turn off the heat. Stir in the corn.

3. Portion the chili into individual containers (such as quart-size leftover takeout containers, glass jars, or silicone soup cubes). Allow the chili to cool completely before freezing.

4. To defrost, remove from the freezer and thaw in the refrigerator for 24 hours. Depending on the shape of the container, you may also be able to run the container under hot water to loosen the chili from the sides. Microwave for 2 minutes or heat on the stovetop until heated through.

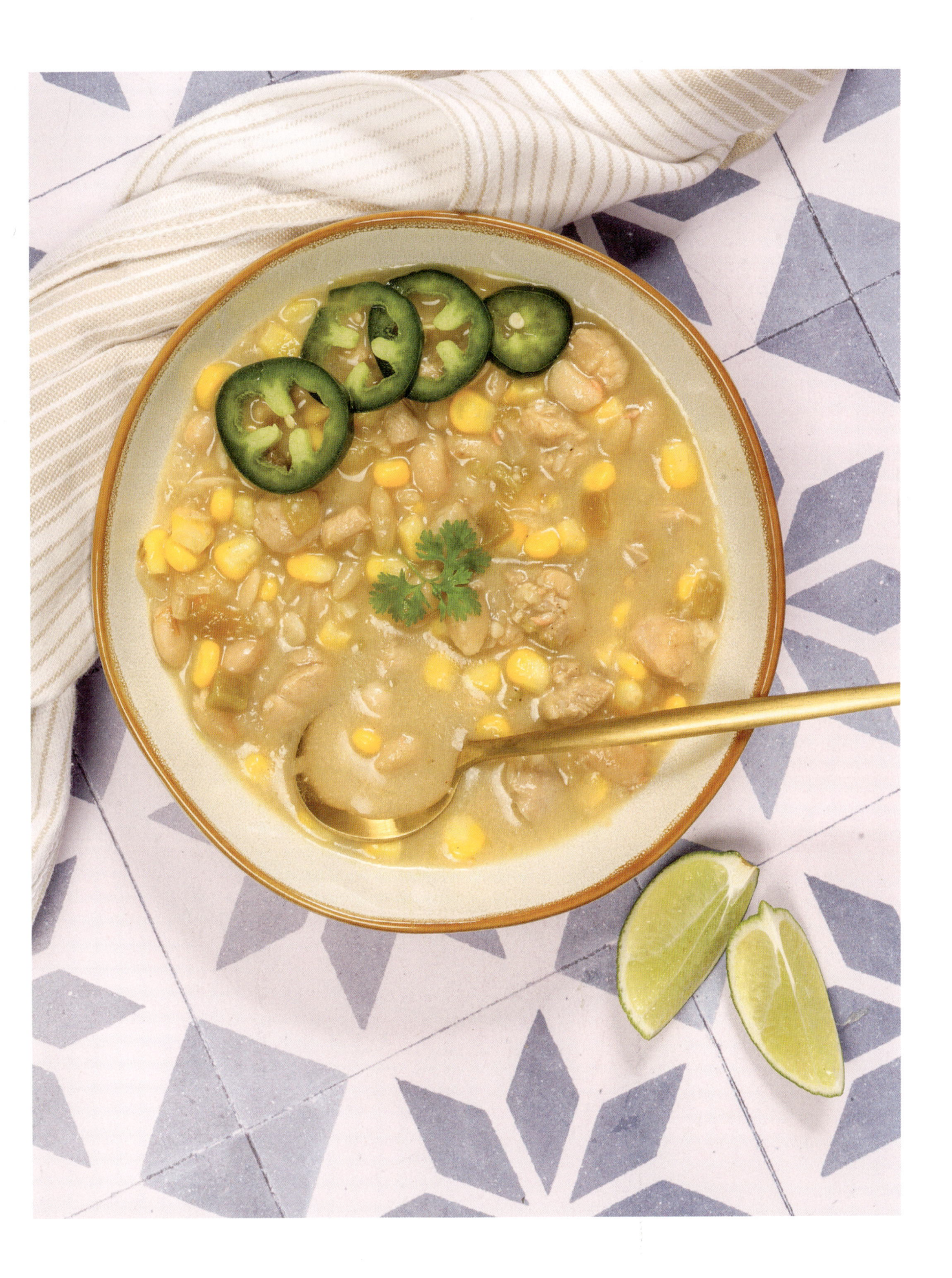

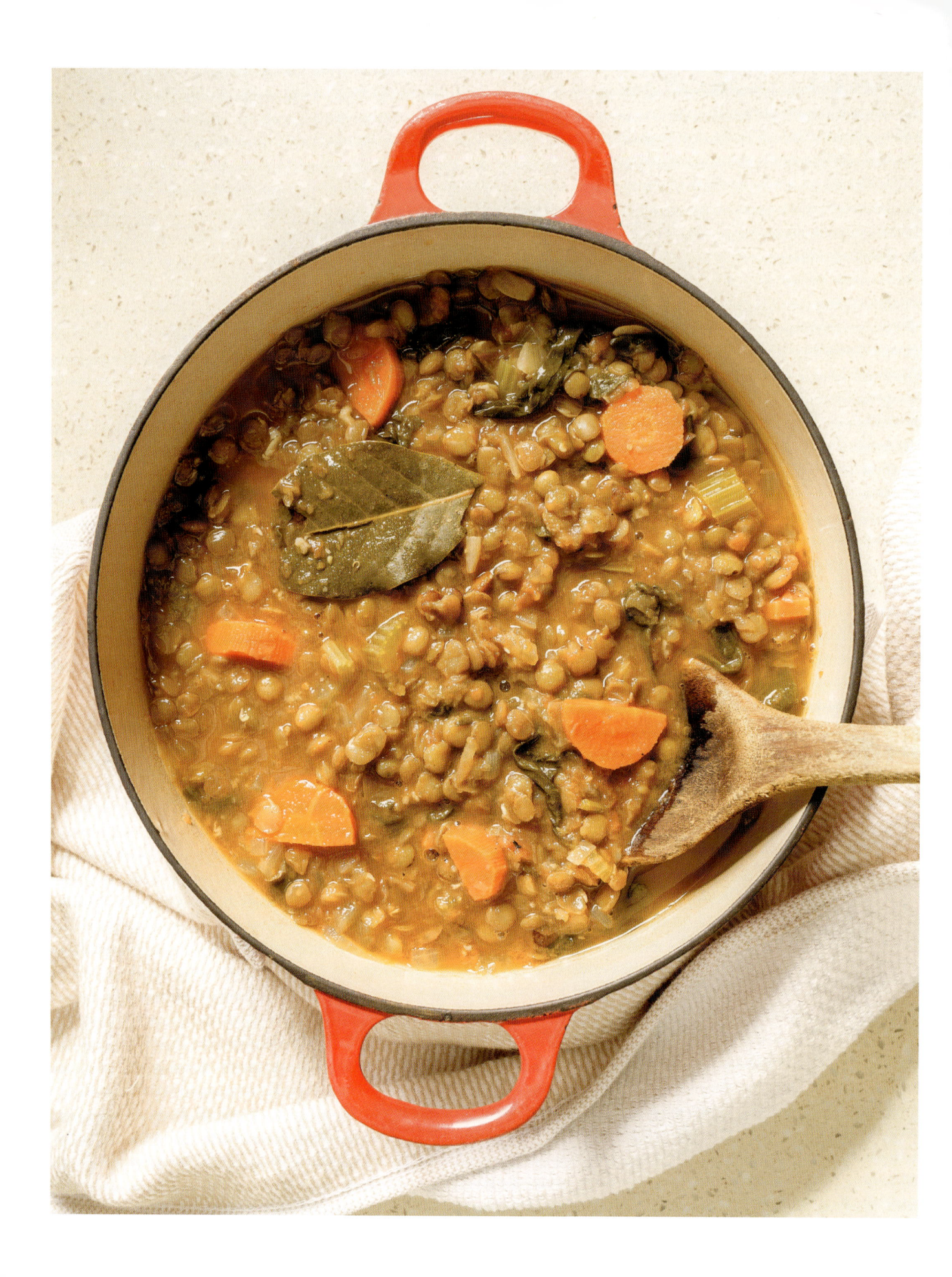

Life-Giving Lentil Soup

SERVES 4
PREP TIME: 10 MINUTES
COOKING TIME: 55 MINUTES

1 tablespoon olive oil

1 medium yellow onion, diced

1 large carrot, chopped

2 celery stalks, chopped

3 garlic cloves, minced

1 ½ cups dried brown or black lentils, rinsed

1 (14-ounce) can fire-roasted crushed tomatoes

4 cups vegetable or chicken broth, plus more for sautéing

1 teaspoon paprika

½ teaspoon ground cumin

½ teaspoon chili powder

1 dried bay leaf

3 cups spinach

1 tablespoon lemon juice

½ teaspoon salt, or more to taste

½ teaspoon black pepper

● **VITAMIN C BOOST**

Pair with our It's A Girl! Smoothie (page 220, +77mg).

● **PROTEIN ADD**

Serve with 3 ounces of shredded meat (+21g) or 3 tablespoons of hemp seeds (+10g).

Per serving: Calories: 243
Fat: 4g | Carbohydrates: 21g
Fiber: 16g | Protein: 14g

Lentils are an excellent plant-based source of both protein and iron, serving 18 grams of protein and 6.6 milligrams of iron (75% of the recommended daily value) per cup. This lentil soup is thick and hearty and a perfect plant-based option during the early postpartum recovery period.

1. Heat the olive oil in a stockpot over low heat. Add the onions, carrots, and celery and sauté for 7–10 minutes, stirring frequently, until the vegetables are soft.

2. Add the garlic and cook for another 2–3 minutes, or until the garlic is soft.

3. Add the lentils, tomatoes, broth, paprika, cumin, chili powder, and bay leaf. Stir.

4. Increase the heat and bring to a simmer. Cover and turn the heat down to medium-low. Simmer for 35–40 minutes, or until the lentils are soft.

5. Remove the bay leaf. To thicken the soup, transfer 1 cup to a blender and blend until creamy, then transfer it back into the pot.

6. Add the spinach and cook for another 1–2 minutes, or until the spinach is wilted.

7. Add the lemon juice, salt, and pepper. To adjust the soup's consistency, add a touch more vegetable broth, if desired.

8. Portion the soup into ziplock bags, reusable silicone bags, or glass containers to freeze. To defrost, place in the refrigerator 1–3 days before you plan to eat it, or run the container under hot water to loosen the soup from the sides. Heat it in the microwave for 2 minutes or in a pot on the stove until heated through.

Ironclad Beef Stew

SERVES 6
PREP TIME: 15 MINUTES
COOKING TIME: 1 HOUR 15 MINUTES

2 pounds beef stew meat, chuck roast, or round roast, cubed into 1-inch pieces

½ teaspoon salt

¼ teaspoon black pepper

1 tablespoon olive oil

1 large onion, diced into large pieces

4 celery stalks, diced into 1-inch pieces

5 large carrots, cut into half-moons

3 large russet potatoes, diced into 1-inch pieces

2 garlic cloves, roughly chopped

1 (28-ounce) can diced tomatoes

1 cup broth (any kind will do)

½ teaspoon dried thyme

2 bay leaves

1 tablespoon cornstarch

2 tablespoons cold water

● **VITAMIN C BOOST**

Have 1 cup of frozen pineapple on the side or for dessert (+79mg).

● **MAKE IT PLANT-BASED**

Try our Life-Giving Lentil Soup on page 73.

Per serving: Calories: 472
Fat: 27g | Carbohydrates: 26g
Fiber: 2g | Protein: 32g

Beef stew is made from tougher cuts of beef that come from muscles that are heavily utilized by the cow and high in collagen. When cooked low and slow (or under the high pressure of an Instant Pot), the collagen in these tough cuts of meat eventually dissolves into the surrounding liquid. When digested, these amino acids can be used to create collagen in your body for the recovery process, or to make any other type of protein in the body.

1. Season the beef with salt and black pepper. Working in two batches in an Instant Pot, select the sauté function, add the oil, and brown the beef for 3–4 minutes on each side. Try not to crowd the pan.

2. Once both batches of beef are browned, return all the beef to the Instant Pot, turn off sauté mode, and add all the remaining ingredients except the cornstarch. Stir, close the lid, and cook under high pressure for 45 minutes. Allow a 15–20 minute natural release.

3. If a thicker stew is desired, mix the cornstarch with the cold water in a small bowl. Add to the stew while it is still very hot. Stir and allow to sit for 5–10 minutes to thicken.

4. Cool completely and place into ziplock bags, reusable silicone bags, or glass containers to freeze.

5. To defrost, place in the refrigerator 1–3 days before you plan to eat it, then reheat in the microwave or on the stovetop. You can also reheat this recipe straight from frozen in the Instant Pot, cooking under high pressure for 4 minutes with a quick release.

NOTE: This recipe can be made in a slow cooker. Just brown the meat in a pan before adding to the slow cooker with the other ingredients (except the cornstarch). Cook on low for 8 hours.

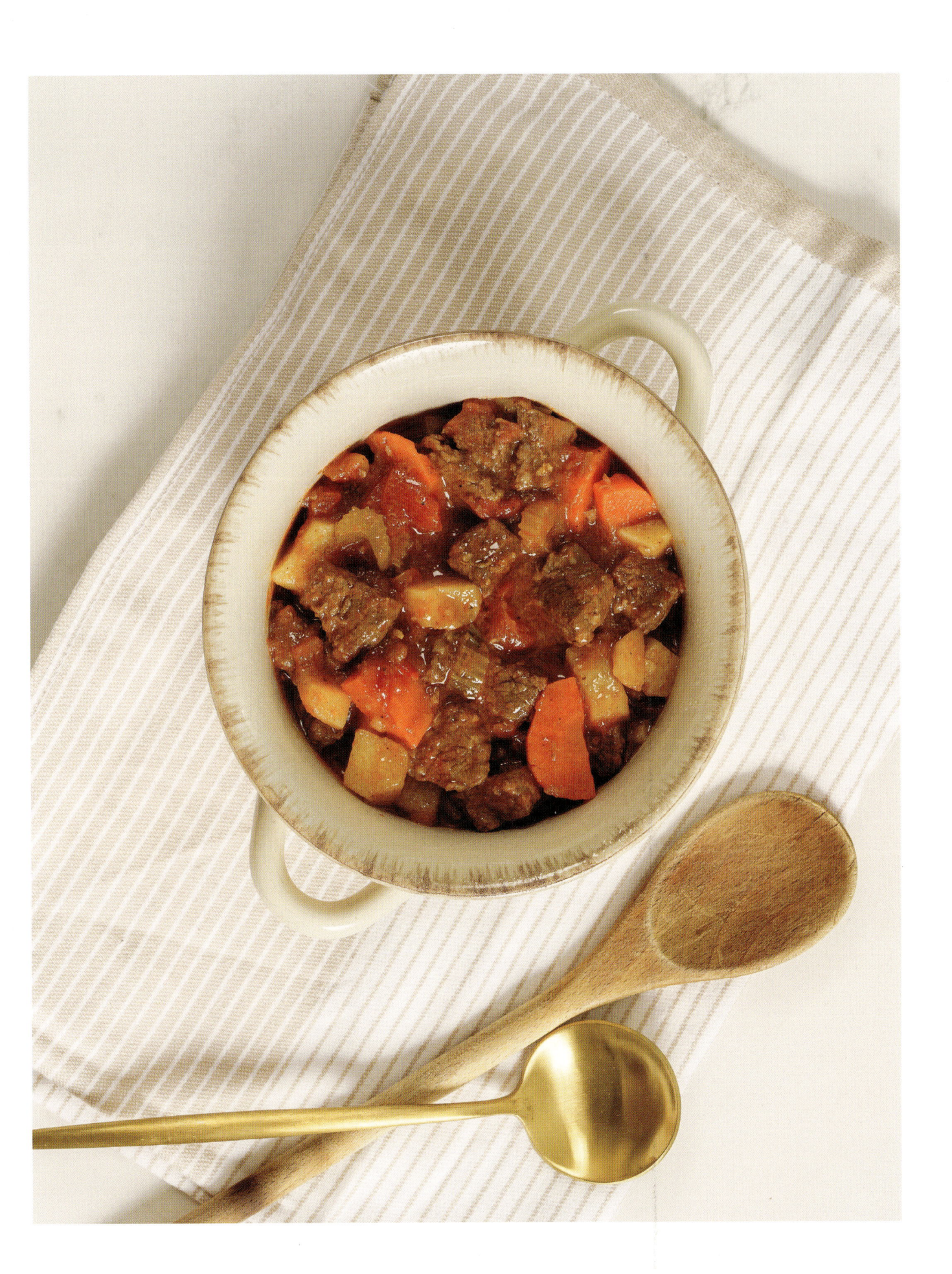

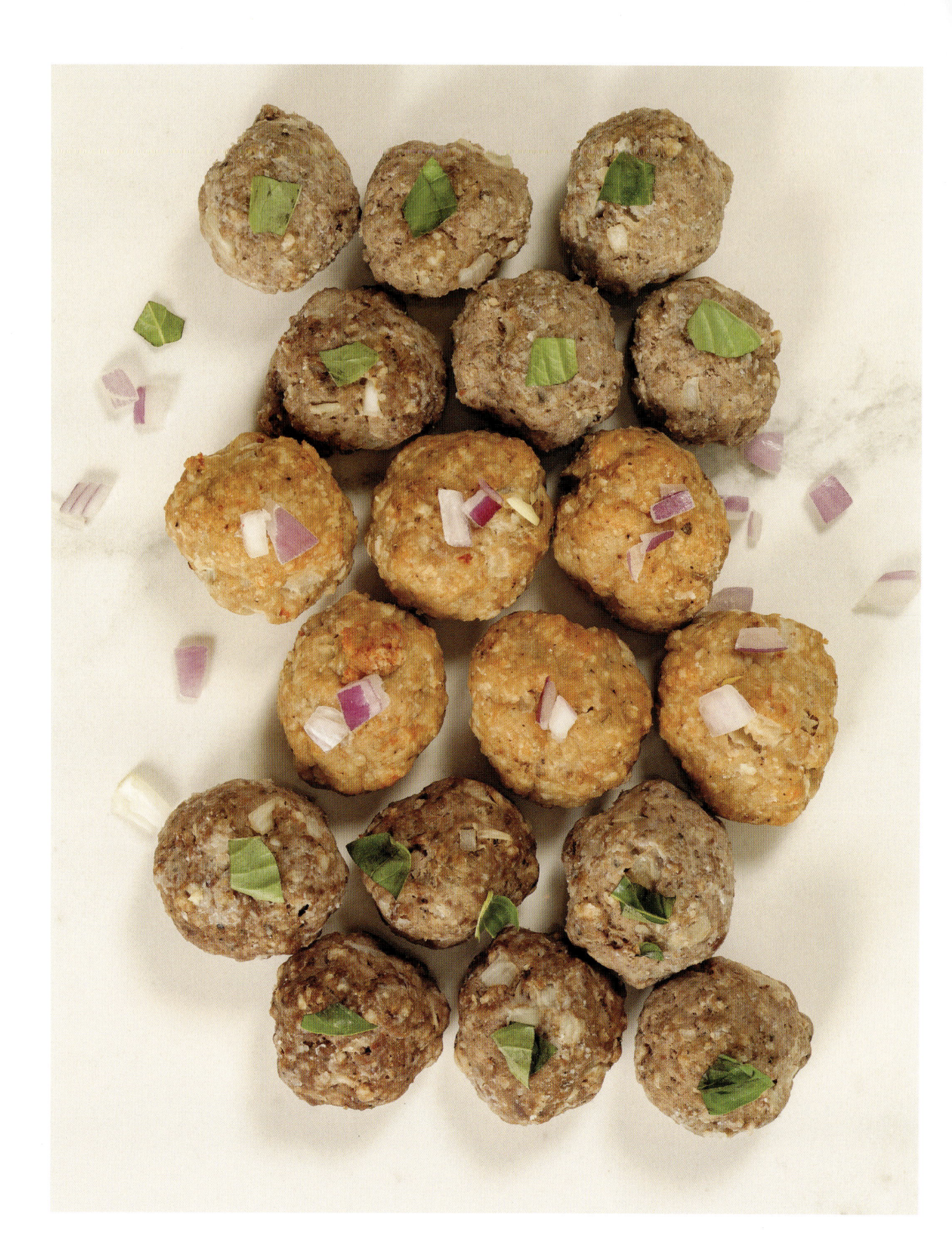

Mighty Miles's Meatballs (3 Ways)

MAKES 32 (1-OUNCE) MEATBALLS PER VARIATION
PREP TIME: 15 MINUTES
OVEN COOKING TIME: 25 MINUTES
AIR FRYER COOKING TIME: 13 MINUTES

PORK

2 slices white bread, torn into small cubes

1 cup milk of choice

½ onion, finely diced

6 garlic cloves, finely chopped

1 teaspoon salt

1 teaspoon black pepper

⅛ teaspoon ground nutmeg

2 pounds ground pork

CHICKEN

2 slices white bread, torn into small cubes

⅔ cup milk of choice

½ onion, finely diced

6 garlic cloves, finely chopped

2 tablespoons poultry seasoning

1 teaspoon salt

1 teaspoon black pepper

1 tablespoon olive oil

2 pounds ground chicken

Continued...

Plain meatballs are a great way to add a protein source to any meal. Each meatball has about 7 grams of protein and is a blank canvas for your creativity. They can be eaten plain on the plate, mixed with sauce, cooked into a recipe (see the pantry recipe ideas on the following page), served over a grain of your choice, or added to a roll for a one-handed lunch. The beef or ancestral blend meatballs are also a great source of iron, an important nutrient to consider during pregnancy and recovery. They have 0.6 milligrams and 0.75 milligrams, respectively.

1. Preheat the oven to 350°F.

2. Combine the torn bread with the milk in a large bowl. Allow to soak for 10 minutes. Using your hands, gently massage the bread to mash it into a paste. Add the onions, garlic, and all the seasonings. Combine with your hands (you can also throw all of this into a blender). Then add the ground meat and thoroughly combine using your hands.

3. To evenly divide the filling, first separate the mixture into four even parts. Then quarter each quarter to make 16 sections, and halve each section again to make 32 meatballs.

4. Place the meatballs on a baking sheet and bake for 25 minutes at 350°F, or until the internal temperature reaches 165°F. You can also air fry them at 400°F for 13 minutes.

5. Cool completely before freezing. The meatballs can be frozen in a reusable or ziplock bag with all the air removed. We recommend freezing 16 meatballs in each bag.

CONTINUED...

BEEF

2 slices white bread, torn into small cubes

1 cup milk of choice

½ onion, finely diced

6 garlic cloves, finely chopped

2 tablespoons Italian seasoning

2 tablespoons grated Parmesan cheese

1 teaspoon salt

1 teaspoon black pepper

2 pounds ground beef or ancestral blend (beef ground with organ meats)

● **VITAMIN C BOOST**

Pair these proteins with other recipes containing vitamin C, such as our smoothies, salads, or mocktails, since meat is not a good source of vitamin C.

● **MAKE IT GLUTEN-FREE**

Substitute the 2 slices of bread for ½ cup of gluten-free rolled oats.

Per meatball: Calories: 30
Fat: 2g | Carbohydrates: 2g
Fiber: 0g | Protein: 7g

6. To reheat: Defrost in the refrigerator overnight. You can also add these straight from the freezer to a sauce such as marinara and heat them through on the stove. Or microwave straight from the freezer for 2 minutes. Allow to cool for 1 minute before eating.

Pantry Recipe Ideas for Meatballs:

Toss with jarred sauces such as marinara, BBQ sauce, or teriyaki sauce.

Hawaiian Beef Meatballs: Blend 1 ½ cups frozen pineapple, 2 tablespoons apple cider vinegar, and ¼ cup water in a blender until a smooth sauce forms. Combine 16 defrosted meatballs, 2 cups frozen pepper-onion mix, and 2 cups frozen brown rice in a large skillet with 1 teaspoon olive oil. Sauté for 3 minutes over medium heat until the pepper-onion mix thaws. Add the blended sauce and cook until the sauce has reduced. Optional: To thicken the sauce further, dissolve 1 tablespoon cornstarch into 2 tablespoons water. Add to the pan and allow to come to a boil.

Pork Swedish Meatballs: Heat 1 tablespoon olive oil in a large skillet over medium heat. Sauté 1 large sliced onion until tender. Add 1 diced clove of garlic, 1 (4-ounce) can of mushrooms (drained) and 1 tablespoon flour. Cook for 2 minutes, then stir in 1 cup broth, ½ teaspoon black pepper, ½ teaspoon salt, and 4 shakes Worcestershire sauce. Allow to bubble and thicken over low heat for 4–5 minutes. Stir in ¼ cup plain yogurt. Add 16 defrosted meatballs and stir to coat. Serve over egg noodles.

Chicken Piccata Meatballs: Sauté 3 cloves of garlic in 3 tablespoons olive oil over low heat. Add 1 tablespoon flour, stir to thoroughly combine with the oil, and cook for 2 minutes. Add ½ cup broth and simmer until the broth begins to thicken. Add 3 tablespoons lemon juice, 2 tablespoons drained capers, and 2 teaspoons dried parsley. Add 16 defrosted chicken meatballs and warm through. Serve over rice or pasta.

Shredded Meat (3 Ways)

SERVES 8 (EACH VARIATION)
PREP TIME: 5 MINUTES
COOKING TIME: 15–50 MINUTES, DEPENDING ON VARIATION

CHICKEN THIGHS

2 pounds boneless, skinless chicken thighs

½ teaspoon salt

½ teaspoon black pepper

½ teaspoon garlic powder

1 cup water

PULLED PORK

2 pounds pork butt or shoulder roast

1 teaspoon salt

½ cup water

SHREDDED BEEF

2 pounds beef chuck or shoulder roast

1 tablespoon olive oil

2 teaspoons salt

½ cup water

● **VITAMIN C BOOST**

Pair these proteins with other recipes containing vitamin C, such as our smoothies, salads, or mocktails, since meat is not a good source of vitamin C.

Per 4-ounce serving:
Calories: 200 | Fat: 12g
Carbohydrates: 0g
Fiber: 0g | Protein: 28g

These recipes got Ashley's husband's vote for best freezer meals during the postpartum stage. They can be added to literally anything and make throwing dinner together a breeze, since carbs, fats, and vegetables don't usually take as much time to cook. Consider these proteins as ingredients for pantry meals.

1. **For chicken thighs:** Place the chicken thighs in a layer on the bottom of an Instant Pot. Sprinkle them with the salt, pepper, and garlic powder. Top with the water. Cook under high pressure for 10 minutes and allow a 5-minute natural release.

2. **For pulled pork and shredded beef:** Remove any large visible pieces of fat from the meat and dice the beef into 2-inch cubes.

3. Place the meat in the Instant Pot, drizzle with olive oil, sprinkle with salt, and pour the water around it into the bottom of the Instant Pot. Cook under high pressure for 40 minutes and allow a 10-minute natural release.

4. Shred and store in a ziplock or reusable silicone bag with all of the air removed. Defrost in refrigerator overnight or add to slow cooker, Instant Pot, or stovetop recipe frozen. Try the chicken thighs in our Pesto Chicken Salad (page 122) and Thai Chicken Salad (page 132), the pulled pork in the Pulled Pork Sandwich (page 171) in our Pantry Meals chapter, and the shredded beef in our Shredded Beef Tacos (page 170) in our Pantry Meals chapter.

NOTE: These recipes can easily be doubled. You can use also serve these meats over pasta, mixed with rice and taco seasoning to fill stuffed peppers, or on bagged salads.

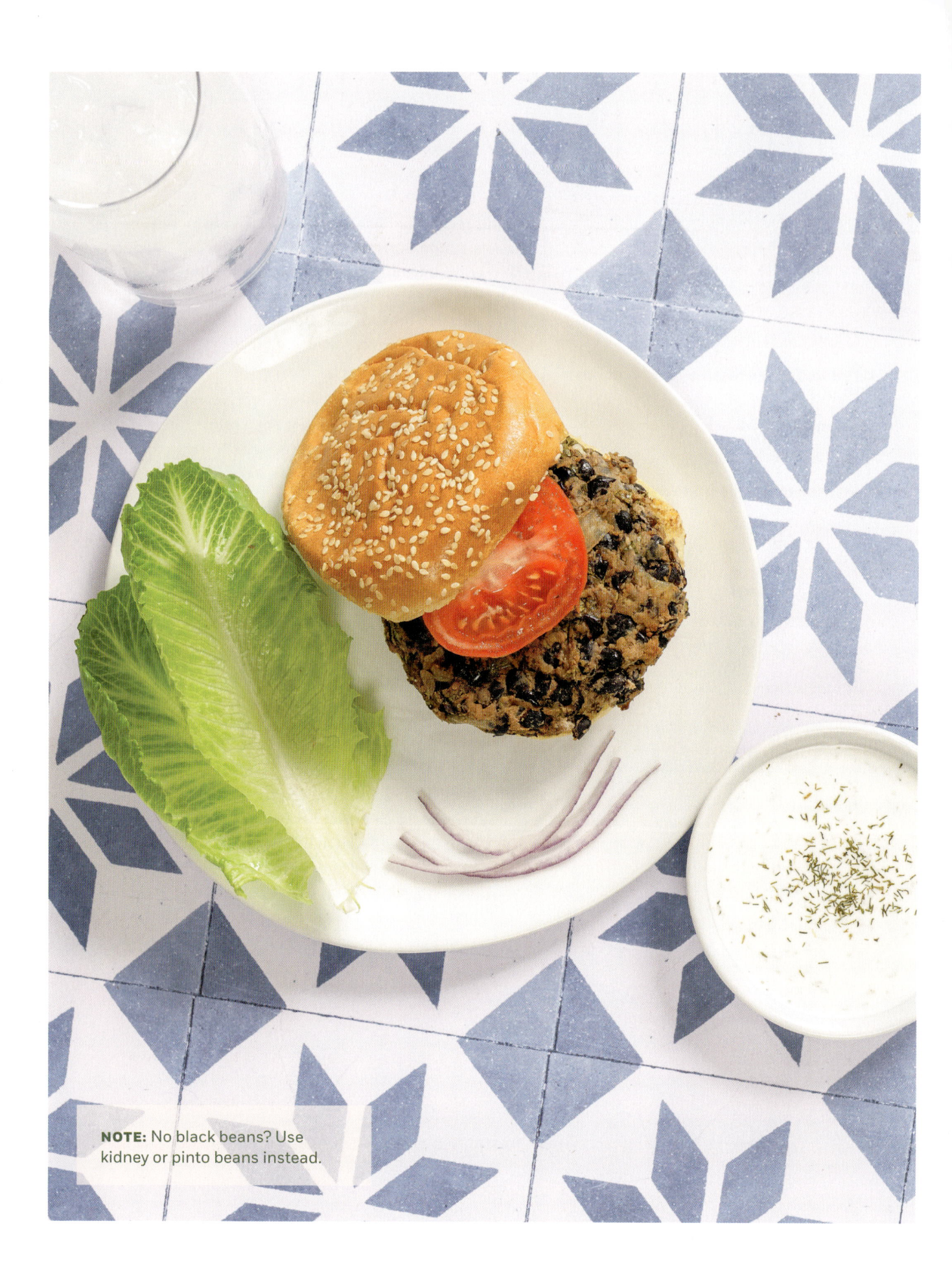

NOTE: No black beans? Use kidney or pinto beans instead.

Mushroom Black Bean Burgers

MAKES 8 PATTIES
PREP TIME: 15 MINUTES
SETTING TIME: 2 HOURS
COOKING TIME: 50 MINUTES

1 tablespoon olive oil

8 ounces mushrooms, chopped

1 yellow or white onion, finely diced

4 garlic cloves, minced

4 cups cooked black beans

1 cup fresh cilantro, chopped

½ cup ground flaxseed

Juice of 2 limes (¼ cup)

2 tablespoons ketchup or mayonnaise

1 teaspoon red pepper flakes

1 teaspoon salt

½ teaspoon black pepper

½ teaspoon ground cumin

● **VITAMIN C BOOST**
Make it into a burger or sandwich and pair with half a ripe tomato (+10mg) and a sliced red bell pepper on the side (+150mg).

● **PROTEIN ADD**
Serve between 2 slices of bread or on a bun (+10g) and add 1 slice of cheddar cheese (+7g).

Per patty: Calories: 205
Fat: 7g | Carbohydrates: 17g
Fiber: 11g | Protein: 11

Filled with black beans and ground flaxseed, these plant-based burgers are rich in fiber and protein. The mushrooms add texture, depth, and additional nutrients to the patties, and the beans are high in zinc to support collagen formation. Better than any store-bought brand, these are sure to become your new favorite bean burger.

1. Heat the olive oil in a large skillet. Sauté the mushrooms and onion over medium heat for 7–9 minutes, or until the onions are translucent. Add the garlic and cook for 1–2 more minutes.

2. Place the beans in a large bowl and mash with a potato masher, leaving some chunks throughout the mixture for texture.

3. Add the mushroom mixture and all the remaining ingredients to the beans. Mix until everything is well combined.

4. Shape the mixture into eight separate balls, then press each one down using the palm of your hand or the bottom of a cup until it forms the shape of a burger patty.

5. Transfer the patties to a freezer-safe container lined with parchment paper. Allow burgers to set for 2 hours in the refrigerator before freezing.

6. When ready to eat, allow them to thaw until they are completely defrosted.

7. Preheat the oven to 375°F. Place the patties on a parchment paper-lined baking sheet and bake for 50 minutes, flipping the burgers at the halfway point.

8. Let cool for 10 minutes before serving.

Mediterranean Turkey Burgers

SERVES 8
PREP TIME: 10 MINUTES
COOKING TIME: 30 MINUTES

1 cup frozen spinach

2 pounds ground turkey

2 eggs

4 ounces feta cheese

12 sun-dried tomatoes, halved and diced (about ⅓ cup diced)

1 tablespoon olive oil, plus more for the pan

½ teaspoon onion powder

½ teaspoon garlic powder

½ teaspoon black pepper

½ teaspoon salt

● **VITAMIN C BOOST**

Serve as a sandwich and pair with a fruit high in vitamin C, such as an orange (+50mg), kiwi (+64mg), or handful of raspberries (+32 mg).

● **MAKE IT PLANT-BASED**

Check out our Mushroom Black Bean Burger recipe on page 81.

Per serving: Calories: 251
Fat: 15g | Carbohydrates: 3g
Fiber: 0g | Protein: 27g

You can pull these turkey burgers from the freezer for a quick lunch option. High in protein and packed with flavor, these will be a staple item in your freezer. Turkey is high in B vitamins and choline, an essential nutrient for baby's brain development. These also make delicious meatballs!

1. Preheat the oven to 350°F.

2. Microwave the frozen spinach for 30 seconds. Allow to cool enough to be handled. Transfer to a paper towel and wring to squeeze out as much water as possible. It will be a surprising amount!

3. Mix all the ingredients together in a large bowl. Section the meat mixture into quarters and then divide each quarter in half to create eight even sections.

4. Brush a baking dish with a thin layer of olive oil. Form eight patties and place on a baking sheet. Bake for 28–32 minutes, until the internal temperature reaches 165°F. For meatballs, roll into 16 even balls and bake for 22–26 minutes or air fry at 400°F for 12 minutes.

5. Allow to cool completely. Wrap each burger in parchment paper and freeze in a ziplock or reusable silicone bag. To reheat, remove from the freezer and microwave for 90 seconds, then let sit for 2 minutes before eating. They can also be defrosted in the fridge and heated for 60 seconds.

NOTE: Ground turkey is high in water content. Don't be alarmed when there is water or white residue on your baking sheet after cooking. This is a type of protein, called albumin, found in high amounts in poultry and fish.

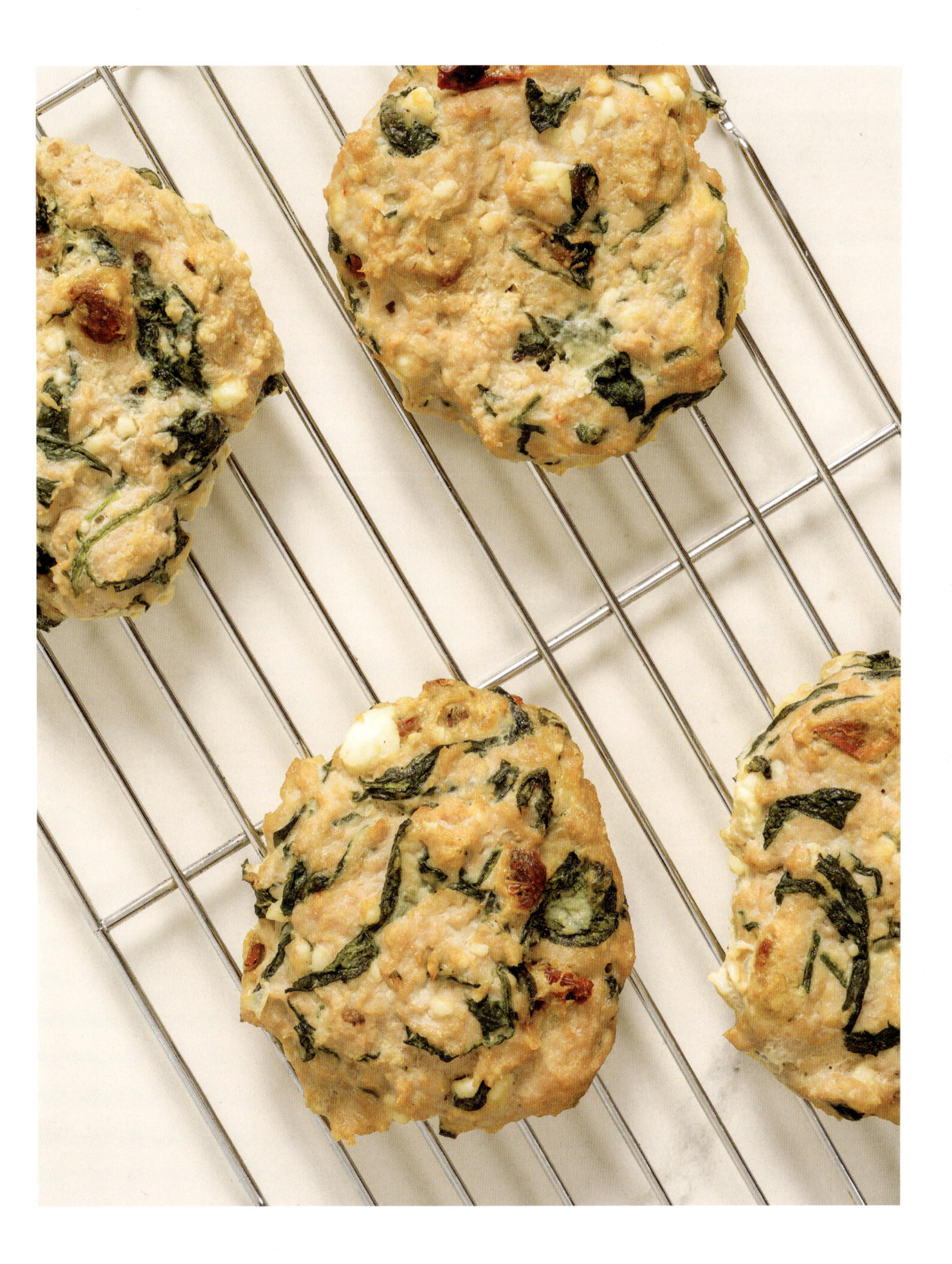

Egg Breakfast Burritos

SERVES 8
PREP TIME: 20 MINUTES
COOKING TIME: 10 MINUTES

1 tablespoon olive oil

12 eggs

⅔ cup salsa

2 (15-ounce) cans black beans, drained and rinsed

4 cups fresh spinach

8 (10-inch) tortillas, flour or whole-wheat

1 cup spreadable sauce (our favorites: cilantro or chipotle Bitchin' Sauce, guacamole crema, chimichurri)

● **VITAMIN C BOOST**

Pair with our Cherry Antioxidant Smoothie (page 223, +51mg).

● **PROTEIN ADD**

Add ¼ cup shredded cheddar (+7g), 2 tablespoons hemp seeds (+5g), 1 chicken sausage link (+9g), or 2 ounces ground turkey (+14g) to the filling.

● **MAKE IT PLANT-BASED**

Check out our Vegan Breakfast Burrito recipe on page 87.

● **MAKE IT GLUTEN-FREE**

Substitute flour tortillas with corn or gluten-free tortillas.

Per serving: Calories: 462
Fat: 21g | Carbohydrates: 51g
Fiber: 4g | Protein: 21g

You'll be thankful to grab these delicious burritos out of the freezer after a long night of interrupted sleep. High in both fiber and protein, as well as choline, these breakfast burritos are a delicious, nutrient-packed breakfast option.

1. Heat the olive oil at medium-low in a large skillet.

2. In a medium bowl, scramble the eggs and salsa together.

3. Add the egg-salsa mixture to the pan and cook, stirring occasionally, until eggs begin to solidify (3–5 minutes).

4. Add the beans and spinach and continue cooking, stirring occasionally, until the eggs are firm (3–5 minutes).

5. Remove the mixture from the pan and allow it to cool.

6. Meanwhile, lay out eight pieces of aluminum foil and spray with nonstick cooking spray. Place one tortilla on each piece of foil. Spread 2 tablespoons of sauce evenly on each tortilla, leaving about 1 inch around the sides. Add one-eighth of the egg mixture to each tortilla.

7. Fold the top and bottom of each tortilla toward the center. Roll from one side until all the filling is contained. Wrap snugly in aluminum foil.

8. These can be placed directly in the freezer.

9. To reheat, remove from the foil and pop straight in the microwave for 3–4 minutes. Allow to sit for 2 minutes before eating. In an air fryer, cook on 375°F for 10–12 minutes. In a toaster oven, cook for 10 minutes in the foil, then remove the foil and cook for an additional 2–5 minutes to crisp the tortilla.

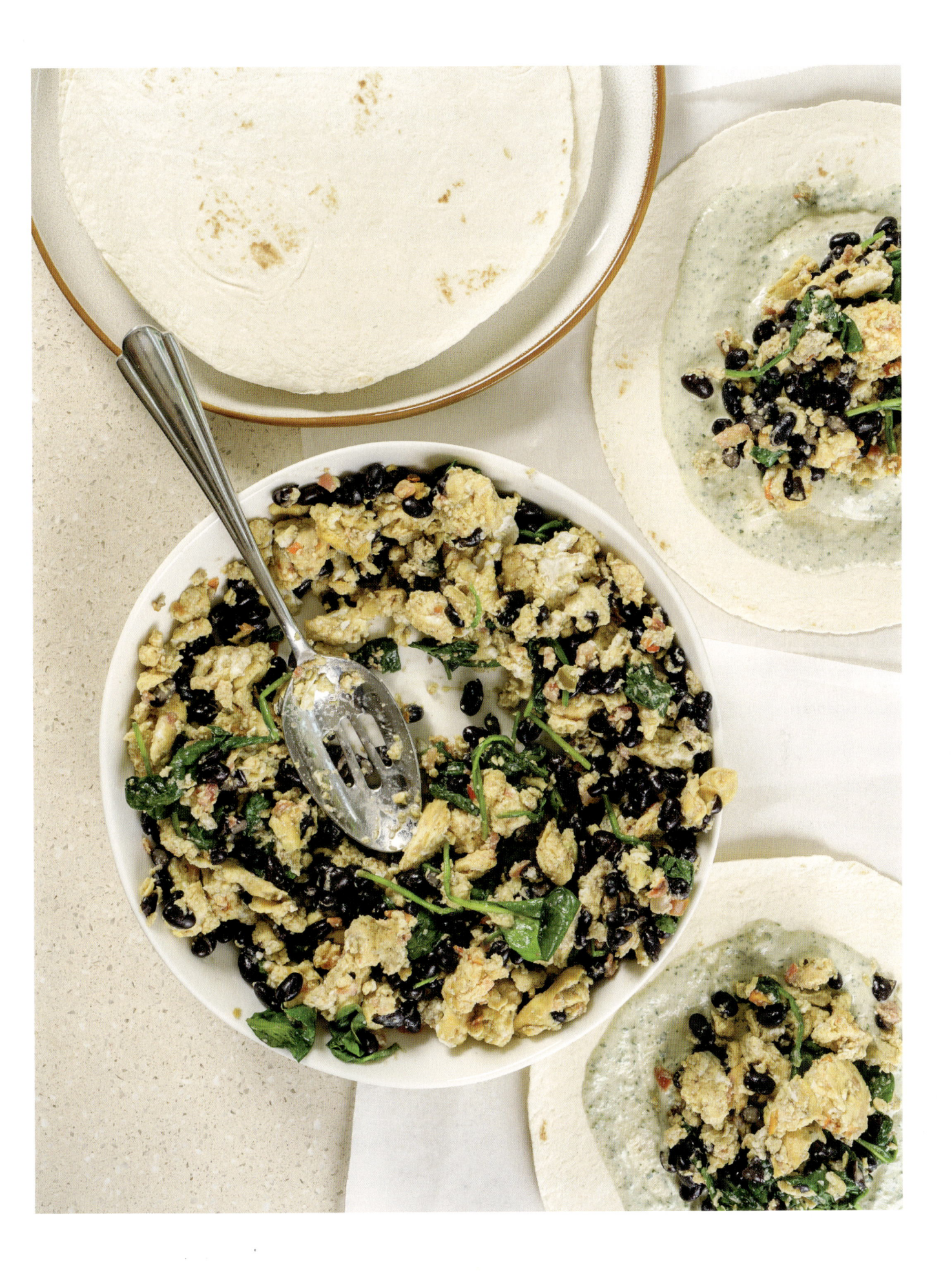

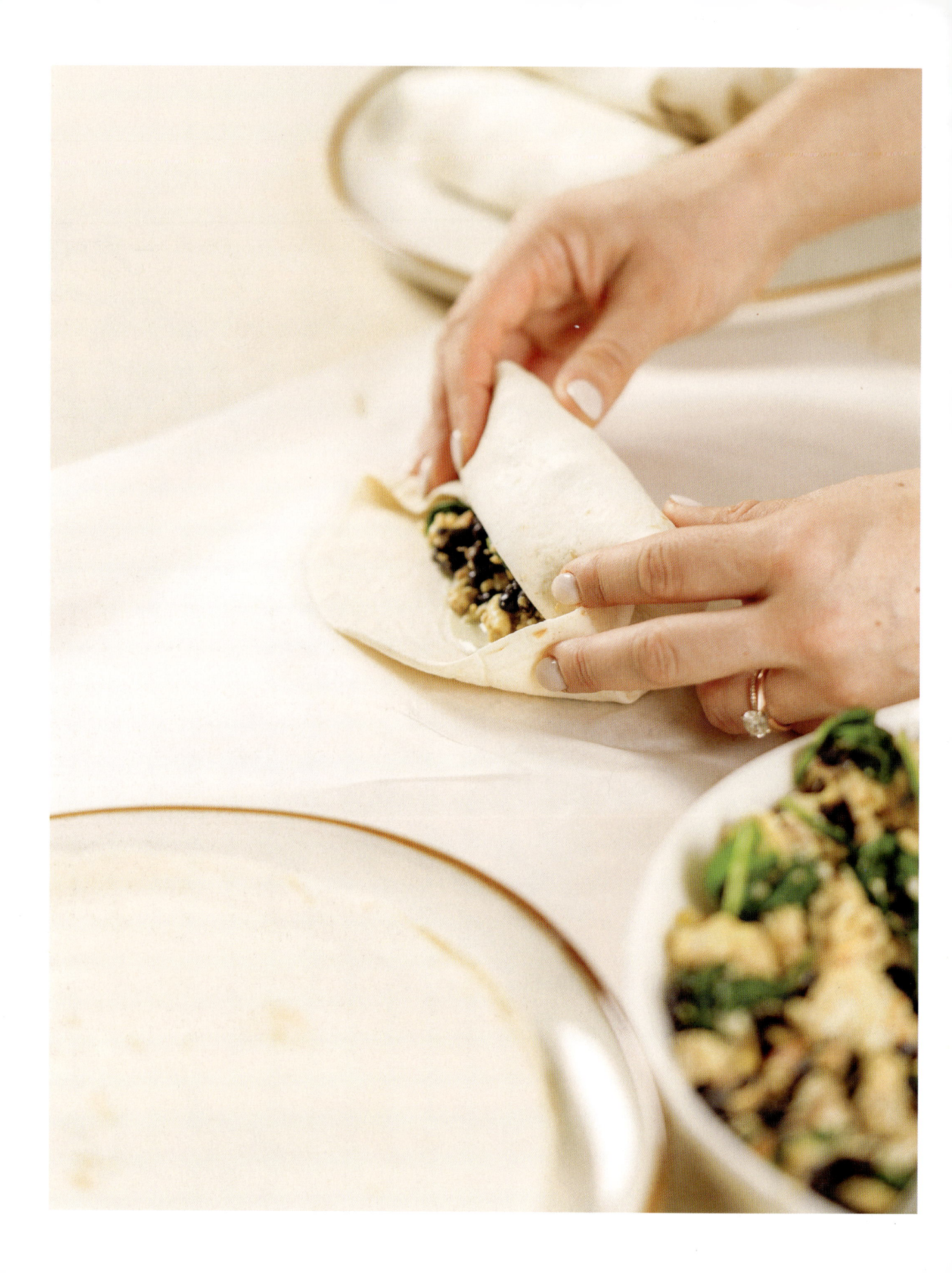

Vegan Breakfast Burritos

SERVES 5
PREP TIME: 10 MINUTES
COOKING TIME: 35 MINUTES

½ large yellow onion, diced

2 garlic cloves, minced

1 (15-ounce) block extra-firm tofu, drained and pressed

1 cup mushrooms, diced

1 (15-ounce) can black beans, drained and rinsed

1 cup salsa

¼ cup nutritional yeast

1 teaspoon chili powder

½ teaspoon ground cumin

Salt and pepper, to taste

2 cups kale or spinach

5 (10-inch) tortillas, flour or whole-wheat

● **VITAMIN C BOOST**

Pair with our Cherry Antioxidant Smoothie (page 223, +51mg).

● **PROTEIN ADD**

Use high-protein tofu (+6g), or add 2 chopped veggie sausage links, such as Tofurky brand (+10g), or ¼ cup hemp seeds (+3g) to the filling.

● **MAKE IT GLUTEN-FREE**

Substitute flour tortillas with corn or gluten-free tortillas.

Per serving: Calories: 395
Fat: 9g | Carbohydrates: 42g
Fiber: 15g | Protein: 24g

This breakfast is a tasty and nutritious plant-based version of our Egg Breakfast Burritos that still provides ample protein and iron, crucial nutrients for acute postpartum recovery.

1. Spray a large skillet with olive oil cooking spray and set over medium heat. Add the onion and cook, stirring, for 5–7 minutes, then add the garlic and cook for another 2 minutes.

2. Crumble the tofu into small pieces and add it to the pan along with the mushrooms. Cook for 10–15 minutes, or until most of the water from the tofu has evaporated.

3. Add in the black beans, salsa, nutritional yeast, and seasonings. Stir to fully incorporate all the ingredients and cook for 5 minutes.

4. Add the kale or spinach and cook for 1 additional minute, or until it has wilted.

5. Remove the mixture from the pan and allow it to cool.

6. Meanwhile, lay out five pieces of aluminum foil and spray with nonstick cooking spray. Place one tortilla on each piece of foil.

7. Build your vegan breakfast burritos by scooping about 1 cup of the filling into the center of each tortilla. Fold the top and bottom of each tortilla toward the center. Roll from one side until all the filling is contained. Wrap snugly in aluminum foil.

8. Store the vegan breakfast burritos in the fridge or freezer. To defrost, place frozen burritos in the oven at 350°F for 15 minutes, or remove from the foil and pop in the microwave for 2–3 minutes.

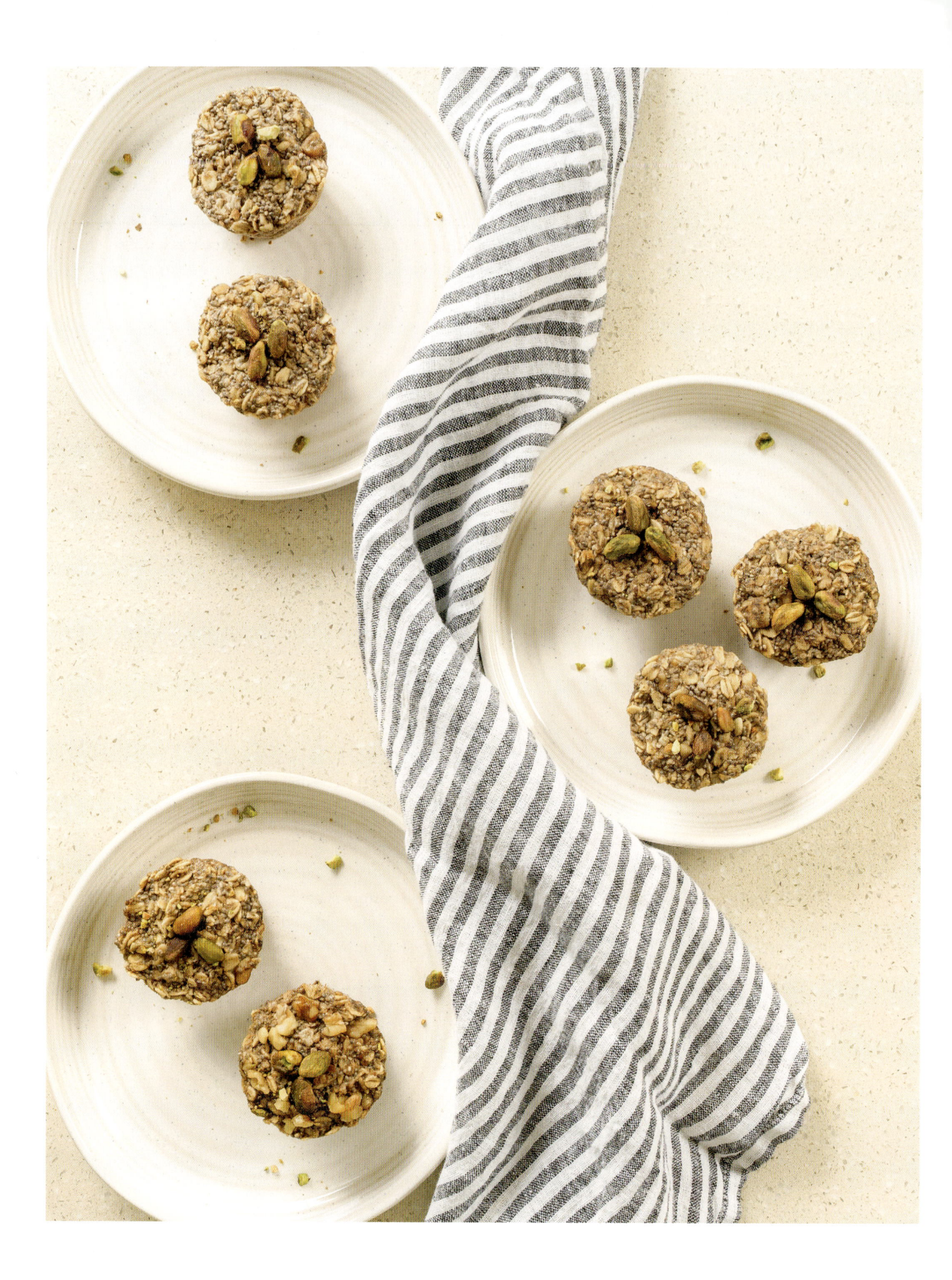

Maple Pistachio Oatmeal Muffins

SERVES 12
PREP TIME: 5 MINUTES
SOAKING TIME: 20 MINUTES
COOKING TIME: 20 MINUTES

2 ¼ cups unsweetened milk of choice

2 eggs or flax eggs (see Note)

½ cup maple syrup

1 ½ teaspoons vanilla extract

1 tablespoon ground cinnamon

½ teaspoon ground nutmeg

½ teaspoon ground ginger

2 cups rolled oats

½ cup chia seeds

½ cup unsalted pistachios or walnuts

🟠 **VITAMIN C BOOST**

Pair with 1 cup of strawberries (+97mg).

🟤 **PROTEIN ADD**

Pair with 2 eggs (+12g), a protein shake (+20g), or ¾ cup Greek yogurt (+20g).

🟣 **MAKE IT NUT-FREE**

Replace pistachios with pumpkin seeds.

Per muffin: Calories: 155
Fat: 5g | Carbohydrates: 22g
Fiber: 2g | Protein: 5g

Enjoy these as a part of your breakfast, an afternoon snack, or a before-bed treat. Oats are high in fiber and may have some milk-boosting properties. Pistachios are a great source of non-marine omega-3 fatty acids, which are critical for a baby's brain development.

1. Preheat the oven to 350°F.

2. In a large bowl, mix together the milk, eggs, maple syrup, vanilla extract, cinnamon, nutmeg, and ginger.

3. Add the oats, chia seeds, and pistachios. Mix until thoroughly combined.

4. Allow to sit for 20 minutes before baking.

5. Line a 12-cup muffin tin and evenly divide the batter among the wells.

6. Bake for 20 minutes, or until the oats are completely set.

7. To freeze, place in a bag and remove all the air. To defrost, leave on the counter for a few hours or thaw overnight in the refrigerator.

NOTE: To make 1 flax egg, combine 1 tablespoon flax meal and 2 ½ tablespoons water. Stir and let sit for at least 5 minutes.

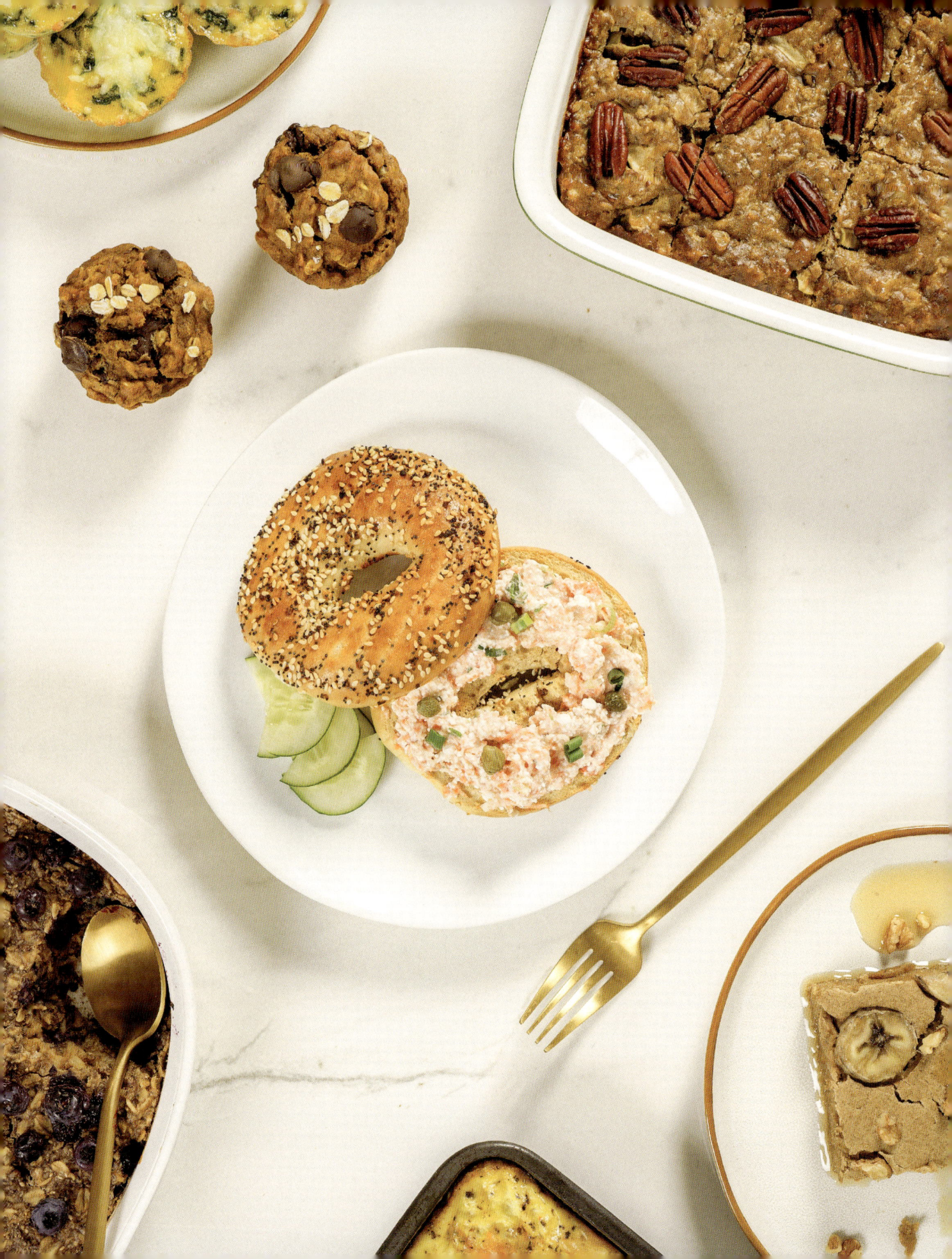

Make-Ahead Breakfasts

Picture this: You've been woken up four times throughout the night to feed your new baby (and maybe a few more to deal with postpartum night sweats). Come morning, you're barely able to stumble to the coffee maker—let alone operate the stove—but your body has been tirelessly producing nourishment for your little one throughout the night, leaving you famished when you wake up. What you need now are essential nutrients, specifically ones to aid in the healing and lactation processes. Luckily, you have breakfast options ready to go in the refrigerator. Starting your day with a nourishing meal will set you on the path to feeling your best all day long.

Apple Cider Oatmeal Bread

SERVES 8
PREP TIME: 15 MINUTES
COOKING TIME: 45 MINUTES FOR 8 X 8-INCH PAN

1 cup rolled oats

1 cup apple cider

1 cup whole-wheat flour

1 teaspoon ground cinnamon

½ teaspoon baking soda

½ teaspoon baking powder

½ teaspoon salt

3 eggs or flax eggs (see Note)

⅓ cup vegetable, avocado, or olive oil

¼ cup maple syrup

1 teaspoon vanilla extract

1 apple, finely diced (unpeeled)

⅓ cup chopped pecans

● **PROTEIN ADD**
Serve with peanut butter (+8g), 2 eggs (+12g), or a protein shake (+20g).

● **MAKE IT GLUTEN-FREE**
Substitute flour with gluten-free flour.

● **MAKE IT NUT-FREE**
Replace pecans with sunflower seeds.

Per serving: Calories: 202
Fat: 5g | Carbohydrates: 31g
Fiber: 4g | Protein: 6g

We encourage you to bake some muffins or quick breads for the freezer to enjoy during those first weeks postpartum when baking just won't be an option. This Apple Cider Oatmeal Bread is a delicious breakfast treat while sipping your morning coffee that will also help you achieve your fiber goal for the day.

1. Heat the oven to 350°F.

2. Combine the oats and apple cider in a saucepan and heat over medium-low until the oats have absorbed all of the liquid. Once absorbed, remove from the heat and set aside.

3. Mix the flour, cinnamon, baking soda, baking powder, and salt in a large bowl. In a smaller bowl, combine the eggs, oil, maple syrup, and vanilla. Add the wet ingredients to the dry ingredients, and mix until thoroughly combined. Stir in the apples and pecans.

4. Grease a shallow 8 x 8-inch baking dish. Transfer the batter to the dish and smooth evenly along the top. Bake for 40–45 minutes, or until a knife comes out clean. For muffins: Transfer to a greased muffin tin and bake for 20–22 minutes; makes 16–18 muffins. For a loaf: Transfer to a greased 8 x 3-inch loaf pan and bake for 55 minutes.

5. To freeze, cut the bread into slices. Freeze slices or muffins in a ziplock bag with all the air removed. To defrost, leave on the counter for a few hours or overnight.

NOTE: To make 1 flax egg, combine 1 tablespoon flax meal and 2 ½ tablespoons water. Stir and let sit for at least 5 minutes.

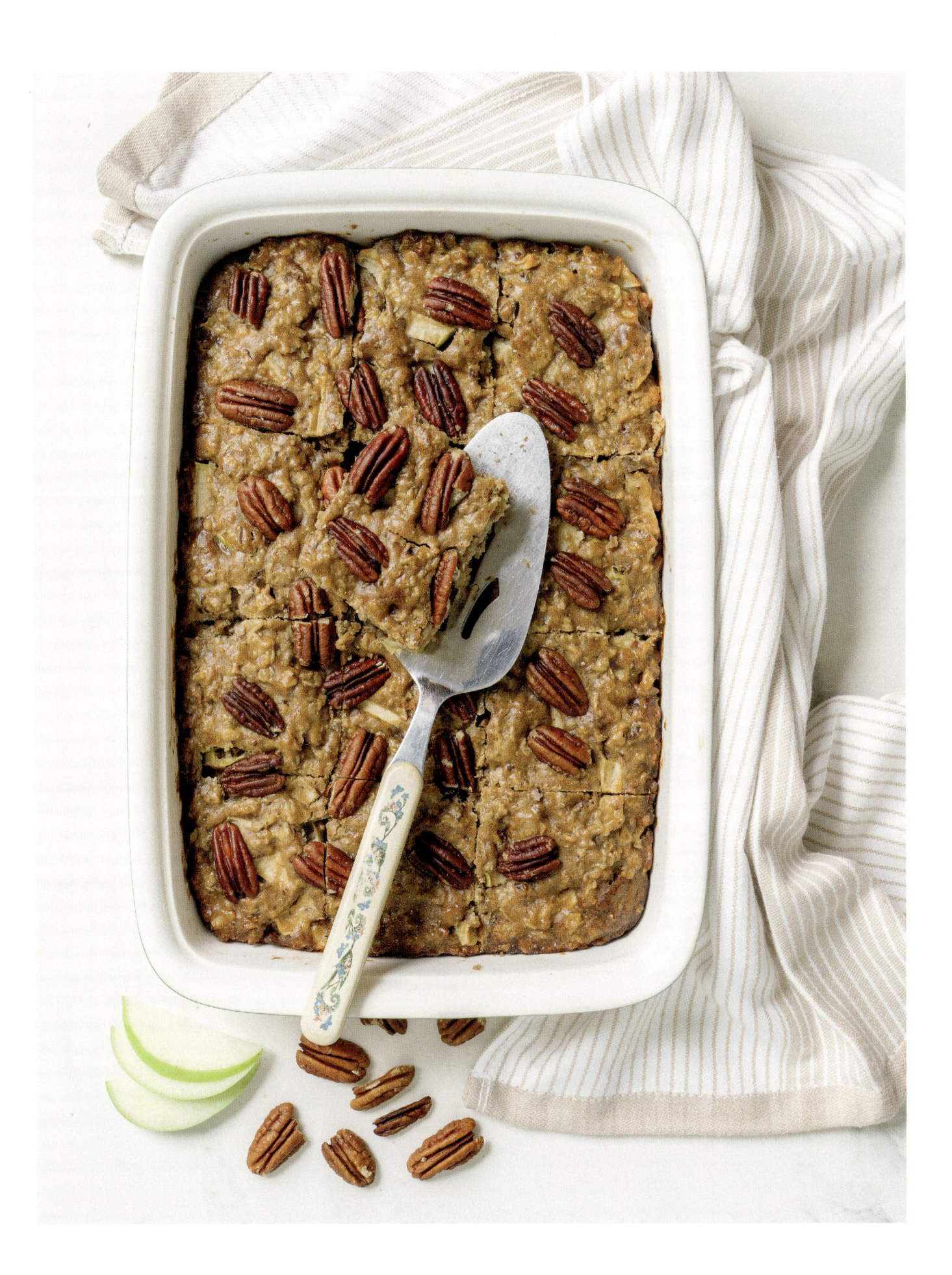

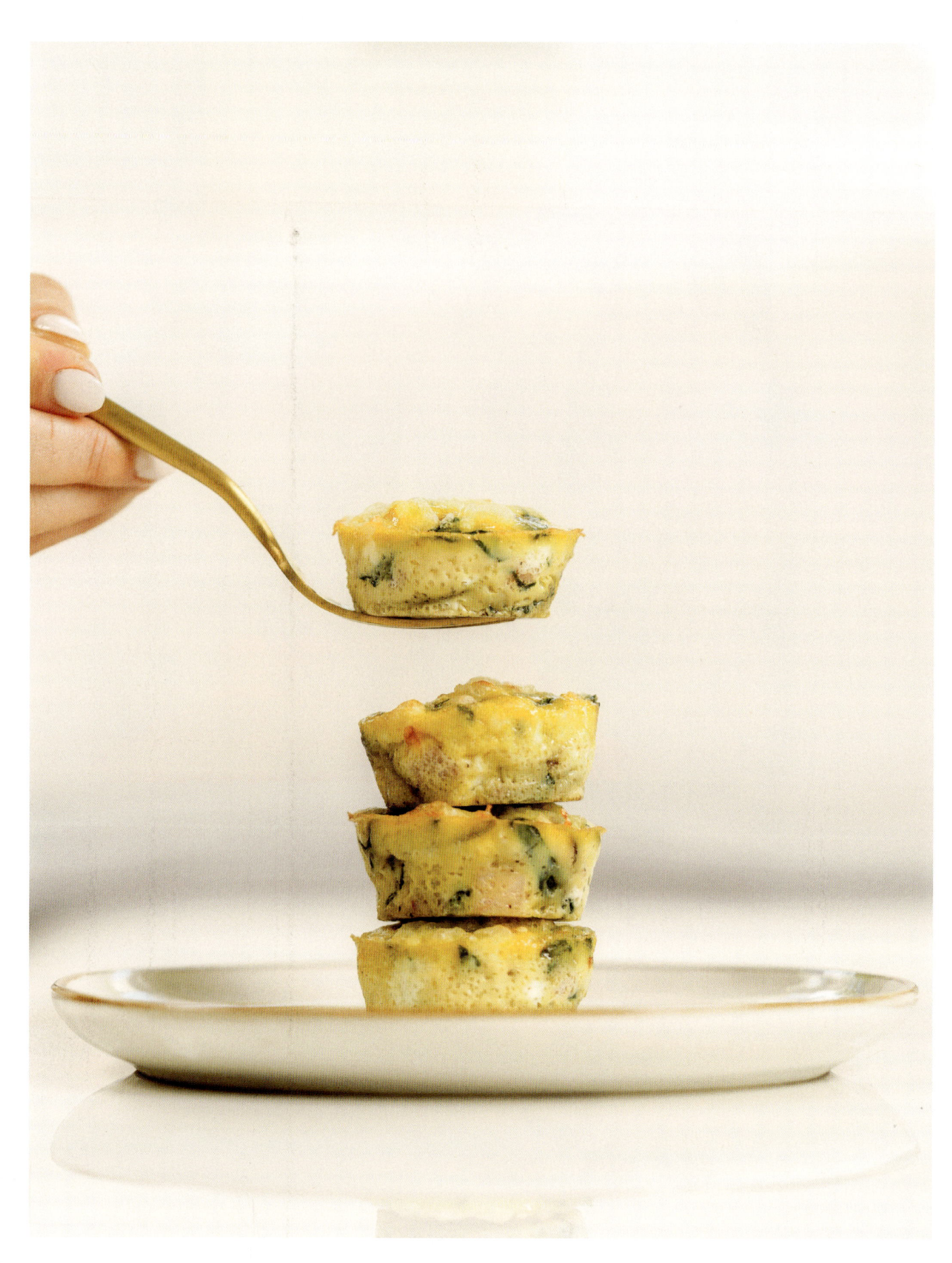

Green Eggs and Ham Cups

MAKES 12 CUPS; SERVES 4
PREP TIME: 10 MINUTES
COOKING TIME: 35 MINUTES

1 tablespoon olive oil

1 small shallot, thinly sliced

4 ounces ham steak, deli ham, or pancetta, finely diced

3 cups fresh spinach, chopped, or ½ cup frozen spinach

¼ teaspoon salt

¼ teaspoon black pepper

¼ teaspoon garlic powder

8 eggs

¼ cup unsweetened milk of choice

¼ cup shredded Gruyère, cheddar, or Parmesan cheese, optional

● **MAKE IT PLANT-BASED**

Check out our Eggless "Egg" Cups recipe on page 96.

Per 3 egg cups: Calories: 234
Fat: 14g | Carbohydrates: 8g
Fiber: 1g | Protein: 20g

These egg cups are a high-protein option that are good for both mama and baby. Their easy-to-consume format ensures mom starts the day with a nourishing, protein-rich meal, while the choline in the egg yolks is a crucial nutrient for the baby's developing brain.

1. Preheat the oven to 350°F.

2. Heat the oil in a pan over medium-low heat. Add the shallots and sauté for 5–7 minutes, or until they soften. Add the ham, spinach, and seasonings. Sauté for 3–4 more minutes until the spinach wilts. Remove from the heat.

3. In a large bowl, whisk together the eggs and milk. Add the ham mixture and stir to combine.

4. Line a 12-cup muffin tin and spray each liner with nonstick cooking spray. Divide the egg mixture evenly among the wells (roughly ¼ cup per well). Sprinkle the cheese on top, if desired.

5. Bake for 25 minutes, or until the eggs are cooked through.

NOTES: Make it a complete meal by pairing with whole-wheat bread and fruit high in vitamin C such as pineapple, oranges, or kiwi.

To freeze these egg cups after baking, wrap them separately in parchment paper and then throw them into a large ziplock bag. To reheat, pop them into the microwave for 1 minute, then continue to heat in 15-second intervals until completely warm.

Eggless "Egg" Cups

MAKES 9 CUPS; SERVES 3
PREP TIME: 10 MINUTES
COOKING TIME: 40 MINUTES

1 (15-ounce) block extra-firm tofu, drained and pressed

½ cup chopped baby spinach

½ bell pepper, finely diced

½ small yellow onion, finely diced

3 tablespoons nutritional yeast

½ teaspoon ground turmeric

½ teaspoon salt

½ teaspoon garlic powder

½ teaspoon onion powder

Black pepper, to taste

● **PROTEIN ADD**

Serve with 2 slices of whole-grain bread (+10g) or 1 veggie sausage link, such as Tofurky brand (+24g).

Per 3 "egg" cups: Calories: 171
Fat: 6g | Carbohydrates: 6g
Fiber: 3g | Protein: 18g

Unlike other egg cup recipes, this version uses tofu to provide protein. Besides providing coloring similar to eggs, turmeric may help fight inflammation, which is often quite high during the early postpartum period. Turmeric contains curcumin, which is an antioxidant compound with anti-inflammatory properties. The black pepper in this dish helps facilitate its absorption, which is usually poor.

1. Preheat the oven to 375°F, and prepare a 12-cup muffin tin by spraying it lightly with olive oil cooking spray or lining it with silicone baking cups.

2. Place the tofu in a blender or a food processor and blend until it turns into a paste.

3. Transfer the blended tofu to a bowl and add the rest of the ingredients. Mix well.

4. Pour the mixture into the muffin tin, dividing it evenly among 9 wells.

5. Bake for 35–40 minutes, or until a skewer inserted into the "egg" cups comes out clean.

NOTE: Make it a complete meal by pairing with whole-wheat bread and fruit high in vitamin C such as pineapple, oranges, or kiwi.

To freeze these "egg" cups after baking, wrap them separately in parchment paper and then throw them into a large ziplock bag. To reheat, pop them into the microwave for 1 minute, then continue to heat in 15-second intervals until completely warm.

Blender Blueberry Muffins

MAKES 10 MUFFINS
PREP TIME: 5 MINUTES
COOKING TIME: 35 MINUTES

3 medium ripe bananas

2 cups rolled oats

¼ cup protein powder, chocolate or vanilla

2 tablespoons chia seeds

1 tablespoon baking powder

Pinch of salt

½ cup unsweetened milk of choice

½ teaspoon vanilla extract

1 cup blueberries, fresh or frozen

● **PROTEIN ADD**
Pair with ½ cup Greek yogurt (+14g), 2 tablespoons nut butter (+8g), or hard-boiled eggs (+6g per egg).

Per muffin: Calories: 129
Fat: 2g | Carbohydrates: 19g
Fiber: 4g | Protein: 6g

Simplify your breakfast routine with these muffins, which only take five minutes to whip up. Unlike typical store-bought blueberry muffins, which are often loaded with added sugar (40 grams on average!), our version is sweetened with bananas and full of health-promoting ingredients such as oats, chia seeds, and blueberries.

1. Preheat the oven to 350°F. Spray a 12-cup muffin tin with nonstick cooking spray or line it with silicone baking cups.

2. In a high-speed blender or food processor, blend all the ingredients except the blueberries together until combined.

3. Transfer the mixture to a bowl and fold in the blueberries. Pour the mixture into the muffin tin, dividing it evenly among 10 wells. Bake for 35 minutes.

4. Allow the muffins to cool for 10 minutes before serving.

NOTES: Change it up: Swap the blueberries for other fruit, or for a dessert muffin, use chocolate chips.

For a sweeter muffin, add 1–2 tablespoons of maple syrup.

You can freeze these in a ziplock bag. Defrost on the counter for about 30 minutes, or pop in the microwave for 1–2 minutes.

NOTES: To make 1 flax egg, combine 1 tablespoon flax meal and 2 ½ tablespoons water. Stir and let sit for at least 5 minutes.

You can freeze these in a ziplock bag. Defrost on the counter for about 30 minutes, or pop in the microwave for 1–2 minutes.

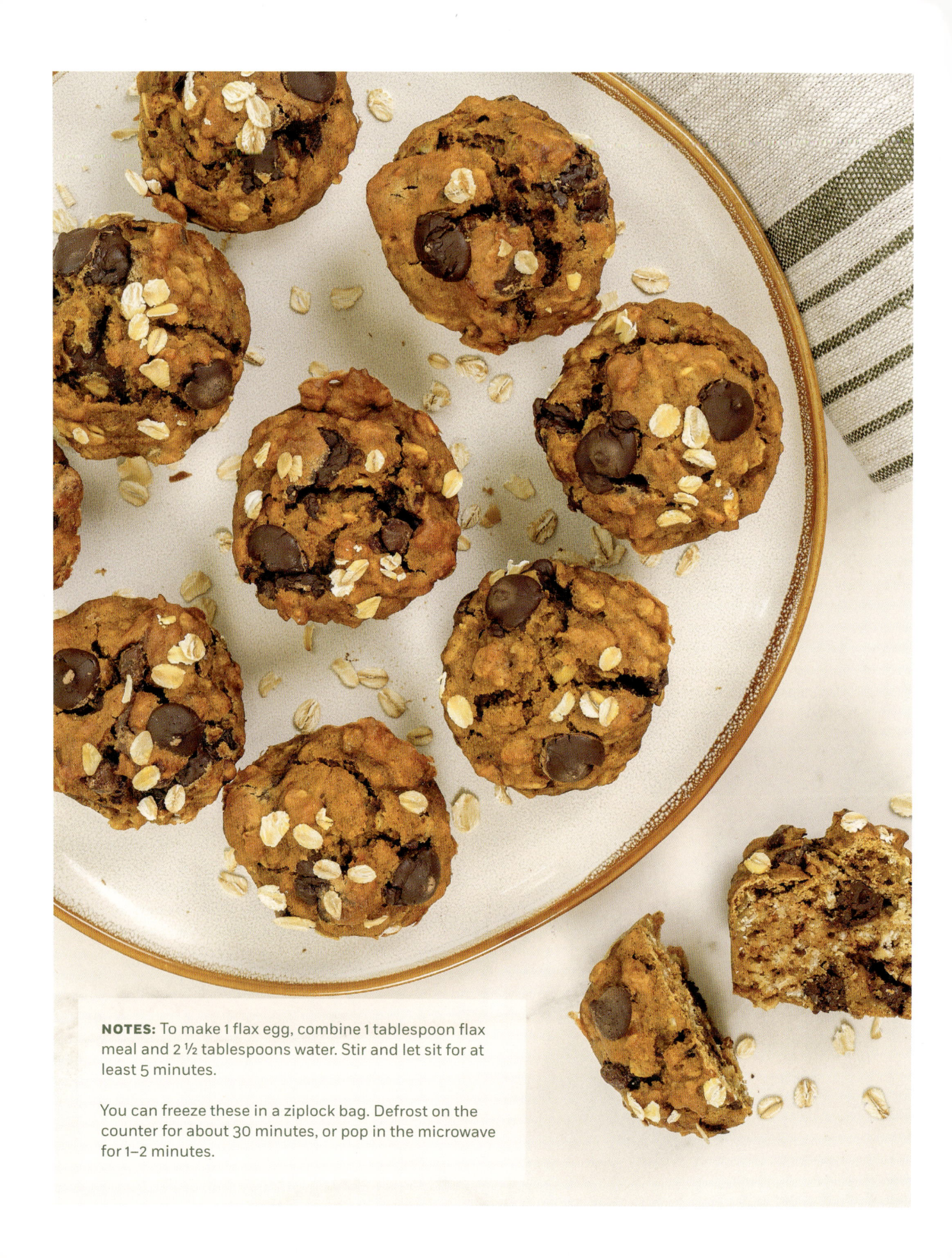

Pumpkin Chocolate Chip Muffins

MAKES 12 MUFFINS
PREP TIME: 5 MINUTES
COOKING TIME: 35 MINUTES

1 cup rolled oats

⅔ cup whole-wheat flour

⅔ cup almond flour

1 tablespoon pumpkin pie spice

1 teaspoon baking soda

1 teaspoon baking powder

¼ teaspoon salt

2 eggs or flax eggs (see Notes)

1 (15-ounce) can pumpkin puree

½ cup maple syrup

⅓ cup unsweetened milk of choice

3 tablespoons vegetable oil or melted coconut oil

1 teaspoon vanilla extract

¾ cup dark chocolate chips, divided

● **PROTEIN ADD**

Pair with ½ cup Greek yogurt (+12g), 2 tablespoons nut butter (+8g), or hard-boiled eggs (+6g per egg).

● **MAKE IT GLUTEN-FREE**

Substitute flour with gluten-free flour.

Per muffin: Calories: 231
Fat: 11g | Carbohydrates: 27g
Fiber: 3g | Protein: 11g

These delicious, satisfying, and potentially milk-boosting muffins are what muffin dreams are made of. Dense and packed with nutrients such as fiber and beta-carotene, an important antioxidant during the recovery period, they are the perfect pairing for any breakfast, snack, or dessert.

1. Preheat the oven to 350°F.

2. In a large bowl, combine the oats, whole-wheat flour, almond flour, pumpkin pie spice, baking soda, baking powder, and salt.

3. In a separate large bowl, mix together the eggs, pumpkin purée, maple syrup, milk, oil, and vanilla extract.

4. Slowly add the dry ingredients to the wet ingredients, stirring while you add them in.

5. Once totally combined, fold in ½ cup of the chocolate chips.

6. Scoop the mixture into a lined 12-cup muffin tin and top the muffins with the remaining ¼ cup of chocolate chips.

7. Bake for 30–35 minutes, or until a toothpick comes out clean.

8. Try to wait 10 minutes for them to cool before serving.

Banana Bread Baked Pancakes

SERVES 6
PREP TIME: 5 MINUTES
COOKING TIME: 30 MINUTES

3 medium ripe bananas

1 ½ cups water

4 eggs or flax eggs (see Note)

¼ cup maple syrup

2 tablespoons olive oil

3 cups rolled oats

½ cup hemp seeds

1 tablespoon baking powder

1 ½ teaspoons ground cinnamon

½ teaspoon salt

¼ teaspoon ground nutmeg

¼ cup walnut pieces or chopped walnuts

● **PROTEIN ADD**

Serve with a side of 2 eggs (+14g), 1 chicken sausage link or patty (+9g), or ½ cup of Greek yogurt (+14g).

● **MAKE IT NUT-FREE**

Replace the walnuts with pumpkin seeds.

Per serving: Calories: 457
Fat: 21g | Carbohydrates: 46g
Fiber: 7g | Protein: 17g

Making pancakes could not be any easier. Toss all of your ingredients into a blender, pour straight into a baking dish, and put in the oven. No flipping or burning the first batch required! Plus, one serving provides roughly 50% of your daily zinc, an important nutrient for collagen formation and tissue repair.

1. Preheat oven to 350°F.

2. In a blender, combine 2 of the bananas with all the remaining ingredients except for the walnuts. Blend until smooth.

3. Spray a 9 x 13-inch baking dish with nonstick cooking spray and pour in the batter, evenly spreading it around the dish.

4. Slice the remaining banana and arrange the slices on top. Sprinkle the walnuts on top as well.

5. Bake for 25–30 minutes, or until a knife comes out clean from the center. Slice in half lengthwise and then into three even sections horizontally. Remove with a spatula.

NOTE: To make 1 flax egg, combine 1 tablespoon flax meal and 2 ½ tablespoons water. Stir and let sit for at least 5 minutes.

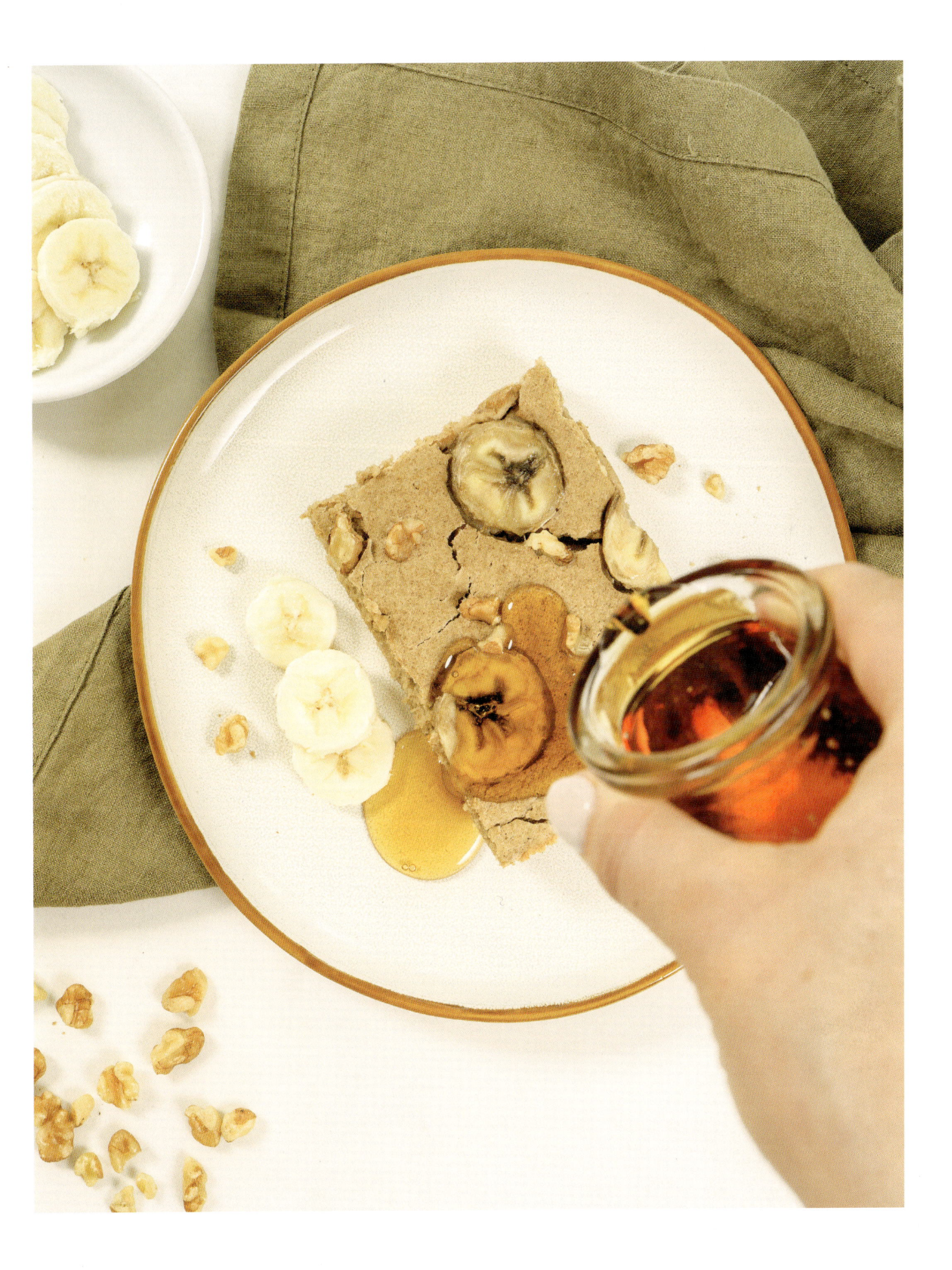

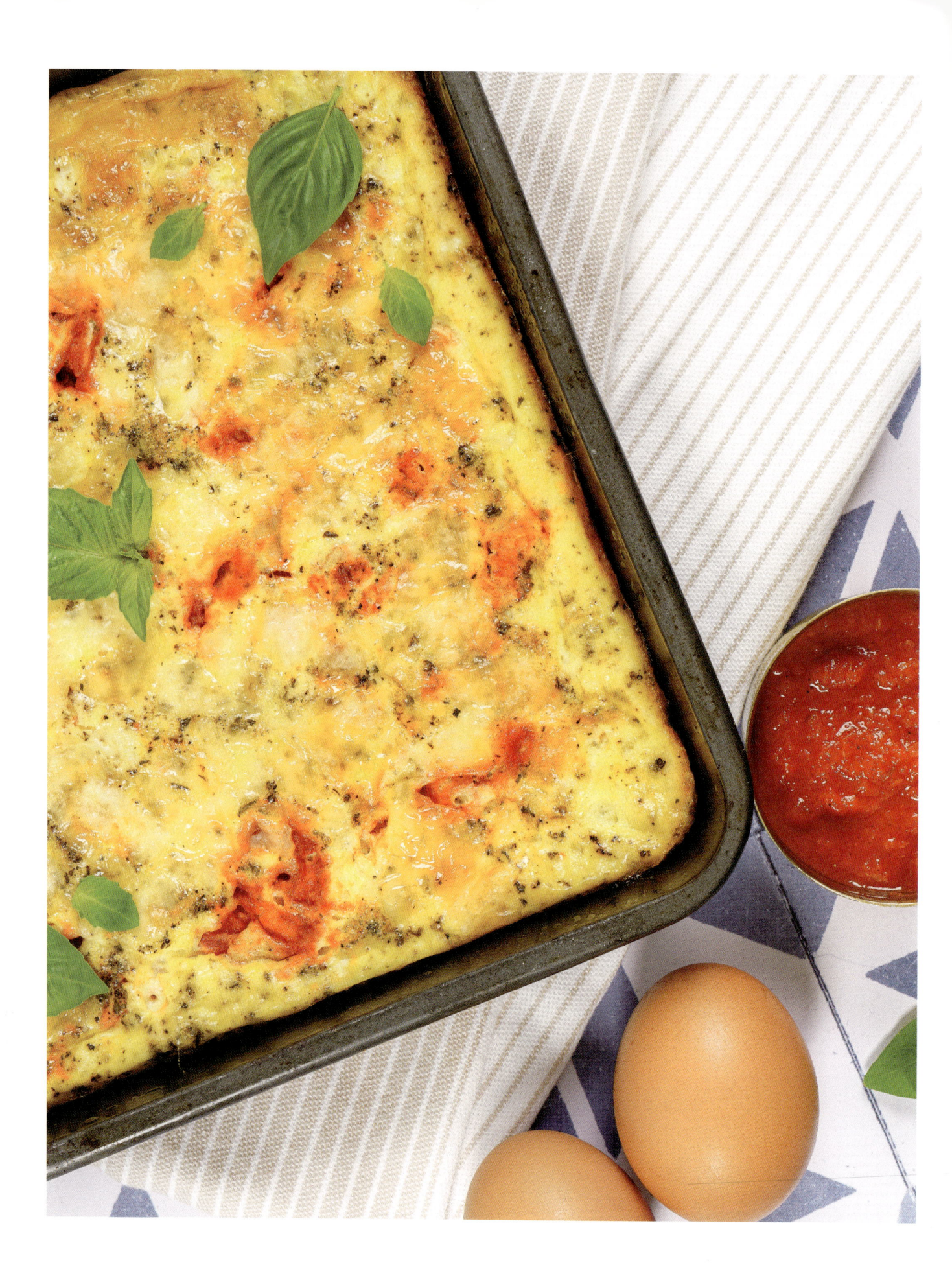

Pizza Eggs

SERVES 4
PREP TIME: 10 MINUTES
COOKING TIME: 30 MINUTES

8 eggs

1 cup cottage cheese

¼ cup water

½ teaspoon Italian seasoning

½ teaspoon garlic powder

½ teaspoon onion powder

¼ teaspoon black pepper

½ cup marinara sauce

¼ cup Italian cheese blend (such as Parmesan, pecorino, mozzarella)

● **PROTEIN ADD**

Top each serving with 8 slices of turkey pepperoni (+5g), 2 ounces cooked Italian sausage (+14g), or 2 ounces deli ham (+7g).

Per serving: Calories: 210
Fat: 12g | Carbohydrates: 6g
Fiber: 0g | Protein: 20g

For us, one pregnancy craving that did not go away after delivery was pizza. Satisfy your pizza cravings with the added benefit of choline, which is found in eggs, to support your baby's brain growth. It's a delicious excuse to have pizza for breakfast, and it tastes even better between two slices of bread.

1. Preheat the oven to 350°F.

2. Mix together the eggs, cottage cheese, water, and seasonings.

3. Spray an 8 x 8-inch baking dish with nonstick spray or coat with olive oil. Pour in the egg mixture. Scatter dollops of marinara sauce on top, then sprinkle with the cheese.

4. Bake for 25–30 minutes, or until a knife comes out clean.

5. Slice into four squares for serving. To reheat leftovers, microwave for 90 seconds.

NOTES: Optional add-ins: These eggs taste great as is, but you can also add any ingredient that you like on your pizza! Just sauté your favorite pizza toppings and allow to cool, then stir into the egg mixture before adding the marinara sauce. Pesto would also be a good topping.

These freeze best when made into a sandwich. Wrap the entire sandwich in parchment paper, then aluminum foil, and freeze. To reheat, allow to thaw overnight, then microwave for 90 seconds.

Overnight Oats (3 Ways)

SERVES 1
PREP TIME: 5 MINUTES
SOAKING TIME: 8 HOURS OR OVERNIGHT

BASE

½ cup rolled oats

2 teaspoons chia seeds

¾ cup unsweetened milk of choice

½–1 tablespoon maple syrup, to taste

½ teaspoon vanilla extract

CHERRY CHEESECAKE

½ cup cherries, fresh, or frozen and thawed, chopped

½ cup unsweetened Greek yogurt

PB&J

½ cup berries

1 tablespoon peanut butter

ZUCCHINI BREAD

½ banana, sliced

½ cup finely shredded or grated zucchini

¼ teaspoon ground cinnamon

● **PROTEIN ADD**

Add 2 tablespoons protein powder before refrigerating (+8g).

● **MAKE IT NUT-FREE**

Replace peanut butter with sunflower seed butter.

Overnight oats take just a few minutes to prepare and require no cooking time, making them an excellent weekday breakfast option. You can even batch-prep these and make seven for the week in under 15 minutes. Overnight oats are also versatile—they're the perfect vehicle for different spices, fruits, and nuts. We've suggested three great flavor combinations here, but the possibilities are endless for keeping your palate excited with every bowl.

1. In a mason jar or glass container, combine all the base ingredients. Add the ingredients for your variation of choice, and stir or shake to mix.

2. Seal the container and place it in the refrigerator for at least 8 hours, or overnight. When ready to eat, microwave it for 1–2 minutes to reheat. Add a few splashes of milk, if needed, to reach your preferred consistency.

Per serving, Cherry Cheesecake:
Calories: 410 | Fat: 9g
Carbohydrates: 50g
Fiber: 9g | Protein: 23g

Per serving, PB&J:
Calories: 440 | Fat: 17g
Carbohydrates: 47g
Fiber: 11g | Protein: 16g

Per serving, Zucchini Bread:
Calories: 421 | Fat: 9g
Carbohydrates: 52g
Fiber: 10g | Protein: 23g

Creamy Chia Seed Pudding

SERVES 1
PREP TIME: 5 MINUTES
SOAKING TIME: 5 HOURS OR OVERNIGHT

½ cup unsweetened Greek yogurt

½ cup unsweetened milk of choice

¼ cup chia seeds

½–1 tablespoon maple syrup, honey, or agave

½ teaspoon vanilla extract

¼ teaspoon ground cinnamon

½ cup fresh berries

● **MAKE IT PLANT-BASED**
Swap the Greek yogurt for a plant-based yogurt.

Per serving: Calories: 398
Fat: 16g | Carbohydrates: 27g
Fiber: 17g | Protein: 21g

Chia seeds are highly nutritious—a ¼-cup serving contains 11 grams of fiber and countless other nutrients. Chia seeds are also one of the richest plant sources of omega-3 fatty acids, a type of fat that is transferred to the baby through breast milk and is essential for promoting optimal development in infants.

1. Combine all the ingredients except the berries in a jar or sealable container. Let sit for 5 minutes at room temperature.

2. Mix once more to ensure there are no clumps. Place in the fridge for a minimum of 5 hours, or overnight.

3. When ready to eat, top with the berries.

NOTE: No yogurt? Double the amount of milk.

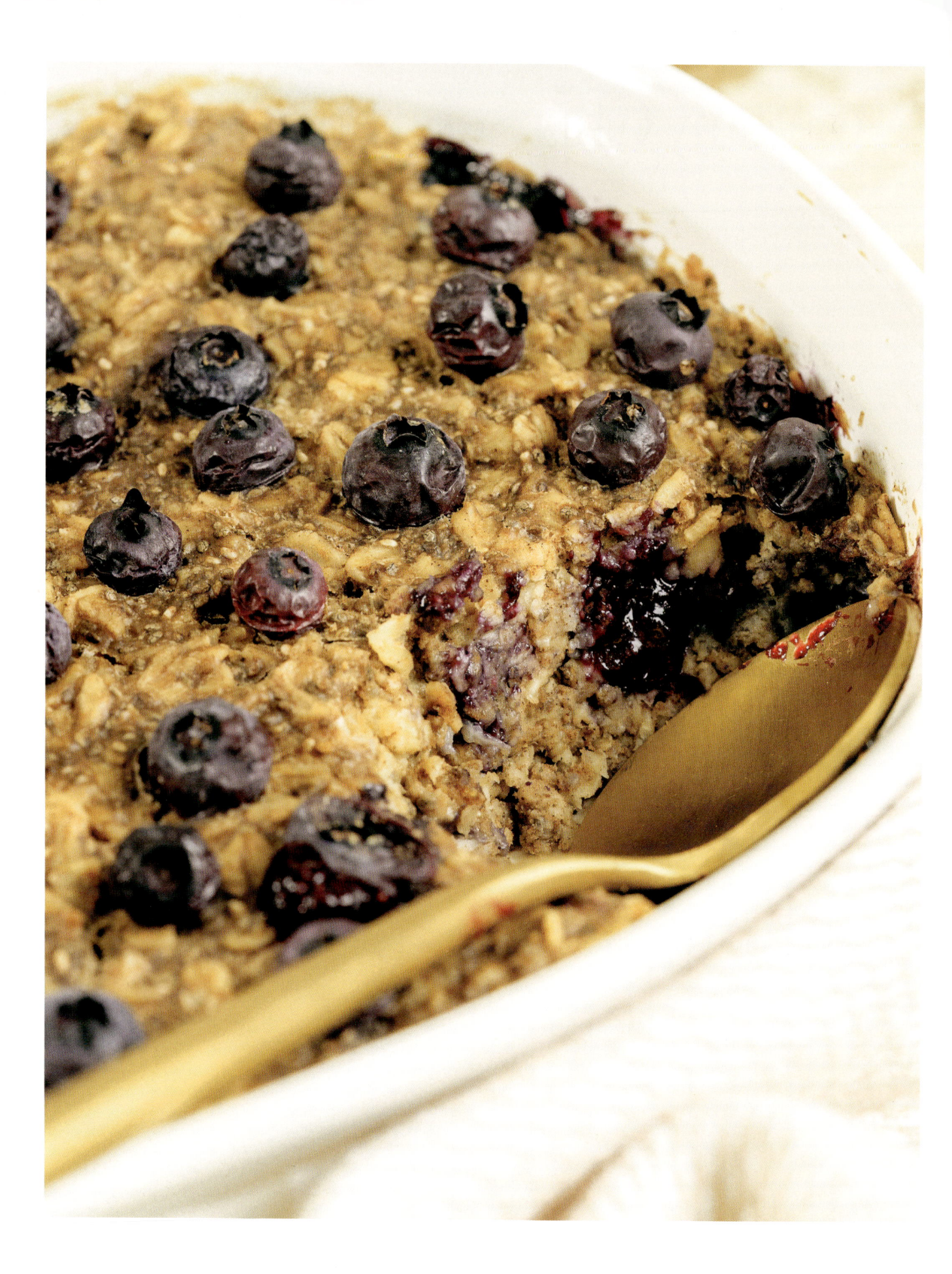

Baked Blueberry Oatmeal

SERVES 5
PREP TIME: 5 MINUTES
SOAKING TIME: 30 MINUTES
COOKING TIME: 35 MINUTES

2 ¼ cups unsweetened milk of choice

2 eggs

½ cup nut butter

¼ cup maple syrup

1 ½ teaspoons vanilla extract

2 cups rolled oats

½ cup chia seeds

1 tablespoon ground cinnamon

2 cups blueberries, fresh or frozen

● **PROTEIN ADD**

Serve with a ¼-cup dollop of Greek yogurt (+7g) or 1 hard-boiled egg (+6g).

● **MAKE IT PLANT-BASED**

Use flax eggs in place of eggs. To make 1 flax egg, combine 1 tablespoon flax meal and 2 ½ tablespoons water. Stir and let sit for at least 5 minutes.

● **MAKE IT NUT-FREE**

Replace peanut butter with sunflower seed butter.

Per serving: Calories: 506
Fat: 24g | Carbohydrates: 45g
Fiber: 13g | Protein: 19g

Packed with fiber and antioxidant-rich blueberries, this is the perfect recovery meal to keep you feeling your best while helping you heal. This recipe literally takes less than five minutes of hands-on work, so you can spend your time with your baby and not in the kitchen.

1. In a large bowl, mix together the milk, eggs, nut butter, maple syrup, and vanilla extract.

2. Add the oats, chia seeds, and cinnamon, and mix until thoroughly combined.

3. Allow to sit for 20–30 minutes before baking. Don't skip this step!

4. Meanwhile, preheat the oven to 350°F. Spray an 8 x 8-inch baking dish with nonstick spray.

5. Evenly spread half of the oatmeal mixture in the bottom of the baking dish. Scatter 1 ½ cups of the blueberries over the top. Cover with the remaining oatmeal mixture, and sprinkle the last ½ cup of blueberries on top.

6. Bake for 30–35 minutes, or until the oats are completely set. Slice and serve.

7. To reheat leftovers in the microwave, either add a splash of milk or cover with a damp paper towel. For a firm texture, reheat slices in a skillet over low heat for 2 minutes on each side.

NOTE: Try different spices, nut butters, toppings, and milks to mix it up. Swap out the blueberries for chocolate chips, use gingerbread-spiced sunflower seed butter instead of peanut butter, try almond eggnog instead of milk, or swap garam masala for the cinnamon.

Smoked Salmon Spread

SERVES 2
PREP TIME: 5 MINUTES
COOKING TIME: 0 MINUTES

4 ounces smoked salmon

1 green onion, roughly chopped

1 cup cottage cheese

⅛ teaspoon black pepper

½ tablespoon capers, optional

● **PROTEIN ADD**

Serve with 2 slices of bread or a bagel (+7g).

Per serving: Calories: 164
Fat: 5g | Carbohydrates: 5g
Fiber: 0g | Protein: 23g

This recipe is just like your favorite "bagel and schmear," but with much more protein and without the trip to the local deli. Swapping cottage cheese for cream cheese brings this recipe in at 25 grams of protein! The smoked salmon also provides nearly half of the omega-3 you need postpartum and about 40% if you are breastfeeding. This is perfection spread over a thick piece of toast or a bagel.

1. In a food processor, pulse the smoked salmon and green onions 5–7 times until they begin to break into small pieces. Add the cottage cheese and black pepper. Pulse 5–7 additional times until thoroughly combined. You want to avoid overmixing and forming a paste, which will still be edible, but less enjoyable.

2. Top with capers, if desired.

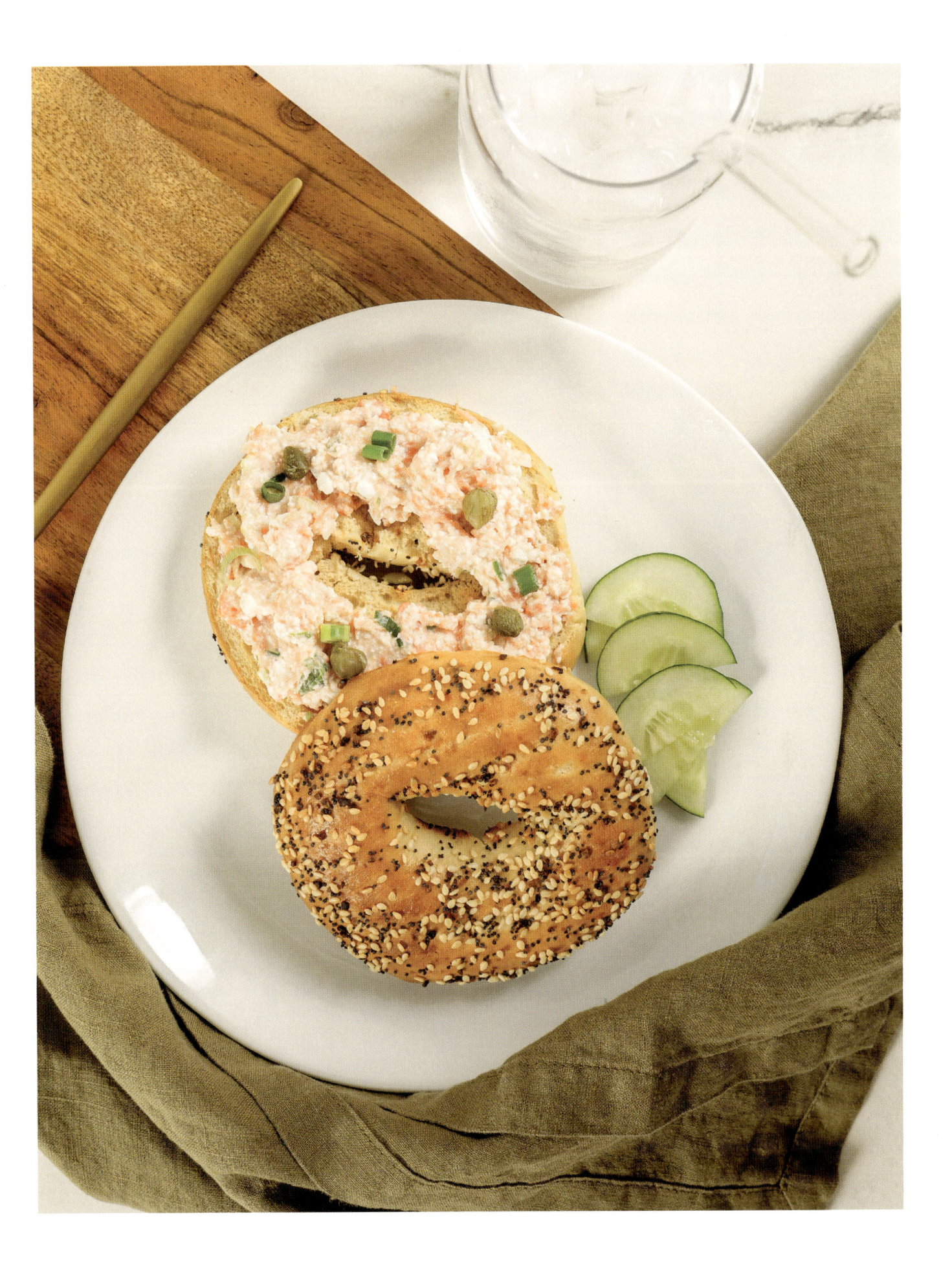

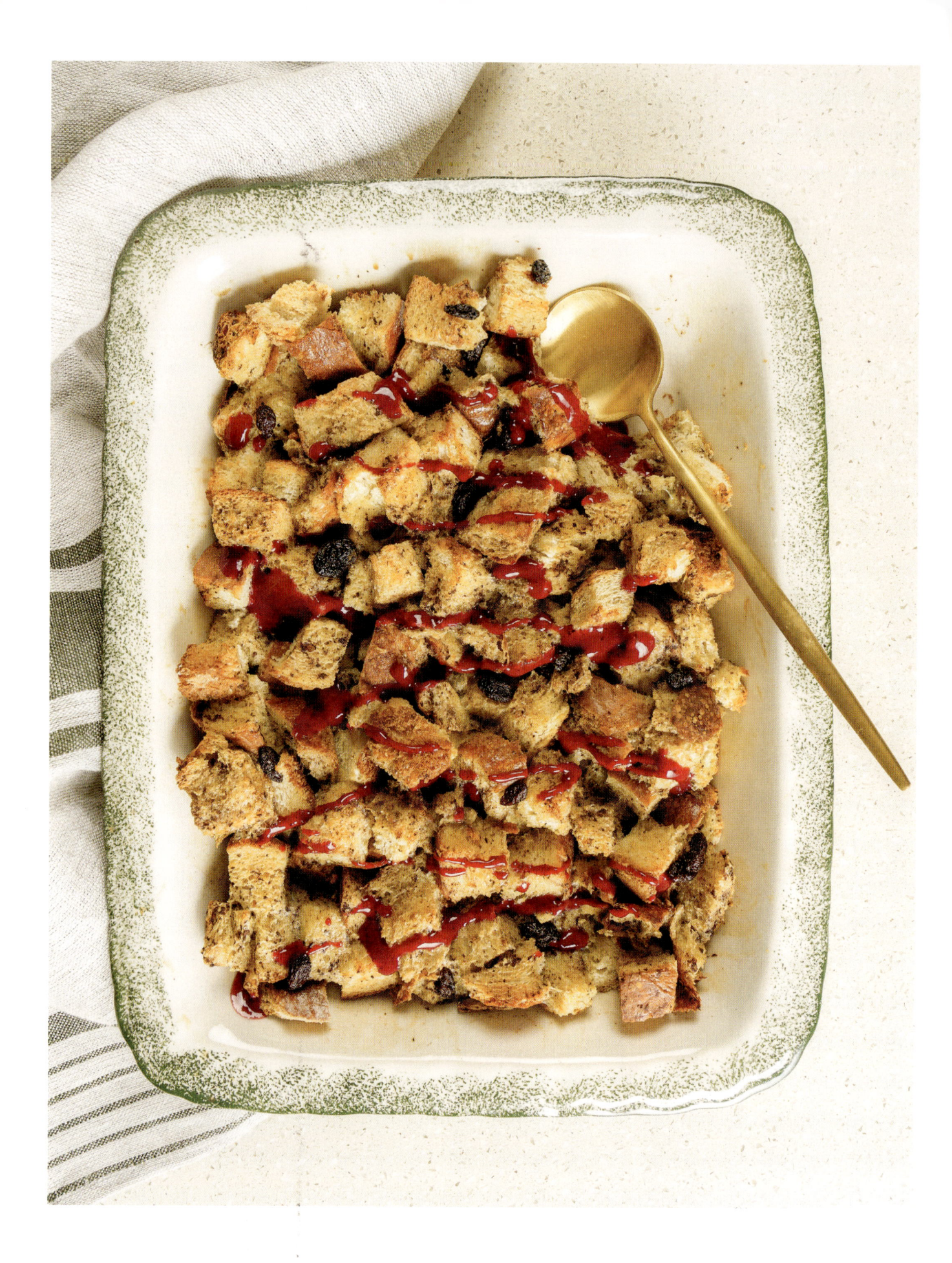

Baked French Toast

SERVES 4
PREP TIME: 10 MINUTES
SOAKING TIME: 30 MINUTES
COOKING TIME: 45 MINUTES

1 (1-pound) loaf crusty, flavorful whole-wheat bread (such as cinnamon-raisin, cranberry-walnut)

8 eggs

1 cup unsweetened milk of choice

¼ cup maple syrup

1 teaspoon vanilla extract

1 teaspoon ground cinnamon

Optional add-ins: fresh or dried fruit, nuts, or seeds

● **PROTEIN ADD**

Top with 2 tablespoons peanut butter (+8g), or serve 1 chicken sausage link on the side (+9g).

Per serving: Calories: 363
Fat: 11g | Carbohydrates: 47g
Fiber: 3g | Protein: 20g

Bring the feeling of a lazy Sunday morning to any day with this baked French toast recipe. This recipe tastes like you have your life together, even though you probably are the most sleep-deprived you've ever been! Each square contains 20 grams of protein and can be easily reheated in the microwave to fuel your postpartum healing and milk production.

1. Cut bread into 1-inch cubes.

2. Mix eggs, milk, spices, and any optional add-ins together.

3. Spray a 9 x 13-inch baking dish with non-stick spray and evenly scatter bread across the pan. Top with the mixture. Press bread down to ensure an even layer, and allow it to sit for 20–30 minutes.

4. Meanwhile, preheat the oven to 350°F.

5. Bake for 35–40 minutes, until eggs are set, or until the temperature reaches 155°F.

NOTES: Making this in a 9 x 13-inch baking dish results in crunchier French toast. If you'd prefer a more moist and custard-like texture, use an 8 x 8-inch dish and bake for 50 minutes.

The ideal bread for this recipe is the type that comes unsliced, with a thick crust, and that you'd usually find in the bakery section of the grocery store. This thicker, artisan bread is ideal for soaking up the eggs and milk and providing texture to the final dish.

Savory Baked French Toast

SERVES 4
PREP TIME: 15 MINUTES
SOAKING TIME: 30 MINUTES
COOKING TIME: 40 MINUTES

1 (1-pound) loaf of crusty, savory bakery bread (such as olive, jalapeño cheddar, rosemary)

8 eggs

1 cup unsweetened milk of choice

¼ teaspoon garlic powder

¼ teaspoon black pepper

Optional add-ins: cheese, herbs, meats, veggies

● **PROTEIN ADD**

Add 1 chicken sausage link (+9g) or ¼ cup shredded cheddar (+7g)

Per serving: Calories: 311
Fat: 11g | Carbohydrates: 33g
Fiber: 2g | Protein: 20g

Similar to our Baked French Toast on page 111, this recipe is a great template that you can customize based on your own preferences. It's easy to make and eat with one hand. Enjoying a nourishing breakfast and getting in 20 grams of protein has never been tastier.

1. Cut the bread into 1-inch cubes.

2. Mix the eggs, milk, spices, and any optional add-ins together.

3. Spray a 9 x 13-inch baking dish with nonstick spray and evenly scatter the bread across the bottom. Top with the egg mixture. Press the bread down to ensure an even layer and allow it to sit for 20–30 minutes.

4. Meanwhile, preheat the oven to 350°F.

5. Bake for 35–40 minutes, until the eggs are set, or the internal temperature reaches 155°F.

NOTES: Some suggested combinations:
- olive bread, mozzarella cheese, ½ teaspoon thyme
- jalapeño-cheddar bread, 1 teaspoon chili powder
- rosemary bread, sun-dried tomatoes, Parmesan cheese

Making this in a 9 x 13-inch baking dish will result in crunchier French toast. If you'd prefer a more moist and custard-like texture, use an 8 x 8-inch dish and bake for 50 minutes.

The ideal bread for this recipe is the type of bread that comes unsliced, with a thick crust, and that you'd usually find in the bakery section of the grocery store. This thicker, artisan bread is ideal for soaking up the eggs and providing texture to the final dish.

Baked Sweet Potato Hash

SERVES 4
PREP TIME: 15 MINUTES
COOKING TIME: 50 MINUTES

2 medium sweet potatoes, chopped

1 large onion, chopped

2 red bell peppers, chopped

1 head cauliflower, broken into florets

2 tablespoons olive oil

1–2 tablespoons creole seasoning (such as Tony Chachere's)

4 fresh turkey, chicken, pork, or veggie sausages

● **PROTEIN ADD**

Use additional sausage (+10–20g each), or top with 1 egg (+6g) or ¼ cup shredded cheddar (+7g).

Per serving: Calories: 400
Fat: 20g | Carbohydrates: 33g
Fiber: 9g | Protein: 19g

Prep this breakfast in advance, and start your day by getting in all of your veggies. High in protein and fiber, this baked hash is the perfect savory breakfast option. Sweet potatoes are high in vitamin A, specifically beta-carotene, and will help you reach your nearly doubled vitamin A requirement during breastfeeding and acute recovery.

1. Preheat the oven to 400°F.

2. Combine all the vegetables on a sheet pan and toss with the olive oil and creole seasoning. Place the whole sausages on top of the vegetables.

3. Bake for 45–50 minutes, tossing halfway through.

Savory Congee Bowl

SERVES: 4
PREP TIME: 10 MINUTES
COOKING TIME: 1 HOUR 30 MINUTES

Congee

6 cups homemade or store-bought bone chicken broth

1 cup white rice

1 teaspoon freshly grated ginger

¼ teaspoon salt

Topping

2 cups shredded cooked chicken thighs

1 cup dried shiitake mushrooms

3 green onions, finely chopped

2 tablespoons dried wakame

2 tablespoons soy or hoisin sauce

1 teaspoon sesame oil

8 fresh basil leaves, torn, optional

● MAKE IT PLANT-BASED

Use vegetable broth and replace the chicken with 1 (15-ounce) block of extra-firm tofu, drained, pressed, and cubed.

Per serving: Calories: 336
Fat: 6g | Carbohydrates: 48
Fiber: 2 | Protein: 21g

Congee is a traditional Chinese porridge often provided for mothers during the postpartum period. It is a great savory option for breakfast that can be made in advance and reheated when desired. Keeping a stash of shredded cooked chicken in the freezer makes it easy to pull the topping together at a moment's notice. Satisfying and warm, this congee bowl provides protein, sodium, carbohydrates, and fiber.

1. Combine all the congee ingredients in an Instant Pot.

2. Cook under high pressure for 30 minutes, and allow a 1-hour natural release.

3. Meanwhile, mix together all the topping ingredients. If preparing ahead, store the topping separately in the refrigerator.

4. Serve the congee topped with the chicken mixture. To reheat, portion one-quarter of the congee into a bowl with one-quarter of the topping mixture and 2 tablespoons of water. Microwave for 60 seconds, then stir and return to the microwave for 30 more seconds.

NOTE: This recipe would also taste delicious with a poached or over-easy egg served on top.

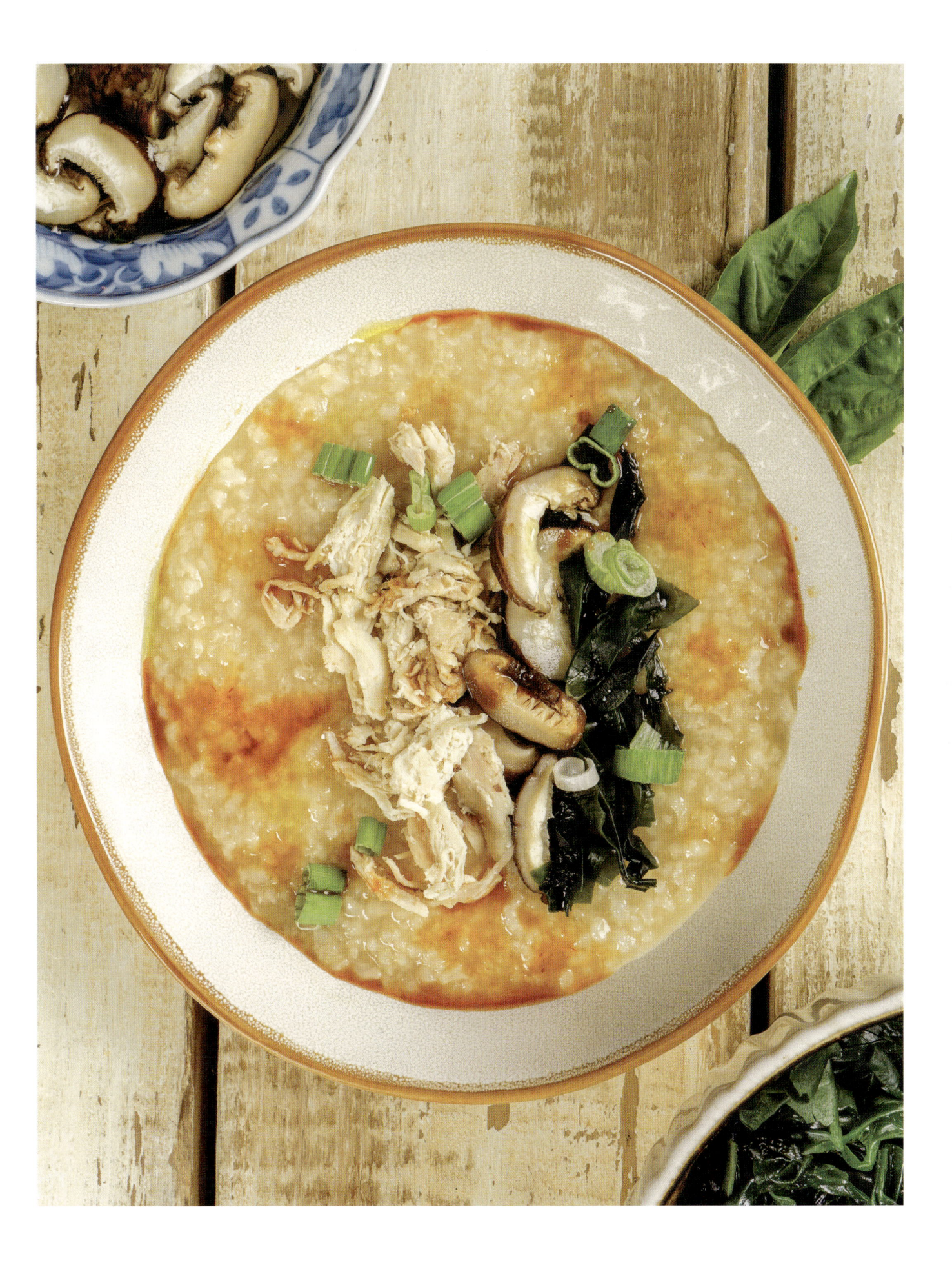

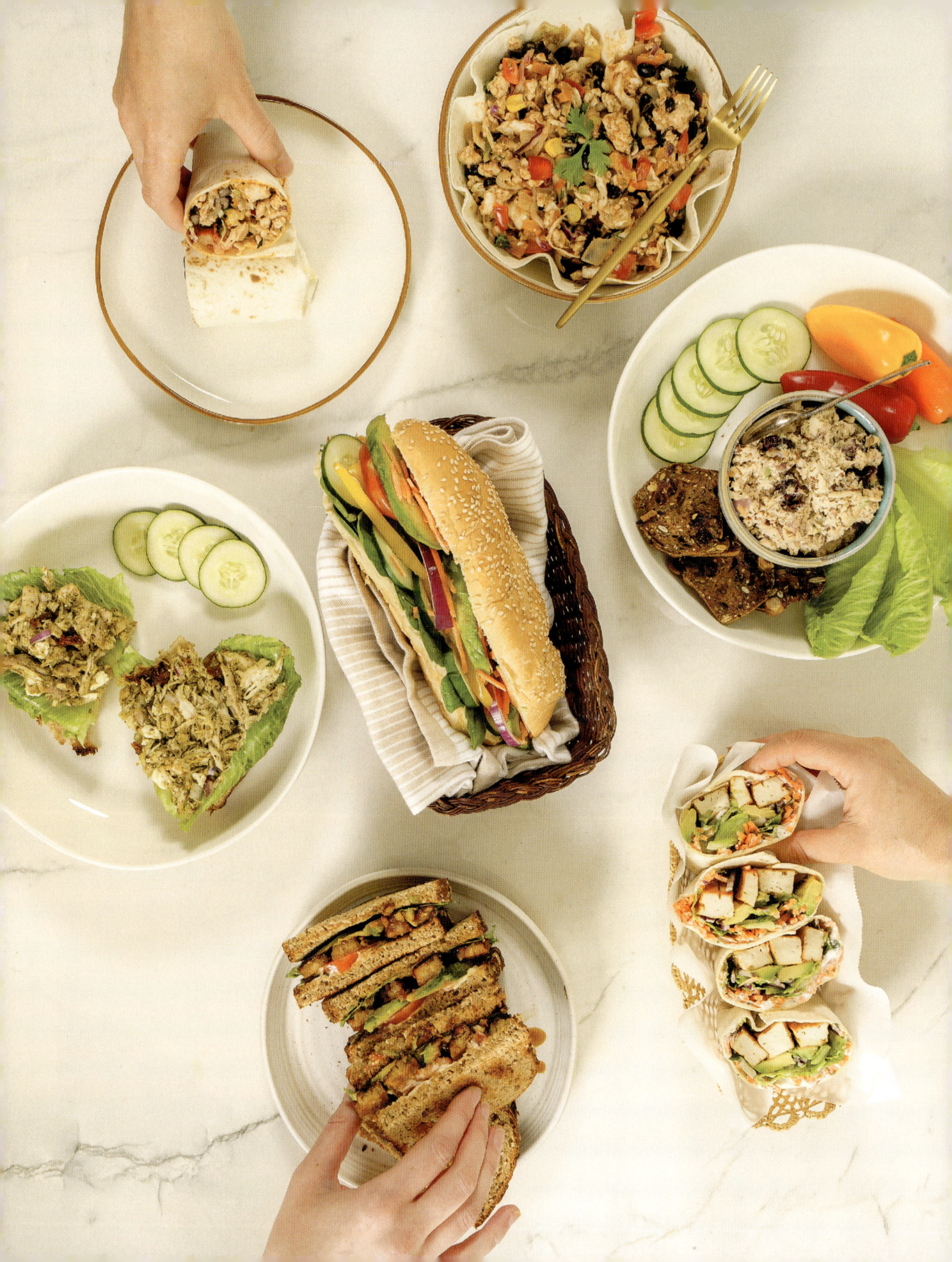

One-Handed Lunches

We love making these recipes, because as moms to two active toddlers, we need our lunches to be portable. There are a wide variety of handheld options in this chapter that don't sacrifice on flavor. Use these recipes in wraps, sandwiches, with crackers, or over a bed of salad greens.

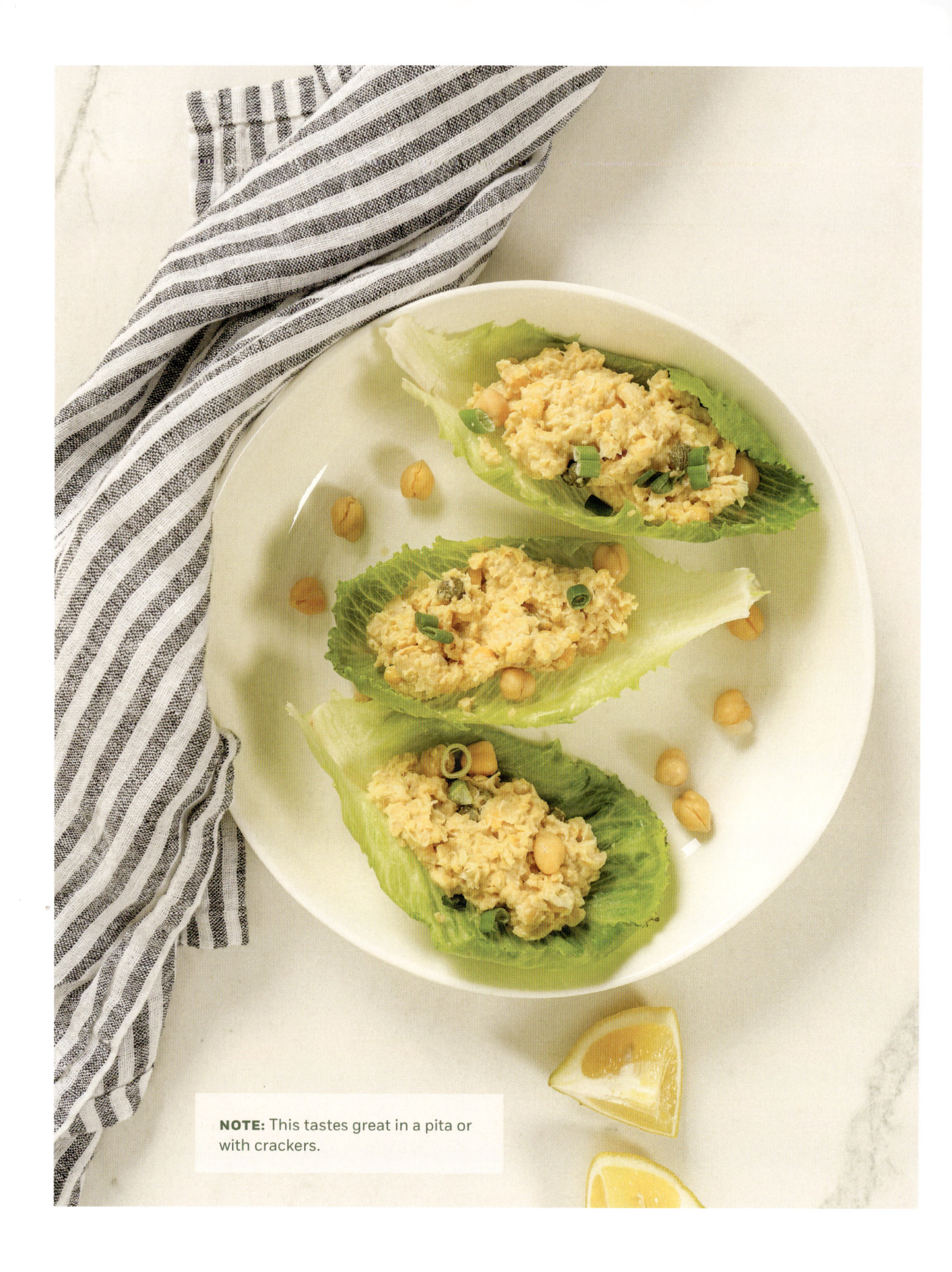

NOTE: This tastes great in a pita or with crackers.

Tuna and Chickpea Salad

SERVES 2
PREP TIME: 5 MINUTES
COOKING TIME: 0 MINUTES

1 (15.5-ounce) can chickpeas, drained and rinsed

2 tablespoons olive oil

Zest and juice of ½ small lemon

1 (5-ounce) can tuna

1 green onion, chopped

½ teaspoon dried parsley

Salt, to taste

● **MAKE IT PLANT-BASED**

Try our Chickpea Toona Salad on page 190.

Per serving: Calories: 389
Fat: 18g | Carbohydrates: 33g
Fiber: 7g | Protein: 25g

This recipe combines high-fiber chickpeas with protein-packed tuna for a well-balanced twist on the classic tuna salad. Extra bonuses: chickpeas are a good plant-based source of choline, while tuna provides omega-3s, both of which are important for a baby's brain development.

1. Combine the chickpeas, olive oil, lemon juice, and lemon zest in a bowl.

2. Using a fork, roughly mash the chickpeas.

3. Add the tuna, green onions, and parsley. Stir to combine. Add salt to taste.

Frito-less Taco Salad

SERVES 4
PREP TIME: 5 MINUTES
COOKING TIME: 20 MINUTES

1 tablespoon olive oil

1 large onion, diced

1 bell pepper, diced

1 pound ground chicken or turkey

2 tablespoons chili powder

1 tablespoon ground cumin

½ teaspoon salt

½ teaspoon black pepper

1 (15.5-ounce) can black beans, drained and rinsed

½ cup salsa

½ cup frozen corn

2 garlic cloves, minced

½ head cabbage, shredded, or 6 ounces shredded cabbage

⅓ cup creamy dressing (such as Bitchin' Sauce, ranch, Thousand Island, or guacamole salsa)

Optional add-ins: hot sauce, chopped tomatoes, avocado, cilantro, shredded cheese

● **MAKE IT PLANT-BASED**

Swap the pound of ground chicken or turkey for 1 (15-ounce) block extra-firm tofu, drained, pressed, and crumbled.

Per serving: Calories: 469
Fat: 19g | Carbohydrates: 41g
Fiber: 16g | Protein: 36g

We love to serve this salad on whole-wheat tortillas for make-ahead tacos that can be eaten with one hand! These remind Ashley of a taco salad she ate often growing up that included Fritos and, suspiciously, always tasted better soggy the next day. Sans the Fritos, this recipe is still a winner that will keep you full for hours, thanks to its high amount of protein and fiber.

1. In a large skillet, heat the olive oil, onions, and bell peppers over medium heat. Cook, stirring, until tender, about 5 minutes, then add the ground chicken or turkey and spices. Cook until the chicken is cooked through (about 8 minutes).

2. Add the beans, salsa, frozen corn, and garlic. Cook for 3–5 more minutes, stirring to thoroughly combine.

3. Transfer the taco mixture to a large bowl and add the cabbage and dressing. Stir to combine.

4. This can be enjoyed hot or cold.

NOTES: This tastes great on its own or wrapped in a 10-inch whole-wheat tortilla.

If you're making this salad ahead, and you prefer crispier cabbage, wait to add it until just before serving.
You can also make your own dressing by blending together ⅓ cup cottage cheese, 1 tablespoon lime juice, and a handful of cilantro, if you have the time!

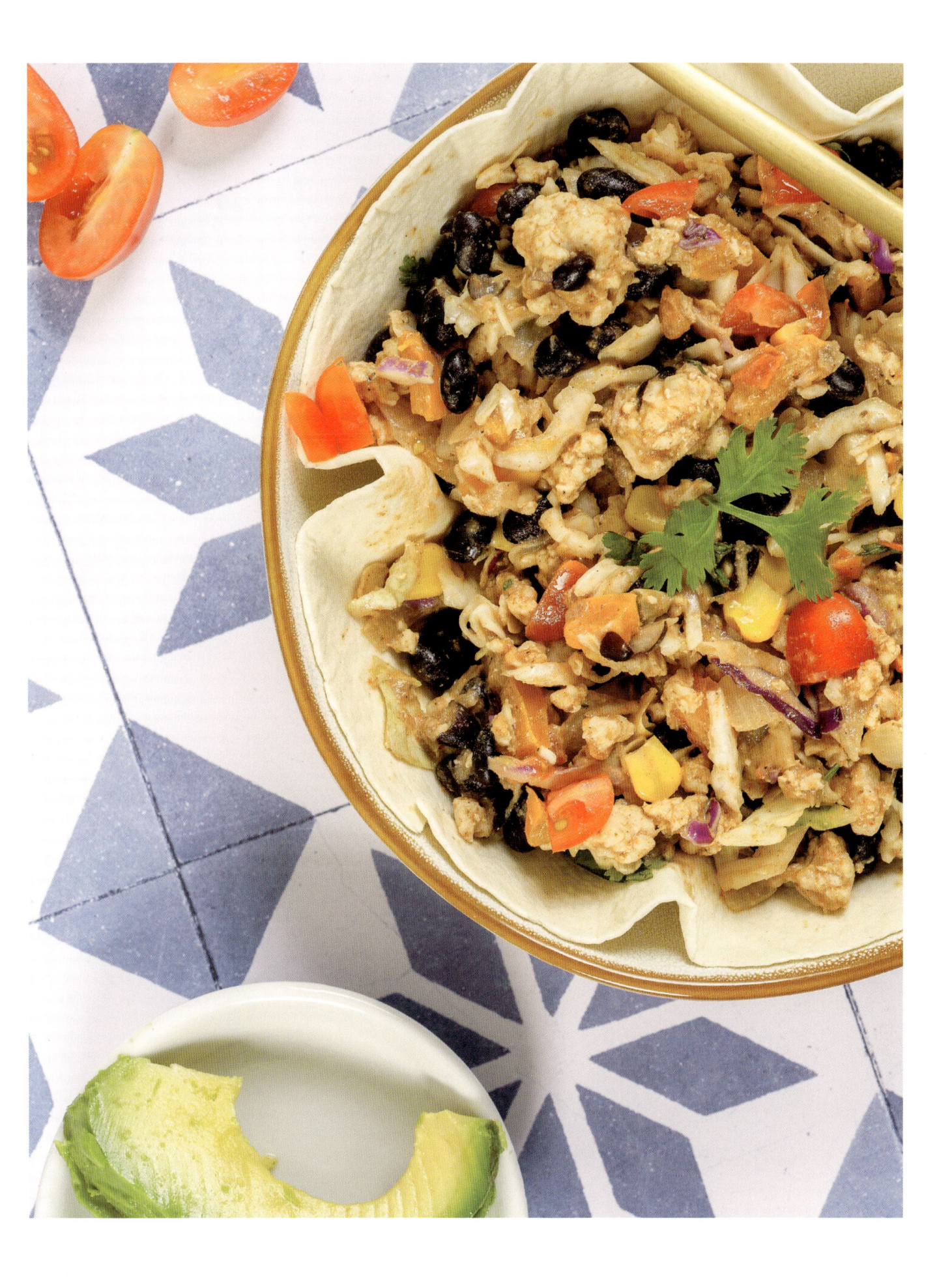

Pesto Chicken Salad

SERVES 4
PREP TIME: 10 MINUTES
COOKING TIME: 0 MINUTES

2 chicken breasts, shredded (about 3 cups)

½ cup pesto

2 ounces crumbled feta

¼ small red onion, finely chopped

16 sun-dried tomatoes (about ½ cup), diced

½ teaspoon garlic powder

¼ teaspoon black pepper

Salt, to taste

Salad greens such as spinach, arugula, or romaine, optional

Per serving: Calories: 396
Fat: 24g | Carbohydrates: 7g
Fiber: 1g | Protein: 39g

Packed with flavor, this one meal can help you make a big dent in your protein needs for the day and can be eaten with just one hand! The mixture of flavors will have you looking forward to lunch, which will reduce the chance of you skipping this important meal.

1. In a large bowl, mix all the ingredients until well combined.

2. Add a handful of green leaves to the chicken salad when ready to serve, if desired (don't add ahead of time or they will wilt).

NOTE: Serve as an open-faced sandwich on crusty bread with the greens on top!

Baby Caesar Salad Wrap

SERVES 1
PREP TIME: 15 MINUTES
COOKING TIME: 0 MINUTES

Sandwich

1 (10-inch) tortilla, flour or whole-wheat

1 cup chopped romaine lettuce

½ cup chickpeas or ½ cup cooked shredded chicken

¼ cup diced cucumber

A few thin slices of red onion

2–3 tablespoons Tahini Caesar Dressing (see below) or bottled Caesar dressing

Sprinkle of Parmesan cheese or nutritional yeast, optional

Tahini Caesar Dressing
(makes ½ cup)

¼ cup tahini

3 tablespoons water

2 tablespoons fresh lemon juice

1 garlic clove

1 teaspoon capers

2 teaspoons caper brine (from the jar of capers)

1 teaspoon Dijon mustard

1 teaspoon nutritional yeast

¼ teaspoon salt

Black pepper, to taste

● **PROTEIN ADD**

For the chickpea version, add 2 tablespoons of hemp seeds (+7g) to the filling.

● **MAKE IT GLUTEN-FREE**

Substitute tortilla with gluten-free tortilla.

This Baby Caesar Salad Wrap can be made completely vegan with chickpeas, nutritional yeast, and homemade Tahini Caesar Dressing, or you can keep it traditional with chicken, Parmesan, and classic Caesar dressing. Either version will hit the spot if you're craving a classic Caesar salad.

1. If using the Tahini Caesar Dressing, combine all the dressing ingredients in a jar or food processor. Shake well, or blend and set aside.

2. Lay the tortilla out and add the romaine, chickpeas or chicken, cucumber, and onion in the center.

3. Top with the dressing and Parmesan or nutritional yeast, if using those.

4. To roll your tortilla, fold the bottom of the tortilla over the filling to meet the top. Tuck in the sides and tightly roll until the tortilla is fully closed and the contents are secure.

5. Optional: crisp up the tortilla by air frying at 400°F for 2 minutes, or grill your tortilla on a grill pan or regular pan for a few minutes for a crisp outer layer.

NOTES: This can be eaten as a salad, too! Skip the tortilla, and increase the amount of romaine lettuce.

Per serving, Chickpea Caesar Salad Wrap: Calories: 379
Fat: 13g | Carbohydrates: 42g
Fiber: 12g | Protein: 16g

Per serving, Chicken Caesar Salad Wrap: Calories: 428
Fat: 25g | Carbohydrates: 23g
Fiber: 5g | Protein: 23g

Elevated PB&J Sandwich

SERVES 1
PREP TIME: 5 MINUTES
COOKING TIME: 1 MINUTE

½ cup frozen berries of choice

1 ½ teaspoons honey, maple syrup, or agave

1 ½ teaspoons chia seeds

1 ½ teaspoons hemp seeds

2 tablespoons creamy or crunchy peanut butter

2 slices whole-wheat bread, toasted

● **PROTEIN ADD**

Serve with our Titi Rita's Horchata (page 231, +7g) or a glass of milk (+8g).

● **MAKE IT GLUTEN-FREE**

Substitute bread with gluten-free bread.

● **MAKE IT NUT-FREE**

Use sunflower seed butter instead of the peanut butter.

Per serving: Calories: 438
Fat: 24g | Carbohydrates: 36g
Fiber: 7g | Protein: 18g

We transformed a regular PB&J sandwich into a more nutritious option. Using actual berries instead of jam slashes the sugar and increases the fiber content, while whole-wheat bread and hemp seeds provide a protein add in this beloved classic. Paired with a cold glass of milk, this sandwich provides nutrient-packed nostalgia.

1. Place the berries in a microwave-safe bowl and heat them in the microwave for 1 minute.

2. Once ready, mash them with a fork and add the sweetener.

3. Add the chia seeds and hemp seeds and mix until well combined.

4. Allow to sit for 2–3 minutes.

5. Spread the peanut butter on one piece of toast and the berry mixture on the other.

6. Put the two pieces of toast together to form a sandwich.

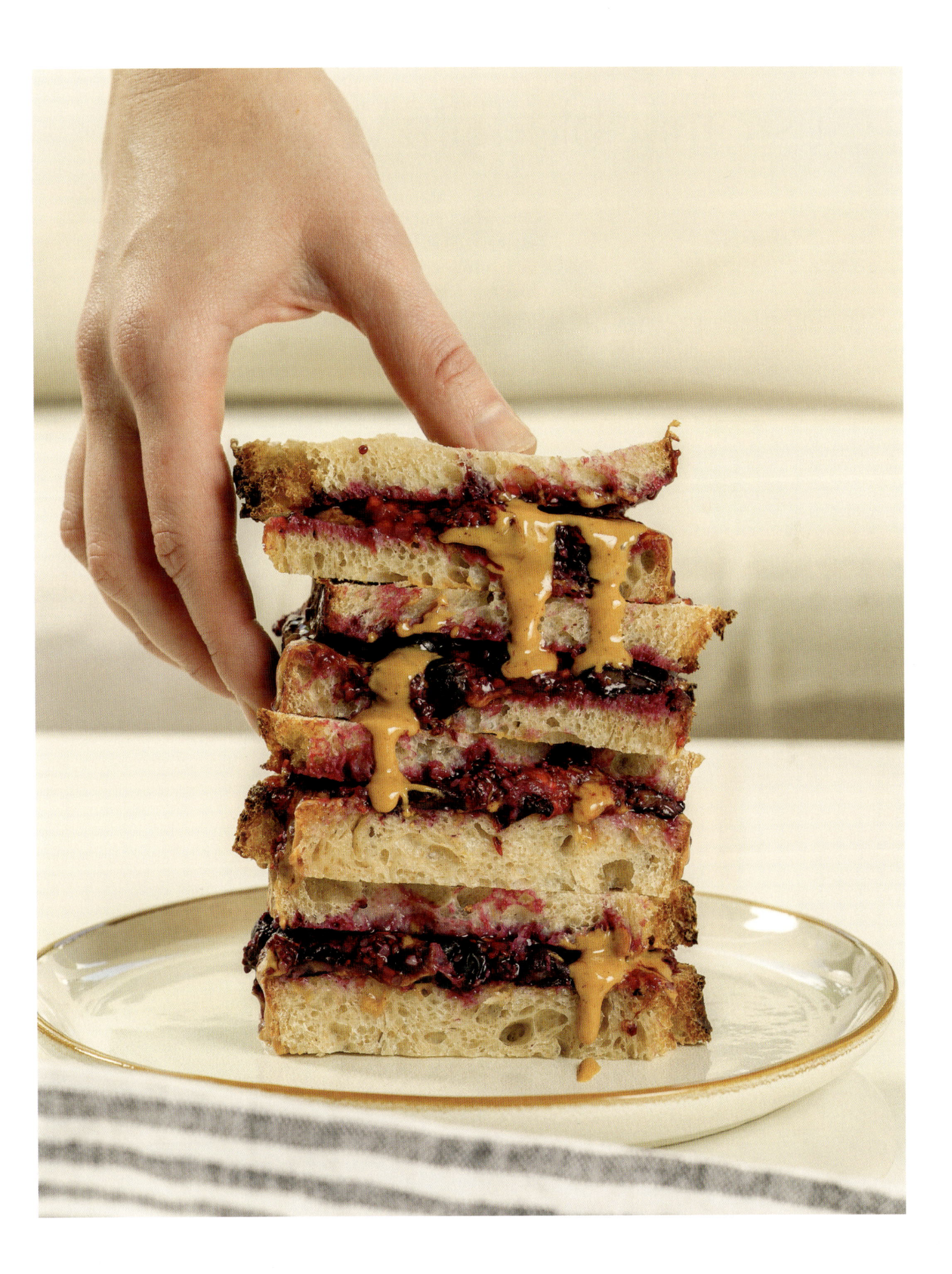

Customizable Tofu Wrap

SERVES 1
PREP TIME: 3 MINUTES
COOKING TIME: 0 MINUTES

1 (10-inch) tortilla, flour or whole-wheat

2 tablespoons hummus

3 ½ ounces baked tofu, sliced

¼ (11-ounce) bagged salad kit (including toppings and dressing)

● **MAKE IT GLUTEN-FREE**
Substitute tortilla with gluten-free tortilla.

Per serving: Calories: 415
Fat: 19g | Carbohydrates: 39g
Fiber: 9g | Protein: 20g

This wrap is more like a template than a structured recipe—after making it once, you'll know the general ingredients and can mix and match in any flavors you'd like. It's a very easy and convenient way to get in proteins, carbs, healthy fats, and fiber.

1. Lay the wrap on a plate and spread the hummus on top.
2. Arrange the sliced tofu down the center of the wrap.
3. Top with the salad greens and garnishes. Add a drizzle of the included dressing.
4. Tuck the top and bottom of the wrap in toward the center, then roll up from one side to form a tight wrap.

NOTE: This recipe can be customized in so many ways: Vary the flavor with different hummus varieties, use different flavors of baked tofu (such as teriyaki, sriracha, and plain), and try different types of bagged salads.

Chicken or the Egg Salad

SERVES 4
PREP TIME: 5 MINUTES
COOKING TIME: 0 MINUTES

3 celery stalks, finely diced

2 green onions, finely diced

¼ cup mayonnaise, or more to taste

2 tablespoons spicy brown mustard

1 tablespoon Old Bay, Season All, or other all-purpose seasoning

2 chicken breasts, shredded (about 3 cups) or 16 hard-boiled eggs

Per serving, chicken: Calories: 271
Fat: 17g | Carbohydrates: 2g
Fiber: 1g | Protein: 36g

Per serving, egg: Calories: 276
Fat: 20g | Carbohydrates: 4g
Fiber: 1g | Protein: 20g

Which one came first? With this recipe, you decide! This staple recipe will never let you down, and both the chicken and egg versions can be whipped together with minimal time and ingredients. This recipe also works great with cooked shrimp!

1. Mix the celery, green onions, mayonnaise, mustard, and seasoning together in a bowl. For the egg salad, remove the yolks and set aside. Finely dice the whites. Mash 8 of the yolks with a fork and mix into the mayonnaise.

2. Add the chicken or egg whites to the bowl and stir until thoroughly combined. If you prefer a creamier salad, add more mayonnaise.

NOTES: Serve in any bread, wrap, bagel, or salad.

Don't throw out your extra yolks. They are an excellent source of choline, which is critical for a baby's brain development. You can add the unused yolks to salads for yourself or mix them your children's food once they are old enough for solids.

Rainbow Hummus Sub

SERVES 1
PREP TIME: 10 MINUTES
COOKING TIME: 0 MINUTES

1 (6-inch) sub roll

¼ cup hummus

2 slices cucumber, cut into half-moons

⅓ cup matchstick carrots

¼ yellow bell pepper, cut into strips

1 handful fresh spinach leaves

A few slices of tomato

A few slices of avocado

● **PROTEIN ADD**

Add 2 ounces of Tofurky plant-based deli slices (+14g) or sliced deli turkey (+10g).

Per serving: Calories: 300
Fat: 13g | Carbohydrates: 29g
Fiber: 10g | Protein: 10g

This colorful hummus sandwich is a quick and easy way to get in your veggies at lunch! The variety of vegetables provides an array of vitamins, minerals, phytonutrients, and antioxidants—all important for postpartum healing.

1. Spread the hummus on the bottom half of the sub roll.
2. Layer all the remaining ingredients over the hummus and top with the other half of the roll.

NOTE: This can also be served on a wrap in place of the sub roll.

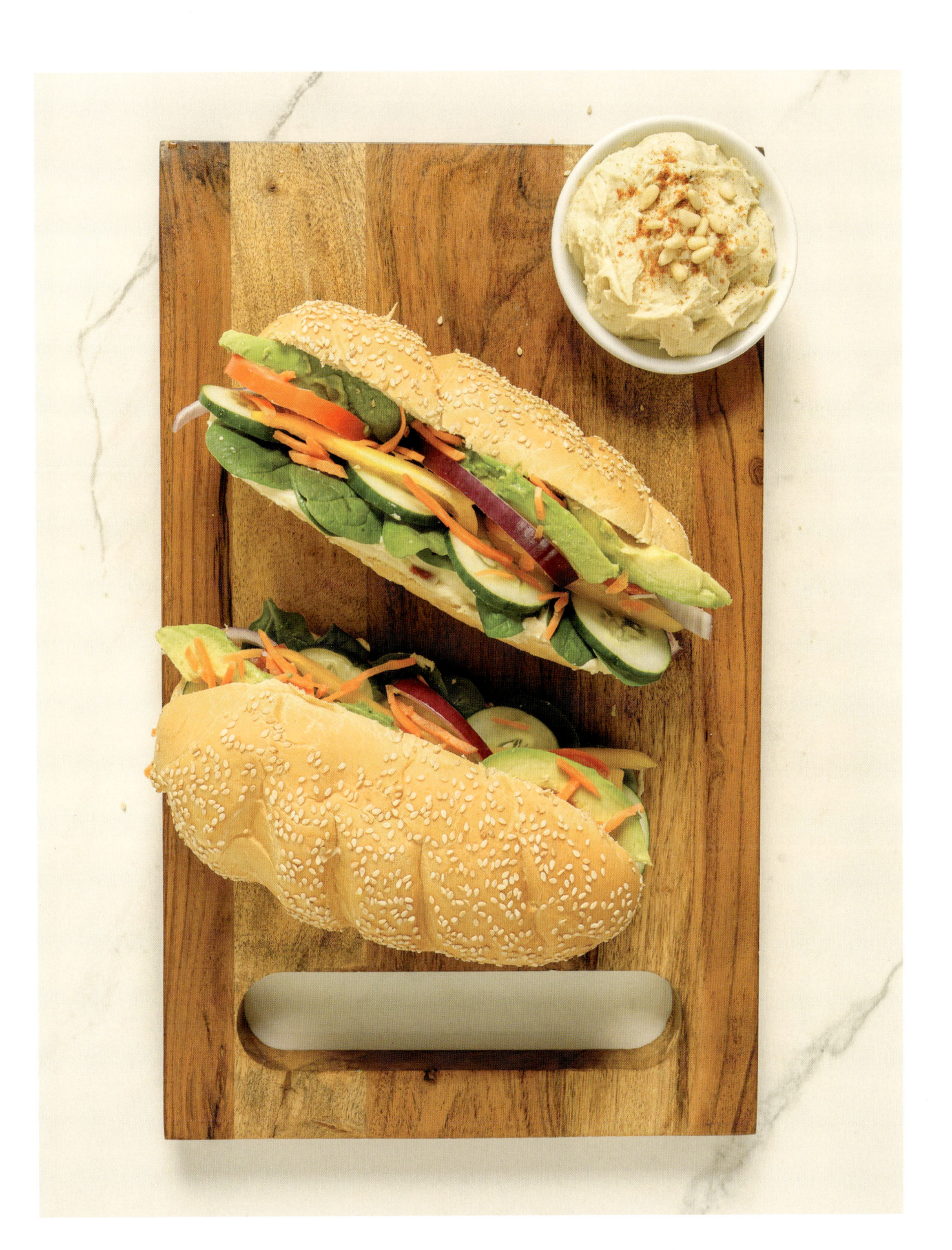

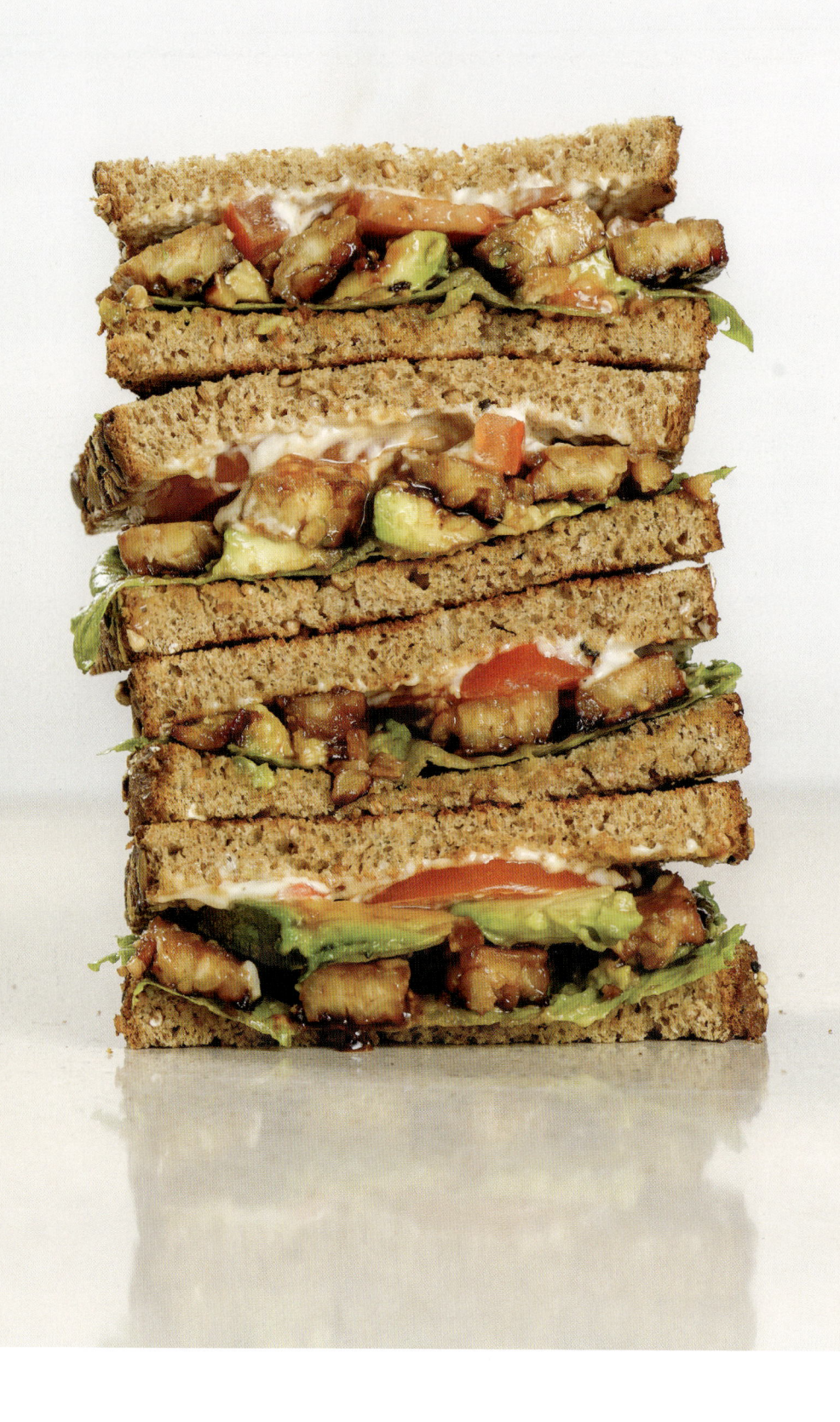

BTLT: BBQ Tempeh, Lettuce, and Tomato

SERVES 2
PREP TIME: 10 MINUTES
COOKING TIME: 10 MINUTES

1 (8.8-ounce) package tempeh

½ cup BBQ sauce

4 slices whole-wheat bread, toasted

2 tablespoons mayonnaise, vegan or regular

4 romaine lettuce leaves

A few slices of tomato

½ avocado, sliced, optional

1–2 teaspoons olive oil

● **MAKE IT GLUTEN-FREE**
Substitute bread with gluten-free bread.

Per serving: Calories: 488
Fat: 24g | Carbohydrates: 43g
Fiber: 5g | Protein: 24g

This sandwich is a plant-based version of the popular BLT (bacon, lettuce, and tomato), only we used BBQ tempeh instead of bacon. Tempeh is made from fermented soybeans, making it an excellent plant-based protein that provides a nutty and earthy flavor.

1. Slice the tempeh into ¼-inch-thick slices.

2. In a large bowl or food storage container, combine the tempeh and BBQ sauce and let it sit for at least 5 minutes for the tempeh to absorb the BBQ sauce.

3. While the tempeh is marinating, begin assembling your sandwiches by spreading mayo on one side of two slices of toast, then layering on lettuce, tomato, and avocado.

4. Heat the oil in a large skillet over medium heat. Once the oil is hot, add the tempeh strips and cook until golden brown, about 5 minutes on each side.

5. Add the tempeh to the sandwiches and top each one with a second slice of bread.

Thai Peanut Chicken Salad

SERVES 4
PREP TIME: 15 MINUTES
COOKING TIME: 0 MINUTES

½ cup creamy peanut butter

¼ cup soy sauce, tamari, or coconut aminos

¼ cup rice wine vinegar

1 tablespoon maple syrup

1 tablespoon sesame oil

2 tablespoons water, or more as needed

3 cups shredded cooked chicken breasts or thighs (about 2 large breasts)

1 (12-ounce) bag coleslaw mix

4 green onions, chopped

1 bunch cilantro, chopped

Optional toppings: chopped peanuts and lime juice

● **MAKE IT PLANT-BASED**

Substitute 2 cups of shelled edamame, 1 (15-ounce) block of baked extra-firm tofu, or a combination of the two in place of the chicken.

Per serving: Calories: 478
Fat: 25g | Carbohydrates: 19g
Fiber: 8g | Protein: 39g

Ready for an updated and delicious twist on chicken salad? Don't skimp on the cilantro; it's absolutely essential for this recipe. Enjoy this mixture on any type of carb vehicle to get it in your mouth as fast as possible!

1. In a large bowl, mix together the peanut butter, soy sauce, vinegar, maple syrup, and sesame oil. Add the water and stir. If the sauce seems too thick, add more water a little at a time until it has a thin consistency that can easily drip off a spoon.

2. Mix in the chicken, coleslaw, green onions, and cilantro.

3. Serve topped with chopped peanuts and a squeeze of lime juice, if desired.

NOTE: This tastes delicious in a sandwich or wrap but can also be enjoyed over rice or ramen noodles.

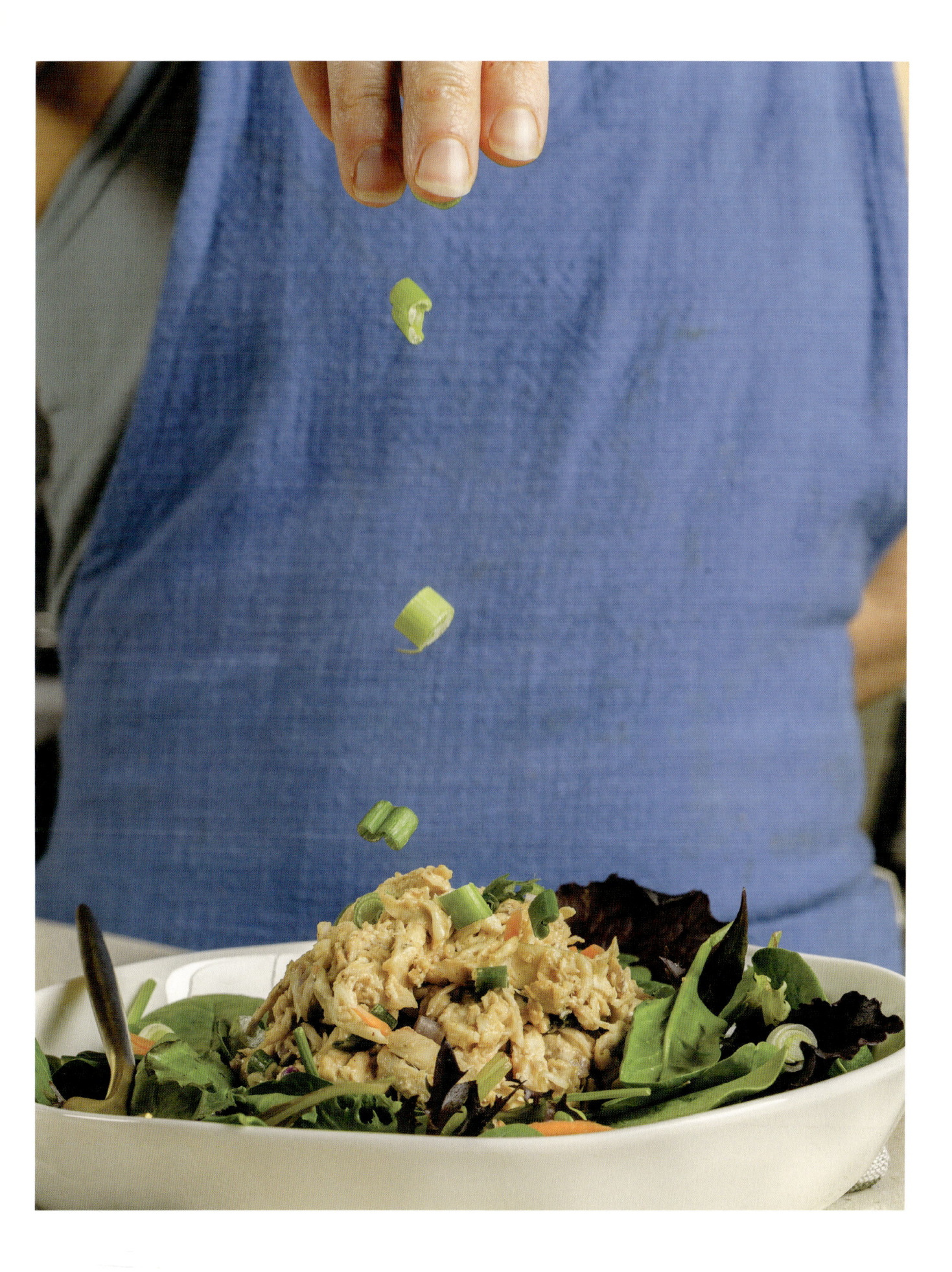

Omega-Boosting Salmon Salad

SERVES 3
PREP TIME: 10 MINUTES
COOKING TIME: 0 MINUTES

Yogurt-Mayo Dressing

¼ cup unsweetened plain Greek yogurt

¼ cup mayonnaise

1 ½ tablespoons lemon juice

1 tablespoon Dijon mustard

1 tablespoon dried parsley

1 tablespoon dried dill

¼ teaspoon garlic powder

⅛ teaspoon salt

⅛ teaspoon black pepper

Salmon Salad

2 (5-ounce) cans salmon

¼ cup finely diced celery

¼ cup finely diced red onion

¼ cup dried cranberries, dried raisins, chopped prunes

¼ cup slivered or sliced almonds

Per serving: Calories: 397
Fat: 25g | Carbohydrates: 12g
Fiber: 3g | Protein: 30g

Salmon is an excellent source of omega-3 fatty acids, a type of fat that's important to both mom's and baby's brain health. In fact, low levels of omega-3s have been linked to the development of postpartum depression. This simple salad provides almost 100% of your omega-3 needs for the day!

1. In a large bowl, mix together all the ingredients for the yogurt-mayo dressing.

2. Add all the salmon salad ingredients and thoroughly combine.

NOTES: No salmon? You can use canned tuna or sardines for this recipe.

Pair with greens or crackers, or eat in a sandwich or wrap.

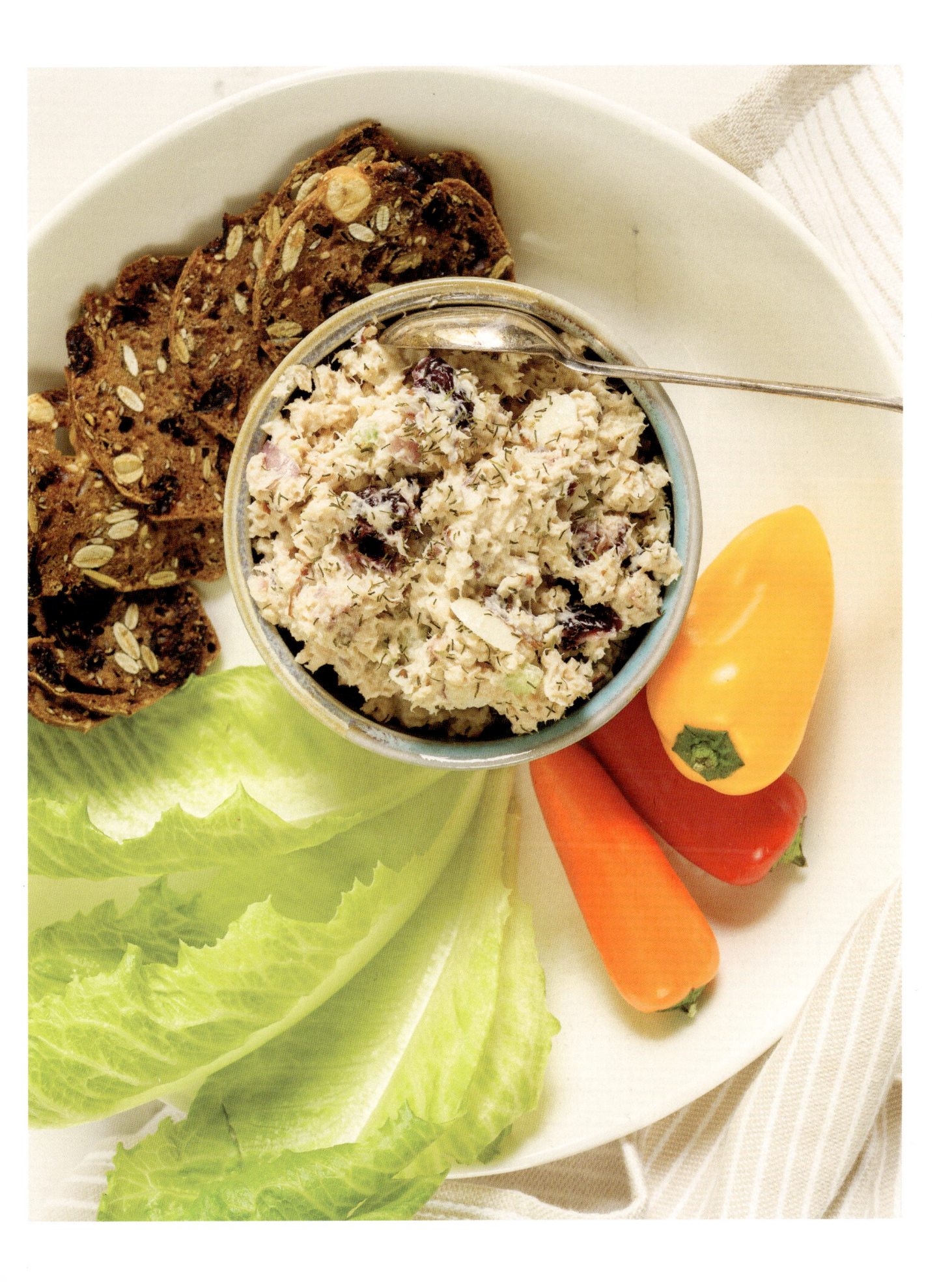

Buffalo Tofu Wrap

SERVES 2
PREP TIME: 10 MINUTES
COOKING TIME: 50 MINUTES

1 (15-ounce) block extra-firm tofu, drained and pressed

1 ½ teaspoons olive oil

½ teaspoon garlic powder

½ teaspoon onion powder

¼ teaspoon salt

⅓ cup buffalo sauce

2 cups chopped romaine

½ cup matchstick carrots

¼ red onion, thinly sliced

½ avocado, sliced

2 (10-inch) tortillas, flour or whole-wheat

¼ cup ranch dressing of choice

● **PROTEIN ADD**

Enjoy another serving of the buffalo tofu (+9g), or substitute 3 ounces of chicken (+21g) for the tofu.

● **MAKE IT GLUTEN-FREE**

Substitute tortillas with gluten-free tortillas.

Per serving: Calories: 491
Fat: 33g | Carbohydrates: 27g
Fiber: 8g | Protein: 16g

Satisfy your cravings for buffalo wings with this mouthwatering plant-based option. This buffalo tofu wrap is an excellent way to try tofu! Plus, the crunchy romaine and carrots with the creaminess of the avocado and ranch dressing provide the perfect texture.

1. Preheat the oven to 400°F.

2. Cut tofu horizontally through the center to form two layers. Then make 3 perpendicular cuts to form 8 individual strips of tofu. Season tofu with olive oil and spices.

3. Layer your tofu pieces evenly on a parchment-lined baking sheet and bake for 45 minutes. (Or air fry at 350°F for 20 minutes.)

4. Place the buffalo sauce in a small bowl and use a fork to dip each tofu piece into the buffalo sauce. Bake for another 5 minutes in the oven (or air fry for 2–3 minutes more).

5. Place half the romaine, carrots, onion, and avocado in the center of each tortilla.

6. Add 4 blocks of buffalo tofu and 2 tablespoons ranch dressing to each wrap.

7. To roll your tortilla, fold the bottom of the tortilla over the filling to meet the top. Tuck in the sides and tightly roll until the tortilla is fully closed and the contents are secure.

8. Optional: crisp up the tortilla by air frying at 400°F for 2 minutes, or grill your tortilla on a grill pan or regular pan for a few minutes for a crisp outer layer.

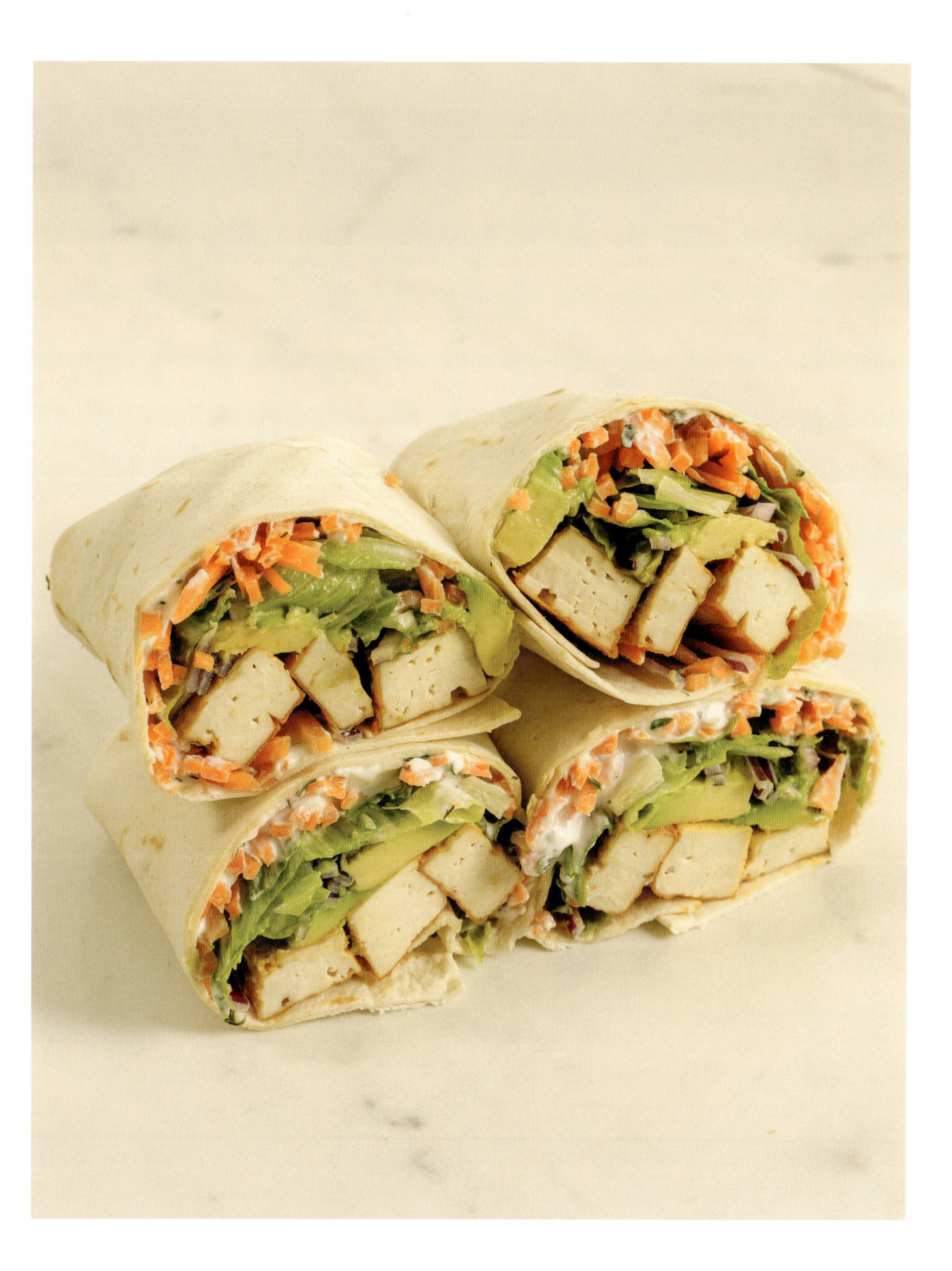

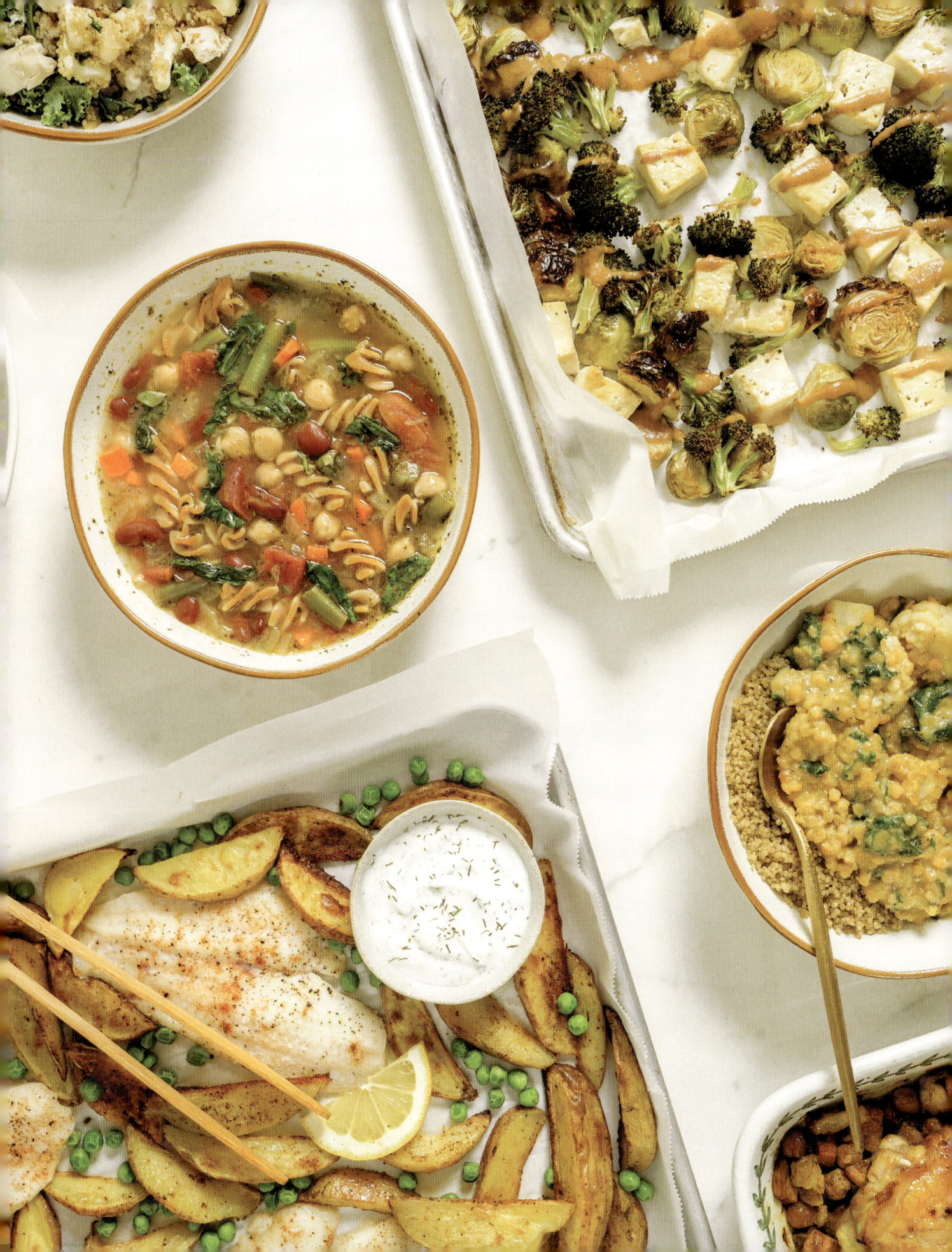

Set-It-and-Forget-It Dinners

All of these dinners involve just one pan, whether it's a sheet pan, Instant Pot, slow cooker, or stovetop pot. You can prepare these meals during a nap earlier in the day, ask a friend or family member to bring them over, or spend a few minutes prepping just before cooking. Then you'll have a few minutes to do other things while dinner cooks without your attention.

Sheet-Pan Fish and Chips

SERVES 4
PREP TIME: 10 MINUTES
COOKING TIME: 25 MINUTES

Chips

4 yellow or 3 russet potatoes, cut into ½-inch wedges

2 tablespoons olive oil, plus more for drizzling

½ teaspoon salt

½ teaspoon garlic powder

½ teaspoon paprika

¼ teaspoon black pepper

Fish

4 white fish filets (such as tilapia, cod, halibut, flounder)

½ teaspoon lemon pepper seasoning

½ teaspoon garlic powder

½ teaspoon paprika

½ teaspoon dried parsley

Salt, to taste

Drizzle of olive oil

Lemon wedges and tartar sauce for serving, optional

Per serving: Calories: 351
Fat: 10g | Carbohydrates: 27g
Fiber: 2g | Protein: 38g

This fish and chips recipe is our healthier and quicker take on the beloved classic British recipe. We even added peas to bring color and more nutrition to this plate. Like other animal proteins, fish is an excellent source of B12, which is an important postpartum vitamin that helps to replenish blood loss following labor and after delivery.

1. Preheat the oven to 450°F. Line two baking sheets with parchment paper and set aside.

2. In a large bowl, combine the potatoes, oil, salt, garlic powder, paprika, and pepper; toss to mix.

3. Transfer the potatoes to one baking sheet and arrange them in one layer.

4. Bake for 15 minutes.

5. Meanwhile, season the fish with lemon pepper seasoning, garlic powder, paprika, dried parsley, salt, and a drizzle of olive oil.

6. Place the fish on the second baking sheet.

7. Once the potatoes have baked for 15 minutes, add the second baking sheet to the oven and roast everything for 8–12 more minutes, or until the fish flakes easily and the potatoes are done.

8. Serve the potatoes and fish with lemon wedges and tartar sauce, if desired.

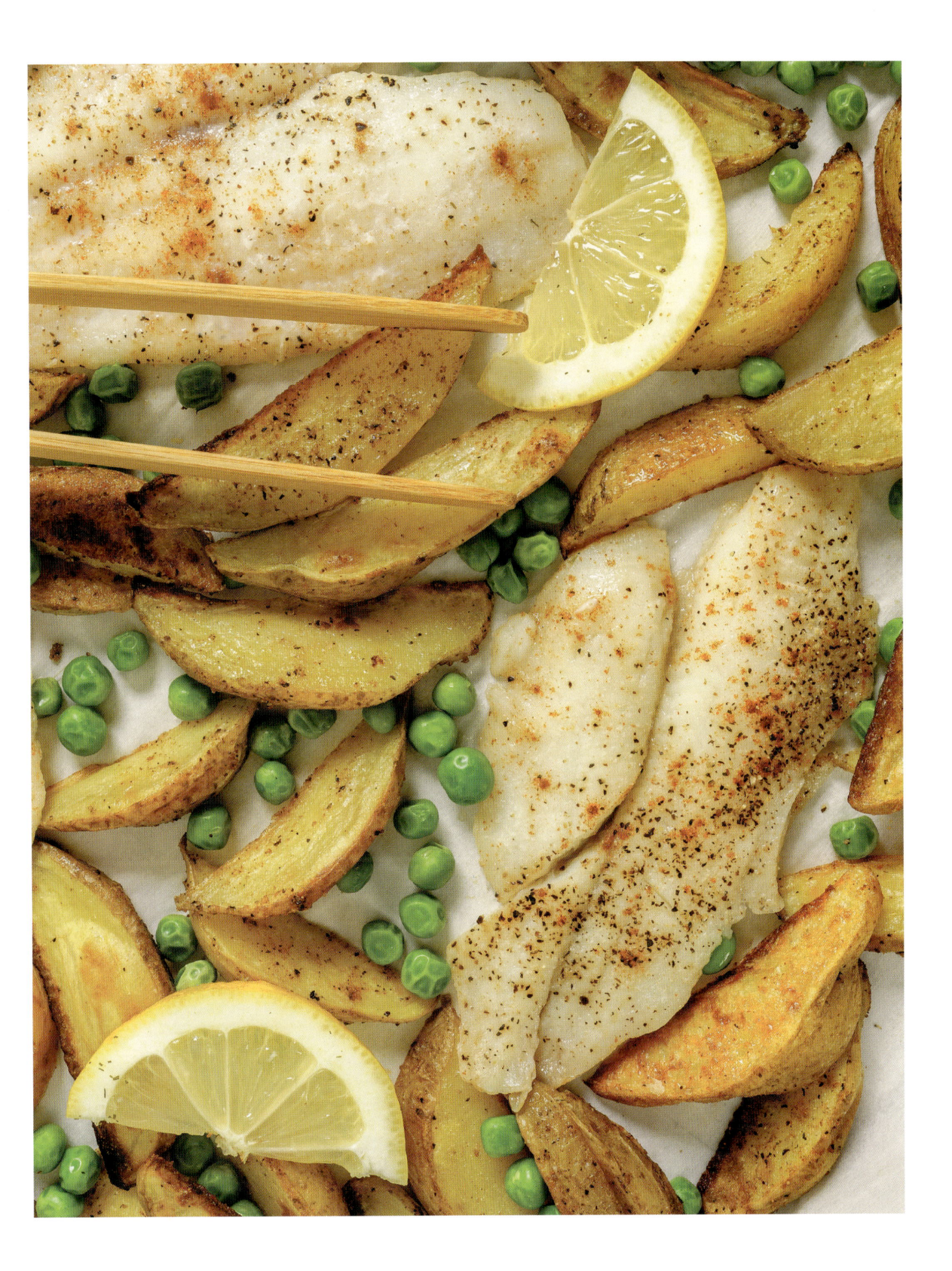

Creamy Chicken Quinoa Bake

SERVES 4
PREP TIME: 15 MINUTES
COOKING TIME: 1 HOUR

Chicken Quinoa Bake

1 pound chicken thighs, cubed

2 cups cauliflower florets

1 bunch kale, chopped (about 2 cups)

1 onion, diced

1 red bell pepper, diced

2/3 cup dry quinoa

3 garlic cloves, chopped

1 teaspoon Italian seasoning

½ teaspoon red pepper flakes

½ teaspoon salt

¼ teaspoon black pepper

1 1/3 cups chicken or vegetable broth

Sauce

2 tablespoons tahini

1 tablespoon warm water

1 tablespoon lemon juice

½ teaspoon salt

● **MAKE IT PLANT-BASED**

Substitute the chicken with 2 (15.5-ounce) cans of chickpeas, drained and rinsed.

Per serving: Calories: 325
Fat: 11g | Carbohydrates: 31g
Fiber: 5g | Protein: 29g

If you aren't usually a fan of quinoa, this dish offers a delicious alternative to how you've likely eaten it before. Cooked in just one pan in the oven and topped with a creamy tahini-based sauce, this recipe includes a lot of flavor with minimal cleanup. Quinoa is a pseudo-cereal offering nearly double the amount of protein and fiber compared to brown rice.

1. Preheat the oven to 375°F.

2. In a large baking dish, combine all the Chicken Quinoa Bake ingredients. Mix together until well combined.

3. Cover the baking dish with foil and bake for 50–60 minutes or until quinoa is tender. Stir after 35 minutes.

4. Meanwhile, in a small bowl, mix together all the sauce ingredients. Drizzle over the chicken quinoa and mix until well combined.

Chicken Drumsticks with Crispy Polenta

SERVES 4
PREP TIME: 15 MINUTES
COOKING TIME: 50 MINUTES

1 teaspoon salt

½ teaspoon black pepper

½ teaspoon garlic powder

½ teaspoon onion powder

½ teaspoon smoked paprika

1 log cooked polenta, cut into 1-inch cubes

1 pound asparagus, broccoli, Brussels sprouts, or zucchini (whatever you have and is in season)

2 tablespoons olive oil

8 chicken drumsticks

Per serving: Calories: 379
Fat: 19g | Carbohydrates: 22g
Fiber: 5g | Protein: 30g

Try this new take on a classic chicken dinner. Baked and then crisped under the broiler, these drumsticks and polenta offer a nice crunch in addition to their flavor. Polenta, made from corn, is a fun substitution for other grains and can be stored in your pantry. Chicken drumsticks are higher in fat than chicken breasts, which makes them more forgiving if you allow them to cook for longer than planned.

1. Preheat the oven to 350°F.

2. Arrange a wire rack atop a large baking sheet. (No wire rack? It's okay to make it without, but your chicken and polenta may not be as crispy.)

3. Mix the salt, black pepper, garlic powder, onion powder, and smoked paprika in a small dish.

4. Combine the polenta and vegetables in a large bowl. Top with the olive oil and half of the seasoning mix. Stir to thoroughly coat with seasoning. Place on one half of the wire rack.

5. Add the drumsticks to the bowl and add the remaining seasoning mix. Toss to evenly coat. Arrange on the other half of the baking dish.

6. Bake for 50 minutes, or until the internal temperature of the chicken reaches 165°F.

7. Not crispy enough? Put under the broiler on high for 5 minutes.

NOTE: This dish also works well in a large air fryer, but each ingredient will have different cooking times. First add the chicken drumsticks and air fry at 375°F for 15 minutes. Then top with the polenta cubes and cook for 5 minutes. Lastly, add the vegetables, and cook for 5 more minutes.

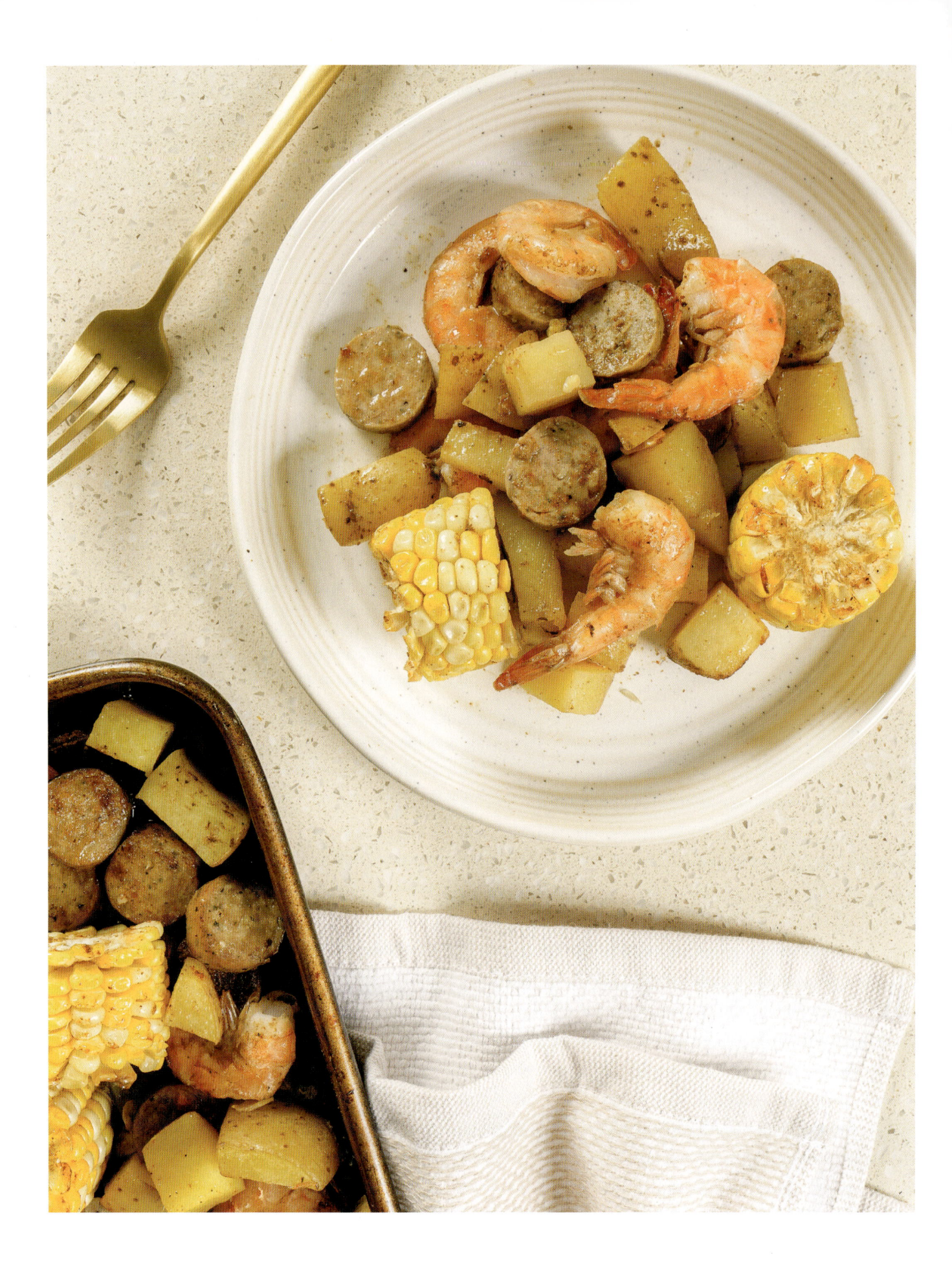

One-Pan Shrimp Boil

SERVES 4
PREP TIME: 10 MINUTES
COOKING TIME: 25 MINUTES

1 pound shrimp, raw

1 (12-ounce) package sweet Italian cooked chicken sausage, thinly sliced

3 medium yellow potatoes, diced into small ½-inch cubes

3 ears corn on the cob, sliced into 2-inch chunks

2 tablespoons olive oil

1 tablespoon Old Bay Seasoning

● **MAKE IT PLANT-BASED**

Omit the shrimp, and substitute chicken sausage with veggie sausage.

Per serving: Calories: 509
Fat: 21g | Carbohydrates: 40g
Fiber: 5g | Protein: 41g

A shrimp boil is a Southern favorite that includes shrimp, potatoes, sausage, and sweet corn all cooked together on a sheet pan. Like other seafood, shrimp is a good source of omega-3 fatty acids, which are essential for both mom and baby. This recipe is a delicious way to eat over 50% of your daily omega-3 requirement.

1. Preheat the oven to 400°F, and line your baking sheet with parchment paper.

2. Place all the ingredients in a large bowl and toss well. Spread everything across the baking sheet in an even layer.

3. Bake in the oven for 25 minutes, or until cooked through.

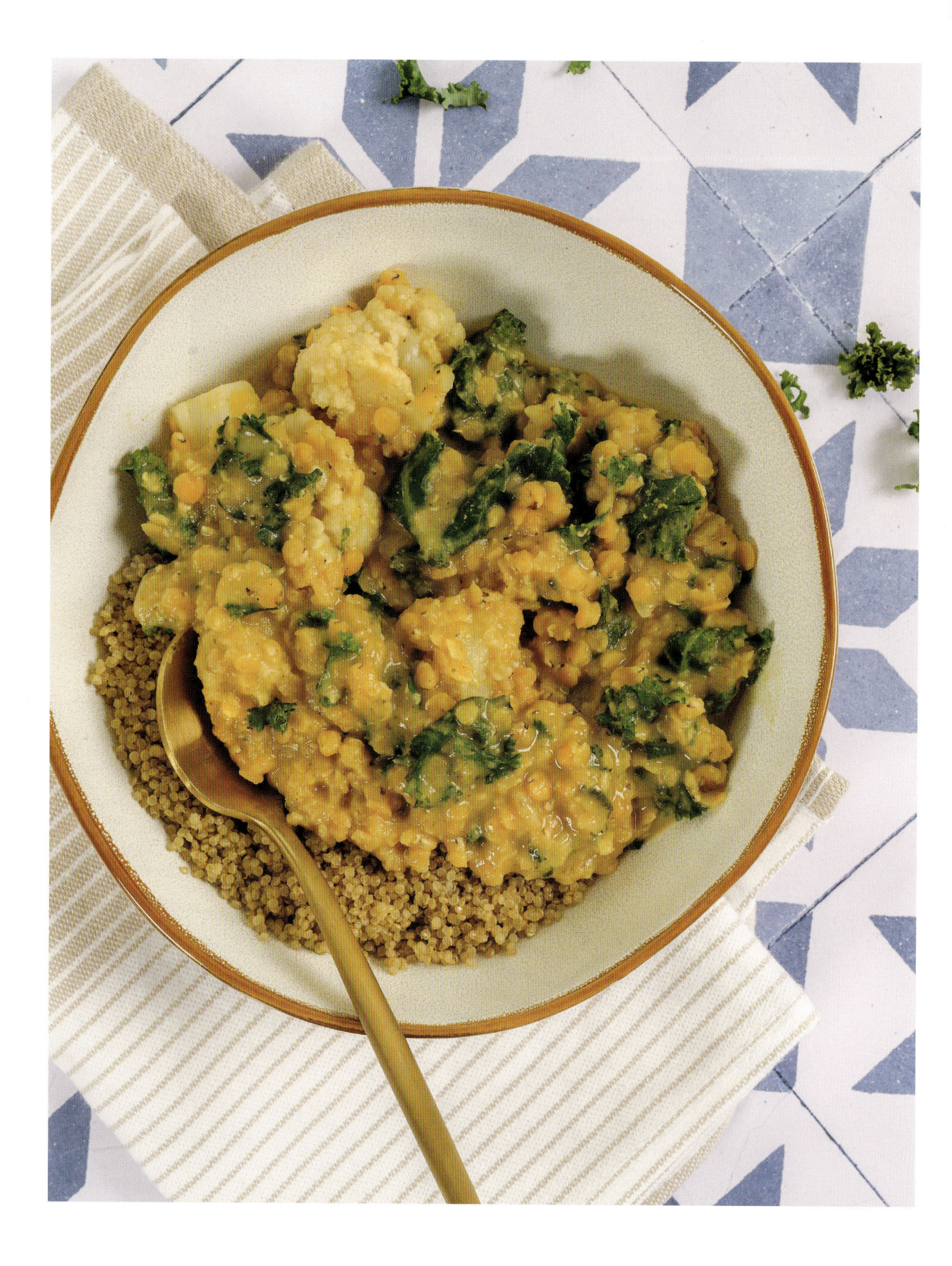

Curried Lentils with Kale and Cauliflower

SERVES 4
PREP TIME: 10 MINUTES
COOKING TIME: 40 MINUTES

1 tablespoon olive oil

½ yellow onion, diced

2 garlic cloves, minced

1 tablespoon curry powder

½ teaspoon garam masala

½ teaspoon sea salt, divided

1 tablespoon tomato paste

3 cups vegetable broth

1 cup light canned coconut milk

¾ cup dried red or green lentils

½ head cauliflower, chopped into small florets

2 cups chopped kale leaves, stems removed

Brown rice or quinoa for serving, optional

● **PROTEIN ADD**

Add in 3 ounces of baked tofu (+15g) or 3 ounces of shredded chicken (+21g) per serving.

Per serving: Calories: 287
Fat: 11g | Carbohydrates: 20g
Fiber: 14g | Protein: 12g

Lentils are a fiber-rich, plant-based protein. This dish mixes them with kale and cauliflower to provide even more fiber to help with healthy digestion. Lentils are also an excellent source of zinc, essential for collagen formation and tissue repair, as well as iron, which helps replenish any blood loss following delivery.

1. Heat the olive oil in a pot over medium-high heat. Add the onions and cook, stirring frequently, until browned (3–5 minutes).

2. Add the garlic, curry powder, garam masala, ¼ teaspoon of the salt, and the tomato paste. Stir for 1 minute.

3. Add broth, coconut milk, and lentils to the pot and bring to a simmer. Cook, uncovered, for 20 minutes, then add the cauliflower florets and cook for 15 more minutes, until the cauliflower is tender.

4. Next, add the kale leaves and cook until they are wilted. Add in the remaining ¼ teaspoon of salt.

NOTE: This meal also freezes well. Freeze leftovers in a freezer bag or airtight container.

3-Bean Chili

SERVES 6
PREP TIME: 10 MINUTES
COOKING TIME: 30 MINUTES

1 tablespoon olive oil

1 yellow onion, diced

1 bell pepper, diced

3 garlic cloves, minced

1 jalapeño, seeded and diced

2 (14.5-ounce) cans diced tomatoes

1 (15.5-ounce) can black beans, drained and rinsed

1 (15.5-ounce) can pinto beans, drained and rinsed

1 (15.5-ounce) can chickpeas, drained and rinsed

1 cup corn, frozen or canned

1 tablespoon tomato paste

1 tablespoon chili powder

½ teaspoon ground cumin

½ teaspoon dried oregano

½ teaspoon garlic powder

½ teaspoon onion powder

½ teaspoon paprika

1 teaspoon salt, or more to taste

½ teaspoon red pepper flakes

¼ teaspoon black pepper

Optional toppings: fresh cilantro, shredded cheese

● **PROTEIN ADD**

Serve with 1 cup of quinoa (+8g) or 3 ounces of shredded pork (+21g).

Per serving: Calories: 263 | Fat: 5g
Carbohydrates: 31g | Fiber: 14g | Protein: 13g

Beans are a plant-based powerhouse due to their high fiber and protein content. Our 3-Bean Chili has three types of beans. What's more, having beans is an excellent way to get in many B vitamins, as well as more potassium than a banana! This dish combines beans with high-potassium tomatoes to keep you hydrated, since potassium is a primary electrolyte, too.

1. Place the olive oil in an Instant Pot and set the cooker to sauté. Add the onion, bell pepper, garlic, and jalapeño, and sauté for 3 minutes.

2. Turn off the heat and add all the remaining ingredients. Stir to combine.

3. Close the Instant Pot and lock the lid. Cook under high pressure for 15 minutes and allow a 10-minute natural release, then manually release any remaining pressure.

NOTE: Double this recipe and freeze your leftovers in two-cup silicone soup cubes for quick and easy lunches. Pop straight from the freezer cubes into a bowl and microwave for 3-5 minutes.

Chicken Barley Stew

SERVES 6
PREP TIME: 10 MINUTES
COOKING TIME: 20 MINUTES

1 pound chicken breast (about 2 breasts)

1 (32-ounce) carton chicken or vegetable broth

1 ½ cups pearled barley, rinsed

8 ounces mushrooms, quartered or sliced

3 carrots, diced

1 large onion, diced

2 celery stalks, diced

3 garlic cloves, chopped

1 tablespoon olive oil

1 teaspoon dried rosemary

1 teaspoon dried thyme

½ teaspoon salt

¼ teaspoon black pepper

● **MAKE IT PLANT-BASED**

Use vegetable broth, and replace chicken with 2 (15.5-ounce) cans of chickpeas, drained and rinsed.

● **MAKE IT GLUTEN-FREE**

Substitute barley with brown rice.

Per serving: Calories: 356
Fat: 7g | Carbohydrates: 45g
Fiber: 9g | Protein 28g

Barley is one of the best sources of soluble fiber, a specific type of fiber that swells when eaten. It plays an important role in healthy digestion, heart health, and blood sugar control.

1. Place all the ingredients in an Instant Pot and stir to combine. Cook under high pressure for 20 minutes and allow a quick release of the pressure.

2. Remove the lid, shred the chicken, and stir to mix.

NOTE: The barley will continue to soak up the liquid as it sits. If you desire more of a stew consistency, add more broth after removing the lid.

Moroccan Chicken, Chickpeas, and Sweet Potatoes

SERVES 6
PREP TIME: 10 MINUTES
COOKING TIME: 45 MINUTES

2 (15.5-ounce) cans chickpeas, drained and rinsed

6 bone-in, skin-on chicken thighs

2 medium sweet potatoes, diced

1 yellow onion, diced

2 tablespoons olive oil

2 teaspoons garlic powder

2 teaspoons paprika

2 teaspoons ground cumin

2 teaspoons ground turmeric

2 teaspoons salt

1 teaspoon ground ginger

½ teaspoon ground cinnamon

● **MAKE IT PLANT-BASED**
Omit the chicken thighs.

Per serving: Calories: 427
Fat: 21g | Carbohydrates: 32g
Fiber: 6g | Protein: 26g

Dive into this sweet, savory, and satisfying dish high in protein and fiber. An added bonus: Many spices, such as those in this dish, also have antioxidant properties and may contribute to the healing process.

1. Preheat the oven to 400°F.

2. Combine the chickpeas, chicken thighs, sweet potatoes, and onions in a 9 x 13-inch baking dish. Toss with the olive oil. In a small bowl, mix together the spices. Add to the baking dish and toss until thoroughly combined. Nestle the chicken thighs on the top of the mixture.

3. Bake for 45 minutes, or until the chicken reaches an internal temperature of 165°F and the sweet potatoes are tender.

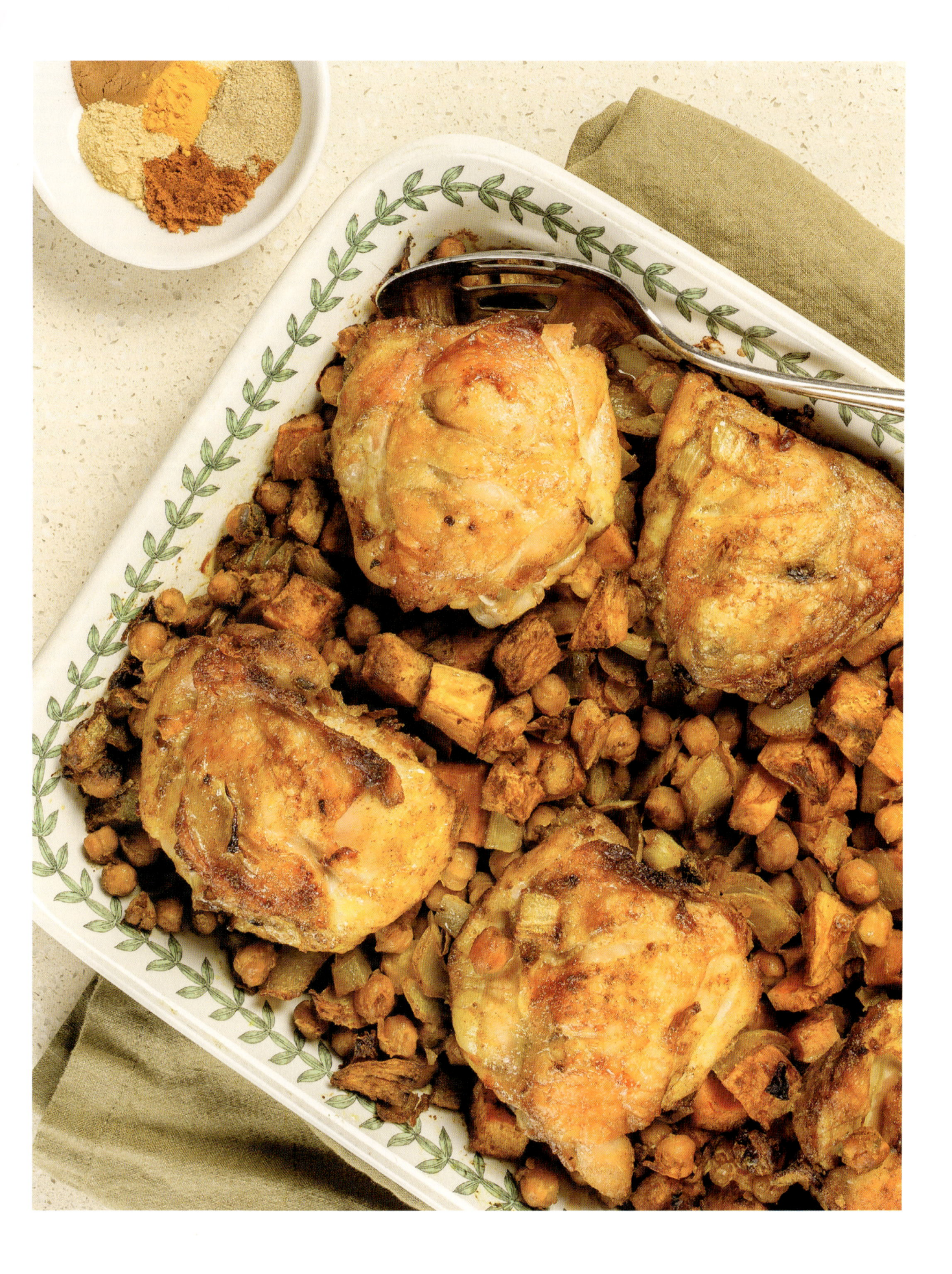

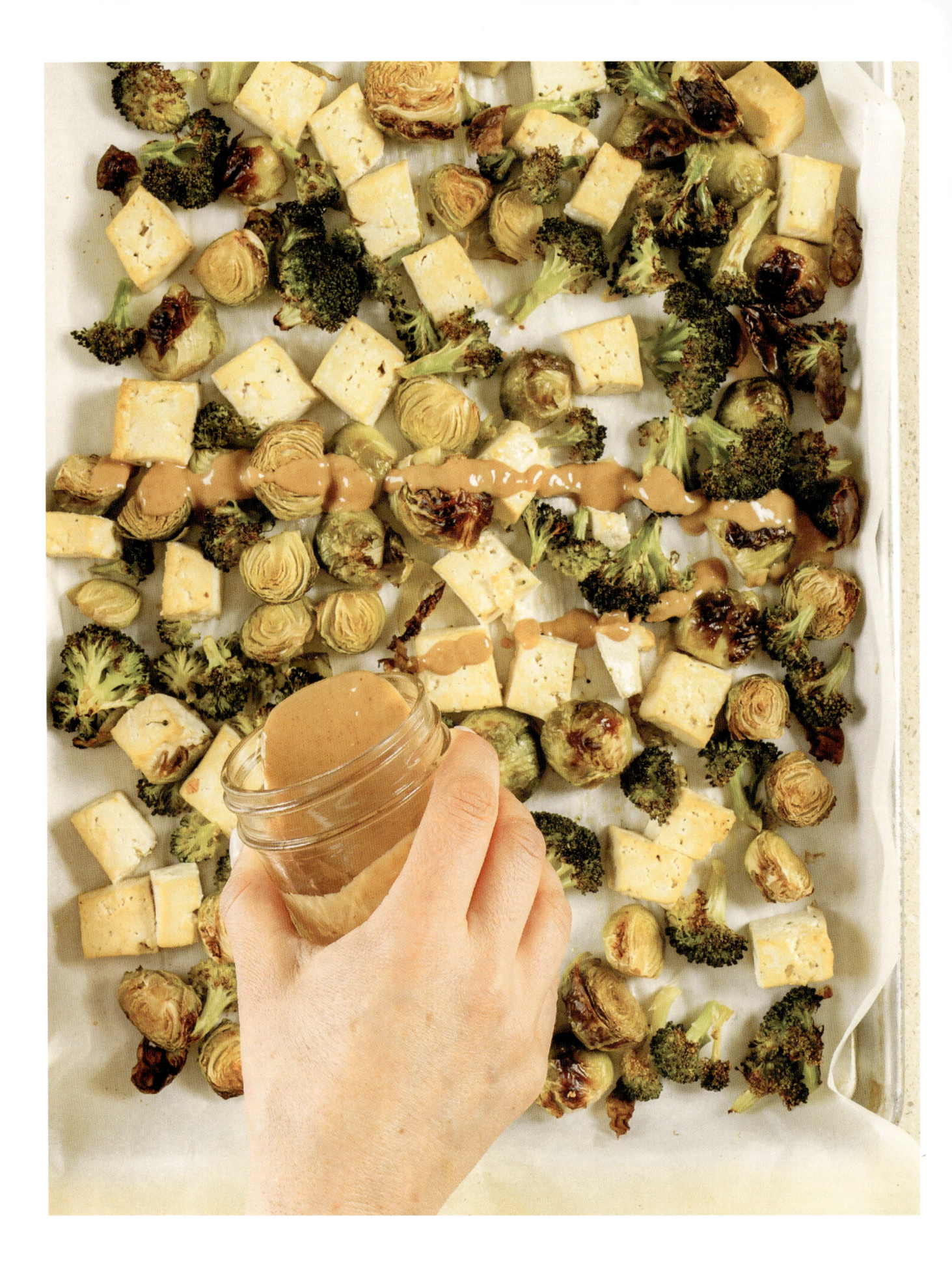

Peanut BBT (Broccoli, Brussels, and Tofu)

SERVES 3
PREP TIME: 15 MINUTES
COOKING TIME: 45 MINUTES

1 (15-ounce) block extra-firm tofu, drained and pressed

2 cups chopped broccoli florets

2 cups halved Brussels sprouts

4 green onions, chopped

1 tablespoon olive oil

¼ cup peanut butter

2 tablespoons soy sauce, tamari, or coconut aminos

1 tablespoon rice vinegar

1 tablespoon maple syrup

1 tablespoon sesame oil

¼ cup hemp seeds

½ teaspoon ground ginger

¼ teaspoon garlic powder

Red pepper flakes or sriracha, optional

● **MAKE IT NUT-FREE**
Replace peanut butter with sunflower seed butter.

Per serving: Calories: 315
Fat: 28g | Carbohydrates: 21g
Fiber: 7g | Protein: 21g

Unlike your basal body temperature, this sheet-pan dinner is always consistent. It is a great source of potassium, vitamins A and C, calcium, iron, protein, and fiber to support your healing and breastfeeding journeys.

1. Preheat the oven to 375°F.
2. Cut the tofu into 1-inch cubes.
3. Toss the tofu, broccoli, Brussels sprouts, and green onions with the olive oil. Transfer them to a baking sheet and bake for 25 minutes.
4. Meanwhile, stir together the remaining ingredients with ¼ cup of water to form a sauce.
5. After 25 minutes, remove the tofu and vegetables from the oven and evenly coat them with the sauce.
6. Return the tofu and vegetables to the oven and bake for 20 more minutes.

NOTE: Pair with a grain, such as brown rice, quinoa, or farro.

Sheet-Pan Steak Fajitas

SERVES 4
PREP TIME: 10 MINUTES
COOKING TIME: 20 MINUTES

1 pound skirt or flank steak, cut into ½-inch-wide slices

2 red bell peppers, thinly sliced

2 green bell peppers, thinly sliced

1 large onion, thinly sliced

2 tablespoons olive oil

1 tablespoon tomato paste

2 tablespoons chili powder

1 tablespoon ground cumin

1 ½ teaspoons ground coriander

1 ½ teaspoons black pepper

1 ½ teaspoons garlic powder

1 ½ teaspoons salt

8 (6-inch) tortillas, flour or corn

Optional toppings: refried beans, guacamole, salsa, sour cream, shredded cheese

Per serving: Calories: 400
Fat: 20g | Carbohydrates: 29g
Fiber: 6g | Protein: 23g

Prep this sheet-pan dinner ahead of time to make mealtime even easier. Try it with different protein sources to keep variety in your menu!

1. Preheat the oven to 400°F.

2. Combine all the ingredients except the tortillas in a large bowl and toss until thoroughly combined. Spread evenly across a baking sheet.

3. Bake for 18–20 minutes until the meat is cooked to your desired doneness.

4. Add the tortillas on top of the steak-veggie mixture during the final 5 minutes to soften.

Protein Source Ideas for Fajitas:

These fajitas work great with different protein sources, but cooking instructions vary slightly:

Chicken breasts or thighs: increase cooking time to 35-40 minutes until internal temperature reaches 165°F.

Shrimp: cook veggies for 10 minutes before adding shrimp. Mix with seasoning and cook for an additional 10-15 minutes.

Fish: cook veggies for 10 minutes before adding fish. Mix with seasonings and cook for an additional 15-18 minutes.

Tofu: cook tofu for 25 minutes, then mix with seasonings and veggies. Cook for additional 25 minutes.

THE POSTPARTUM NUTRITION COOKBOOK

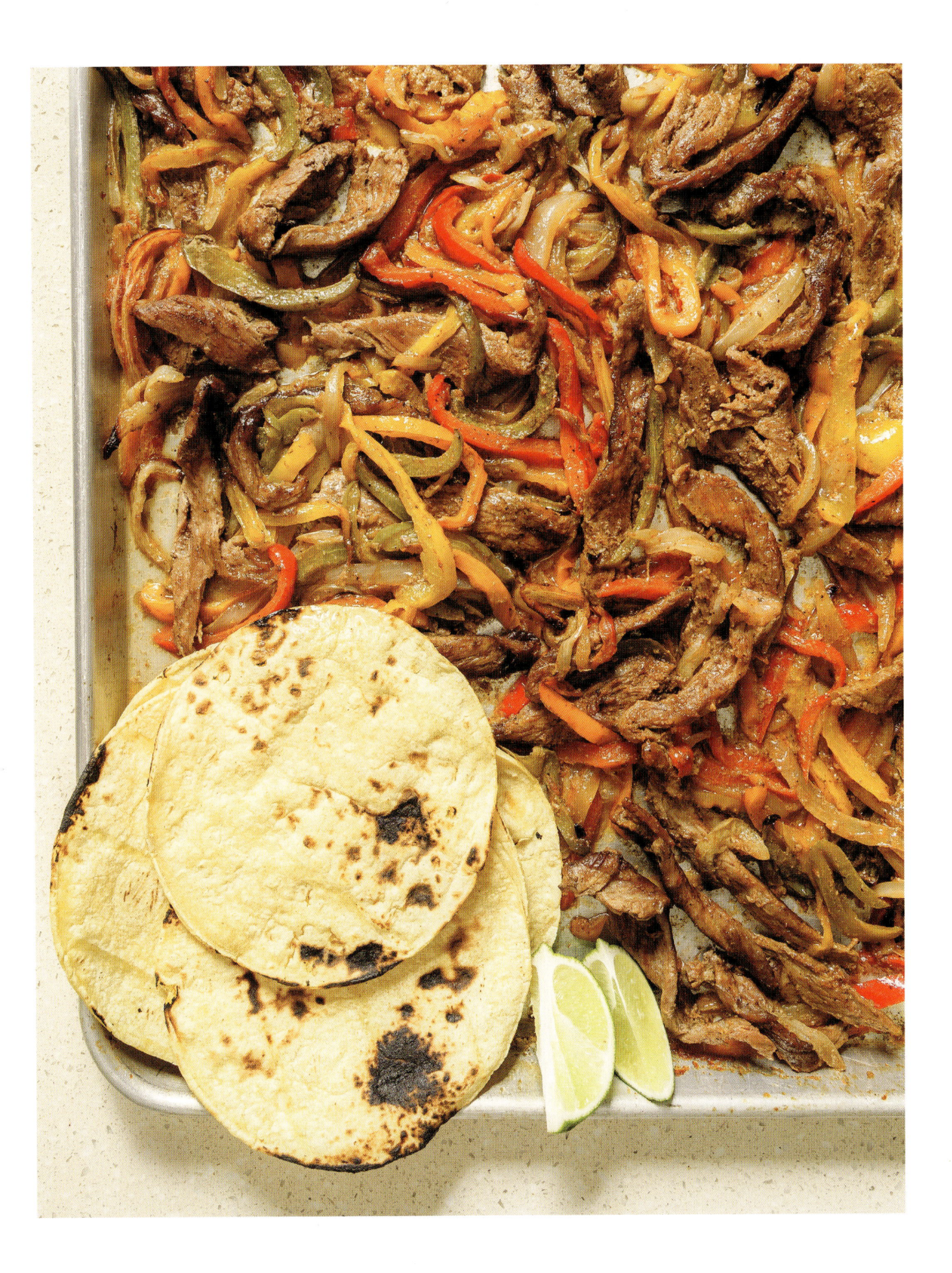

Pressure Cooker Cashew Chicken

SERVES 4
PREP TIME: 5 MINUTES
COOKING TIME: 15 MINUTES

1 ½ pounds chicken thighs, chopped into bite-sized chunks

6 green onions, sliced

½ cup unroasted, unsalted whole cashews

1 (6-ounce) can sliced water chestnuts, drained

4 garlic cloves, finely chopped

¼ cup hoisin sauce

2 tablespoons soy sauce, tamari, or coconut aminos

1 tablespoon rice vinegar

1 tablespoon sesame oil

¼ teaspoon black pepper

2 teaspoons cornstarch

1 tablespoon cold water

Optional: white rice

Per serving: Calories: 336
Fat: 13g | Carbohydrates: 21g
Fiber: 2g | Protein: 35g

Make your favorite takeout meal even faster at home! This dish is higher in protein than what you'd get from your usual takeout spot, can be paired with a frozen vegetable to boost the vitamin C content, and tastes great over fluffy homemade rice.

1. Combine all the ingredients except the cornstarch and water in an Instant Pot. Cook under high pressure for 8 minutes and allow a quick release.

2. Stir together the cornstarch and water in a small bowl. Once the cornstarch is dissolved, add it to the Instant Pot. Stir thoroughly to combine and let sit for 5 minutes. Stir again. Serve over rice if desired.

NOTES: No hoisin? Substitute an equal amount of BBQ sauce plus 1 tablespoon of soy sauce.

Spanish Chicken and Rice

SERVES 4
PREP TIME: 10 MINUTES
COOKING TIME: 8 MINUTES

1 pound chicken thighs, cubed

6 carrots, thinly sliced into rounds, or about 20 baby carrots, thinly sliced

1 large onion, diced

3 garlic cloves, minced

1 (15.5-ounce) can chickpeas, drained and rinsed

1 (14.5-ounce) can diced tomatoes

¾ cup white rice

½ cup pitted green olives, halved

½ cup water

1 ½ teaspoons smoked paprika

1 teaspoon salt

1 teaspoon black pepper

Per serving: Calories: 453
Fat: 9g | Carbohydrates: 61g
Fiber: 8g | Protein: 31g

Prep the ingredients ahead of time and enjoy a siesta before dinner! This one-pot meal makes hearty servings that will fill you up while making you feel like you are on a Spanish vacation. You may even have most of these ingredients in your pantry.

1. Combine all the ingredients in an Instant Pot and mix well.

2. Cook under high pressure for 8 minutes, then allow a quick release until all the steam is out.

NOTE: To make jambalaya, add celery and bell pepper instead of the carrots, and use 2 tablespoons of creole seasoning instead of paprika.

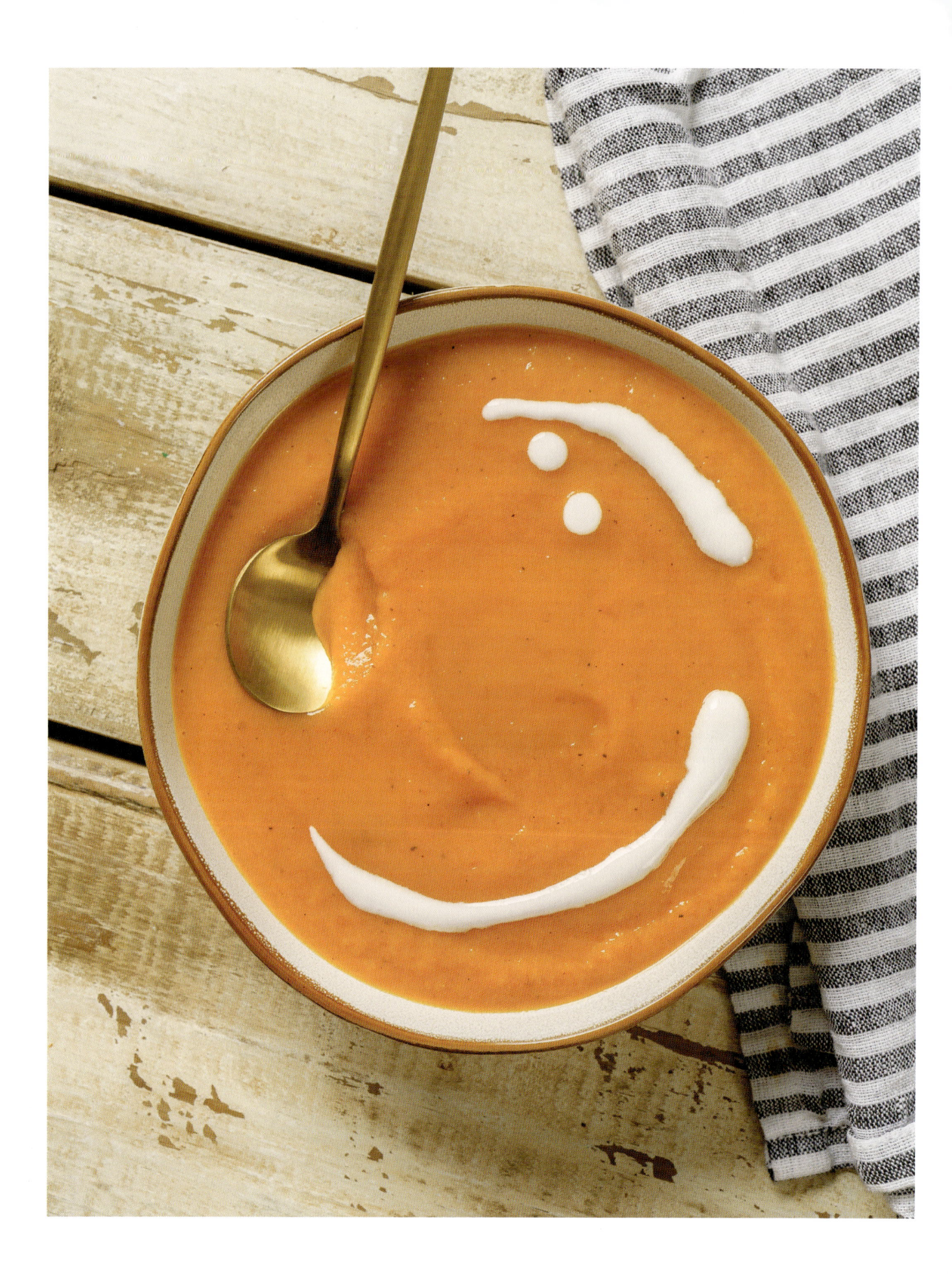

Butternut Squash Soup

SERVES 4
PREP TIME: 15 MINUTES
COOKING TIME: 45 MINUTES

1 butternut, acorn, or kabocha squash, or one (12-ounce) container peeled and cut squash

1 head garlic

4 carrots, peeled with tops removed

2 red bell peppers, halved

1 onion, peeled and halved

2 tablespoons olive oil

½ teaspoon salt

½ teaspoon black pepper

1 (15.5-ounce) can cannellini beans, drained and rinsed

3 cups vegetable or chicken broth

● **PROTEIN ADD**

Add fresh boneless, skinless chicken thighs (+21g per 3-ounce serving) or chicken sausage (+12g per link) to the sheet pan, and bake with veggies. Do not blend. Shred and add to blended soup.

Mix in a block of drained, firm tofu (+9g per serving) while blending the soup.

Per serving: Calories: 300
Fat: 7g | Carbohydrates: 52g
Fiber: 11g | Protein: 10g

This creamy, dreamy soup is made in the oven and blended to perfection. It is jam-packed with almost 1,000% of your vitamin A requirement to help meet your increased needs during recovery and breastfeeding.

1. Preheat the oven to 350°F.

2. Cut the butternut squash in half and scoop out the seeds. Cut off the entire top of the head of garlic. Place the squash, garlic, carrots, bell peppers, and onion on a baking sheet. Coat everything with the oil, salt, and pepper.

3. Bake for 45 minutes, or until the vegetables are soft. Remove the skin of the squash. Squeeze the head of garlic to remove the cloves from the skins.

4. Transfer half of the roasted ingredients, half of the can of beans, and 1 ½ cups of broth to a high-powered blender (it will all fit in a 64-ounce blender). Blend until mixture is smooth and creamy. Repeat with the second batch of roasted vegetables, beans, and broth.

NOTE: This also makes a great freezer meal. Portion soup into individual containers (either leftover takeout quarts, glass jars, or silicone soup cubes). Allow the soup to cool completely before freezing.

Creamy Tomato-Feta Pasta Bake

SERVES 4
PREP TIME: 5 MINUTES
COOKING TIME: 50 MINUTES

2 cups whole cherry tomatoes

1 (8-ounce) box chickpea pasta

1 tablespoon olive oil

2 teaspoons minced garlic

2 teaspoons dried basil or Italian seasoning

¼ teaspoon black pepper

1 (8-ounce) block feta cheese

2 cups vegetable broth

2 cups unsweetened milk of choice

2–3 cups chopped spinach

Red pepper flakes, optional

● **MAKE IT PLANT-BASED**
Use plant-based feta.

Per serving: Calories: 451
Fat: 22g | Carbohydrates: 35g
Fiber: 10g | Protein: 27g

We created our own version of the viral tomato-feta pasta bake but simplified it a step further—just toss all the ingredients into a baking dish, and voilà! You'll have a calcium-rich, comforting dish.

1. Preheat the oven to 400°F.

2. Combine the tomatoes and uncooked chickpea pasta in a 9 x 13-inch baking dish. Add the olive oil, garlic, basil, and pepper. Toss to combine.

3. Place the feta in the center.

4. Pour the veggie broth and milk over the top, ensuring that all the pasta is submerged.

5. Cover with aluminum foil, crimping it tightly around the edges of the pan so that no steam can escape.

6. Transfer to the oven and bake until the pasta is tender (about 50 minutes).

7. Once done, remove it from the oven, add the spinach, and mash the cheese and tomatoes with a fork to break everything down. Mix until well combined. Top with red pepper flakes, if desired.

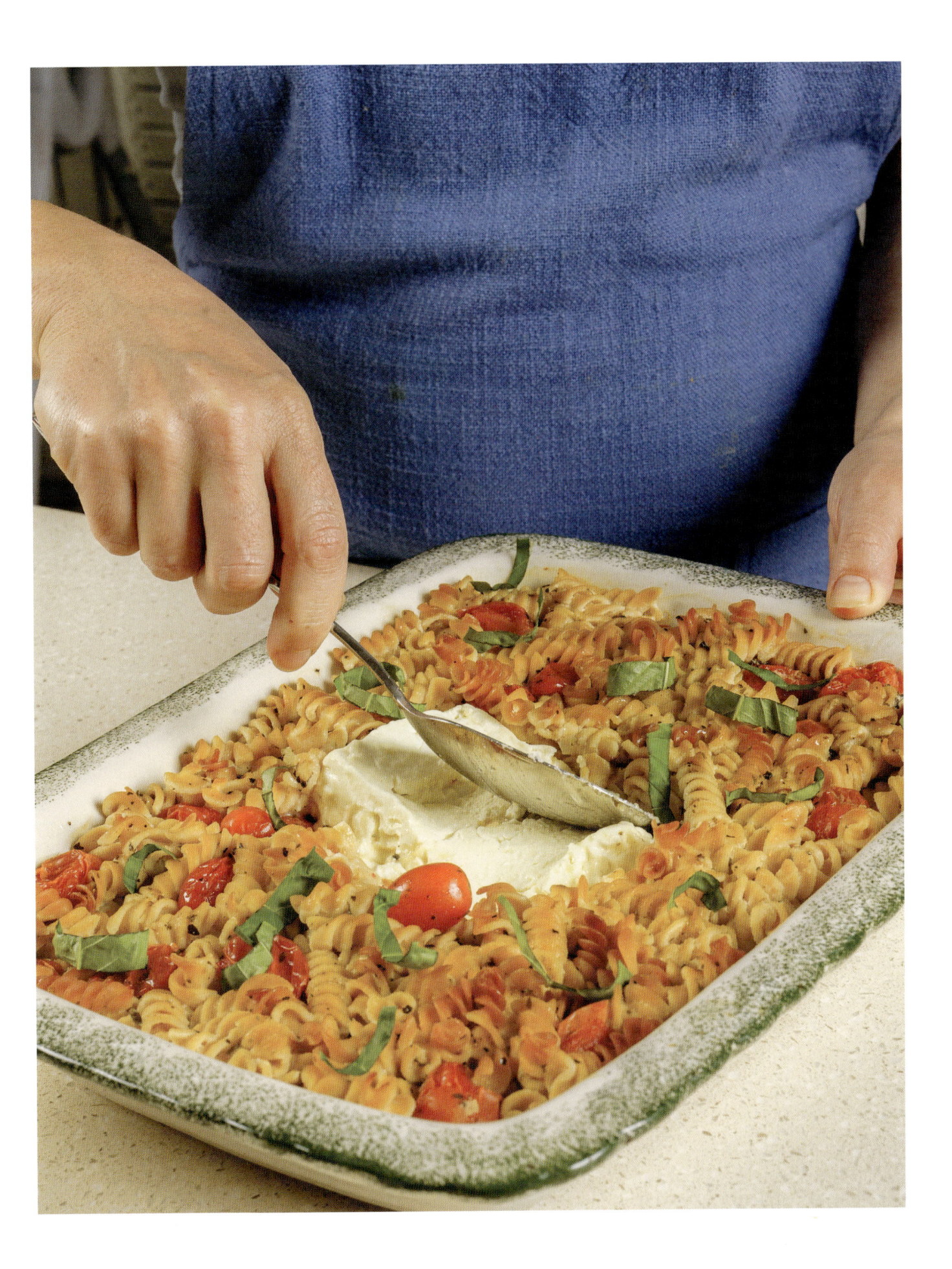

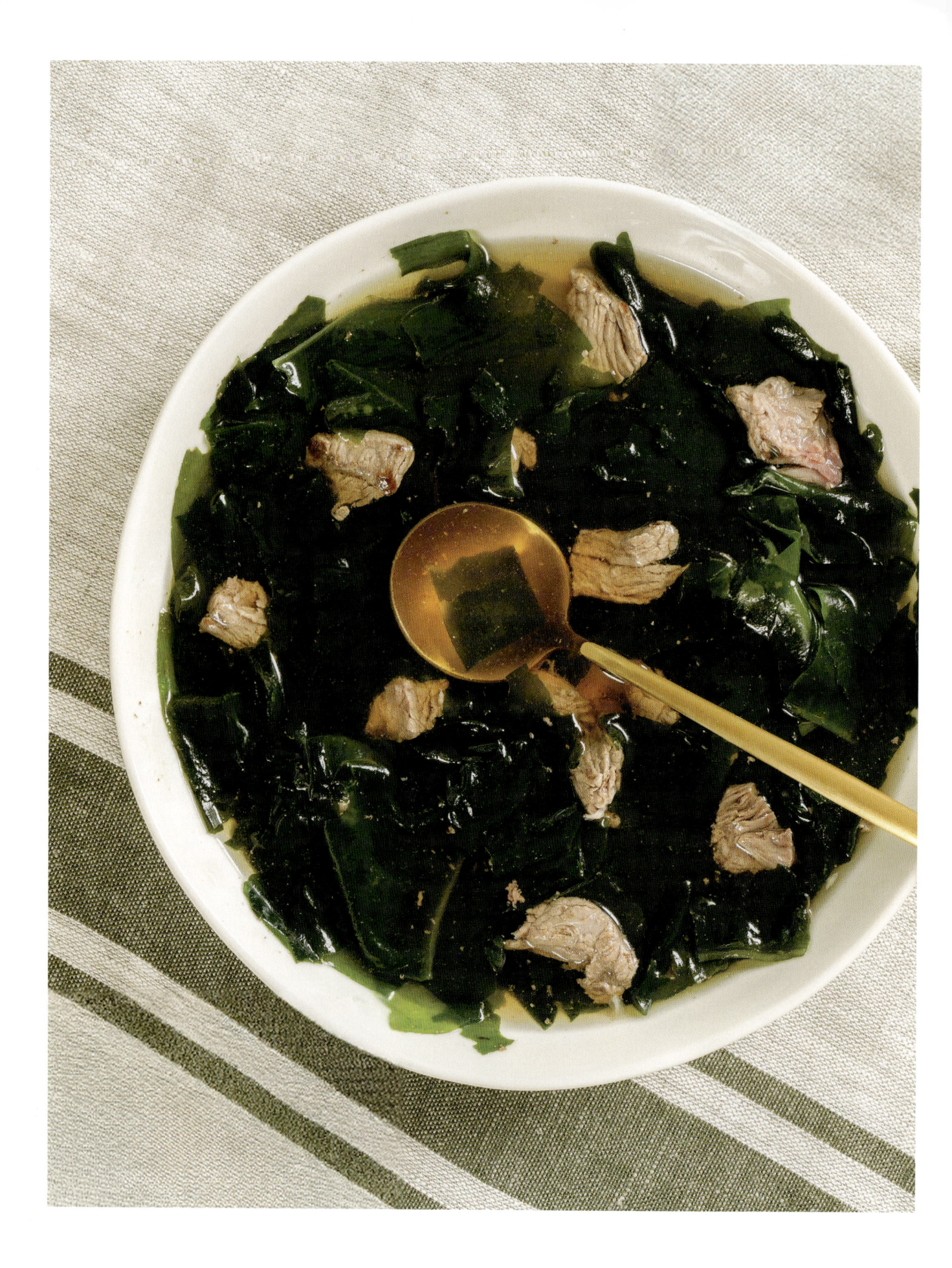

Seaweed Stew (Miyeok Guk)

SERVES 6
PREP TIME: 10 MINUTES
COOKING TIME: 20 MINUTES

10–15 grams dried seaweed (Korean miyeok or Japanese wakame); about 2 cups when rehydrated

½ pound beef chuck or round steak, cut into bite-sized pieces

½ teaspoon salt

¼ teaspoon black pepper

2 tablespoons sesame oil

2–3 garlic cloves, minced

10 cups water

3 tablespoons soy sauce

● **MAKE IT PLANT-BASED**
Swap the meat for ½ (14-ounce) block of soft or silken tofu.

Per serving: Calories: 139
Fat: 7g | Carbohydrates: 8g
Fiber: 1g | Protein: 12g

This stew is a popular dish given to new moms in South Korea. The main ingredient is seaweed, one of the richest food sources of iodine. Iodine requirements notably increase during lactation to support the cognitive development of the baby.

1. Soak the dried seaweed in cold water for 5–10 minutes to allow it to expand. Drain the water, rinse the seaweed, and squeeze out excess liquid.

2. Cut the seaweed into bite-sized strips (or purchase pre-cut seaweed).

3. Season the beef with salt and pepper.

4. In a medium pot over medium heat, combine the sesame oil, garlic, and beef. Cook, stirring frequently, until the beef is partly cooked (3–5 minutes).

5. Add the seaweed, water, and soy sauce. Stir.

6. Cover the pot and boil over medium to medium-high heat for 10–15 minutes.

NOTE: You can find seaweed at most Asian markets or on Amazon.

Spinach Artichoke Pasta

SERVES 3
PREP TIME: 5 MINUTES
COOKING TIME: 15 MINUTES

1 (8-ounce) box bean-based pasta

1 tablespoon olive oil

3 garlic cloves, chopped

1 (15-ounce) can quartered artichoke hearts, drained

½ (16-ounce) bag frozen spinach

1 cup cottage cheese

¼ cup shredded Parmesan cheese

¼ teaspoon black pepper

● **MAKE IT PLANT-BASED**

Swap the cottage cheese for 1 cup silken or soft tofu and omit the Parmesan cheese.

Per serving: Calories: 461
Fat: 13g | Carbohydrates: 60g
Fiber: 14g | Protein: 26g

Whip together this delicious dish when you are running low on supplies. High in fiber, it's a winner for your taste buds and digestion. Artichokes are a surprisingly great source of soluble fiber, the type of fiber that plays an important role in healthy digestion, heart health, and blood-sugar control.

1. Boil the pasta according to the package instructions.

2. Reserve ¼ cup of the cooking liquid, then drain the pasta in a colander.

3. While the pasta is in the colander, add the olive oil and garlic to the cooking pot. Sauté for 2 minutes until the garlic softens.

4. Add the artichokes and frozen spinach. Stir until the spinach wilts completely.

5. Stir in the cottage cheese, Parmesan, black pepper, and reserved cooking water. Mix until a cohesive sauce is formed.

6. Add the pasta back to the pot and stir until thoroughly coated in the sauce.

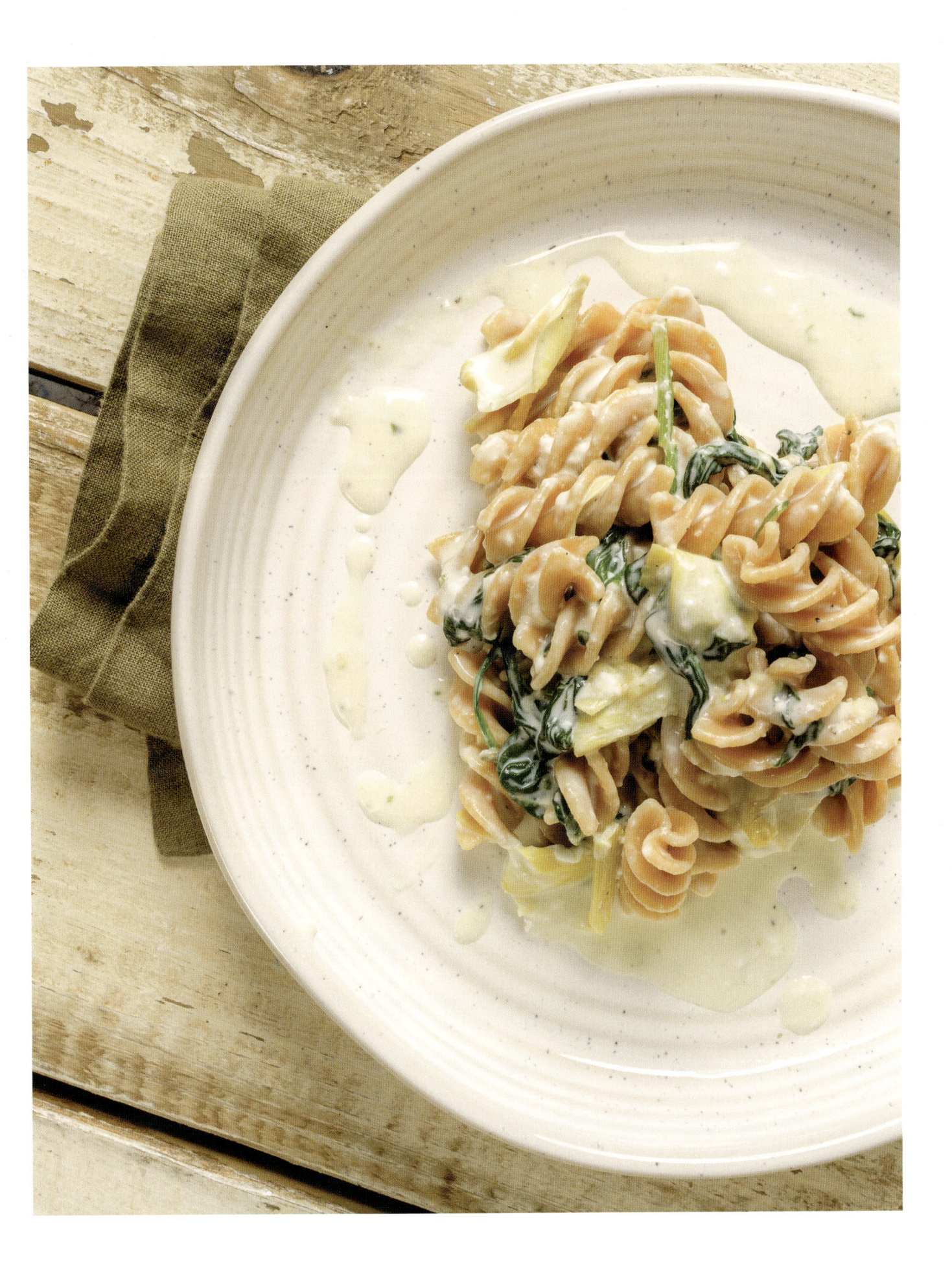

Shredded Beef Tacos

SERVES 4
PREP TIME: 5 MINUTES
COOKING TIME: 15 MINUTES

1 pound frozen Shredded Beef (page 79)

2 cups frozen pepper-onion mix

½ cup salsa

½ teaspoon ground cumin

½ teaspoon salt

¼ teaspoon garlic powder

Salt, to taste

4 (10-inch) tortillas, corn or flour

● **MAKE IT PLANT-BASED**

Substitute 2 (15.5-ounce) cans of black beans, drained and rinsed, for the beef.

Per serving: Calories: 317
Fat: 14g | Carbohydrates: 26g
Fiber: 2g | Protein: 21g

It doesn't get much easier than taking things from the freezer and pushing a few buttons to get dinner on the table. And what makes these shredded beef tacos even better? They're high in iron that can help to replenish your iron stores post-delivery.

1. Place the shredded beef straight from the freezer into an Instant Pot. Add the frozen pepper-onion mix, salsa, and seasonings.

2. Cook under high pressure for 5 minutes and allow a quick release.

3. Serve on the corn or flour tortillas, and feel free to add whatever toppings you have available, such as avocado, cilantro, jalapeños, or chipotle sauce.

Pulled BBQ Pork Sandwich

SERVES 4
PREP TIME: 2 MINUTES
COOKING TIME: 15 MINUTES

1–1 ½ pounds of frozen Pulled Pork (page 79)

½ cup BBQ sauce, plus more for serving

¼ cup water

4 rolls or 8 slices of bread

● **MAKE IT GLUTEN-FREE**
Use gluten-free rolls or bread.

Per serving: Calories: 373
Fat: 7g | Carbohydrates: 46g
Fiber: 4g | Protein: 32g

A normal pulled pork sandwich from your favorite BBQ restaurant takes over 12 hours to make on the smoker. You can enjoy the same meal with just five minutes in the Instant Pot! Using pulled pork from your freezer, this comes together super quickly for an easy weeknight meal. Pork is also high in B vitamins, protein, and zinc.

1. Place the shredded pork straight from the freezer into an Instant Pot. Add the BBQ sauce and water.

2. Cook under high pressure for 5 minutes and allow a quick release until all the steam is out.

3. Serve on bread or rolls topped with additional BBQ sauce, if desired.

NOTE: This is the perfect meal to serve with a bagged salad on the side or with precut raw veggies such as carrots, celery, and red bell peppers for added vitamin C.

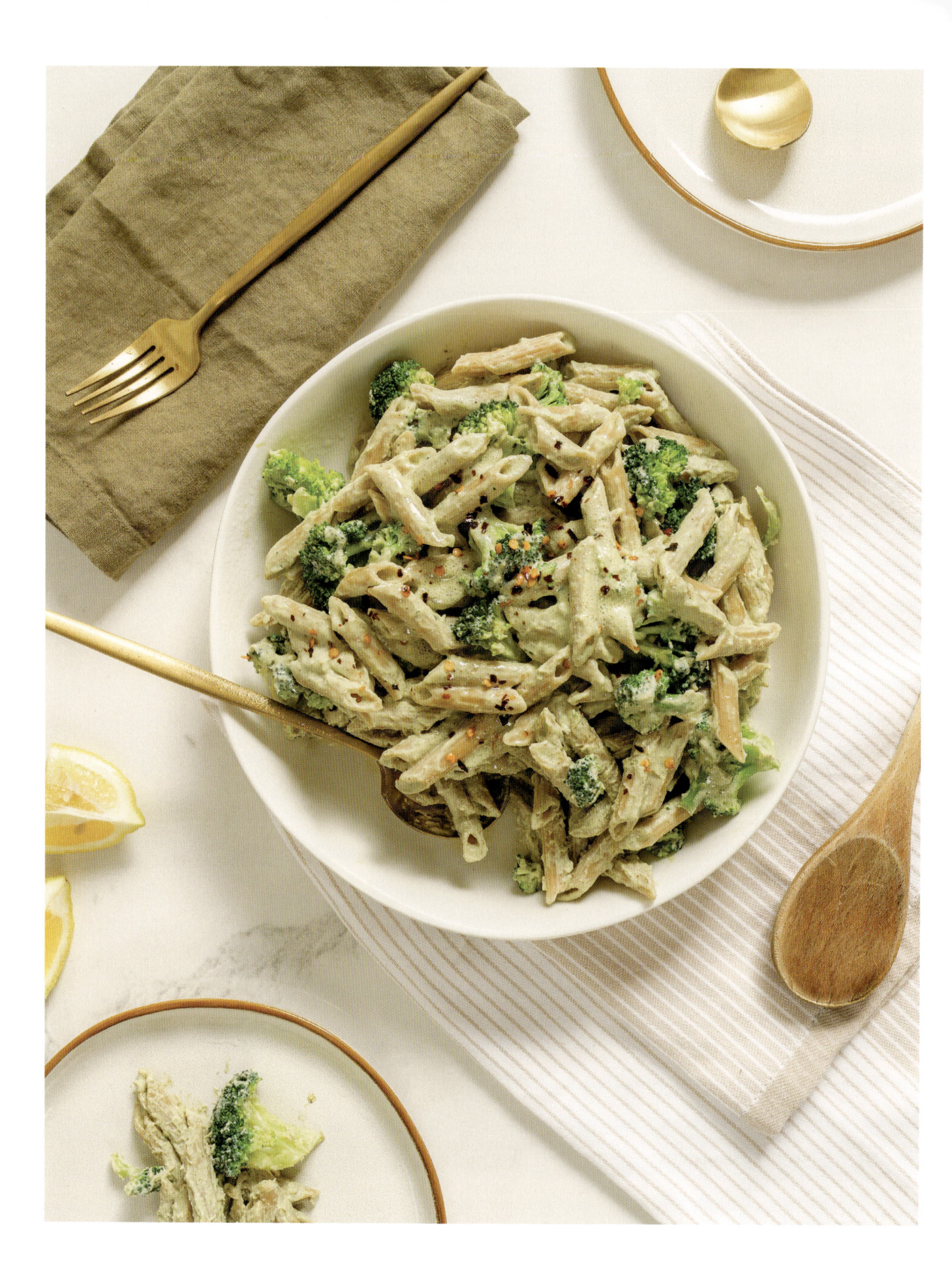

Creamy Pesto Pasta

SERVES 3
PREP TIME: 5 MINUTES
COOKING TIME: 15 MINUTES

1 (8-ounce) box bean-based pasta

½ (8-ounce) bag frozen broccoli

½ (15-ounce) block silken or soft tofu

½ cup pesto

½ teaspoon garlic powder

¼ teaspoon black pepper

Salt, to taste

¼ cup Parmesan cheese or nutritional yeast, optional

Per serving: Calories: 515
Fat: 26g | Carbohydrates: 52g
Fiber: 8g | Protein: 28g

Bean-based pastas are an excellent pantry ingredient since they have much more protein and fiber than typical pasta. This recipe pairs bean pasta with a creamy pesto sauce to elevate pasta night without a ton of ingredients or hassle. Frozen broccoli adds a boost of vitamin C.

1. Boil the pasta according to the package instructions. During the last minute of cooking, add the frozen broccoli and cook until the pasta is done.

2. Meanwhile, combine the remaining ingredients in a blender and blend until smooth.

3. Drain the pasta, return it to the pot with the burner off, and add the sauce.

4. Stir for 5 minutes until the pasta and sauce are combined and the sauce is warmed through.

NOTE: This can be made with any firmness of tofu, but if you use firm or extra-firm, the sauce will be thicker and may require some water to thin.

PANTRY MEALS

173

Grandma's Tomato Soup and Grilled Cheese

SERVES 1
PREP TIME: 5 MINUTES
COOKING TIME: 10 MINUTES

Soup

1 (14.5-ounce) can pureed or diced tomatoes

½ cup canned cannellini or Great Northern beans

½ cup chicken or vegetable broth

2 tablespoons tomato paste

1 teaspoon olive oil

½ teaspoon Italian seasoning

¼ teaspoon onion powder

¼ teaspoon garlic powder

¼ teaspoon salt

Grilled Cheese

2 slices whole-wheat bread

2 (1-ounce) slices white cheddar cheese

● **MAKE IT PLANT-BASED**

Use plant-based cheese in the grilled cheese sandwich.

● **MAKE IT GLUTEN-FREE**

Substitute bread with gluten-free bread.

Per serving: Calories: 516
Fat: 16g | Carbohydrates: 68g
Fiber: 14g | Protein: 26g

This soup has the perfectly creamy, stick-to-your-grilled-cheese, big-tomato flavor that you remember straight from the can. If you prefer a thinner soup, add a bit more broth. Paired with a grilled cheese sandwich, it brings back memories, but with a few more nutrients.

1. Combine all the soup ingredients in a blender or food processor. Blend until smooth.

2. Pour the soup into a pan and heat over medium-low for 5–10 minutes until it comes to a gentle bubble.

3. While the soup is cooking, heat a pan over medium heat. Spray with nonstick spray and add one slice of bread. Top the bread with the cheese, then with the second slice of bread. Cook on each side until the bread is crispy and cheese is melted.

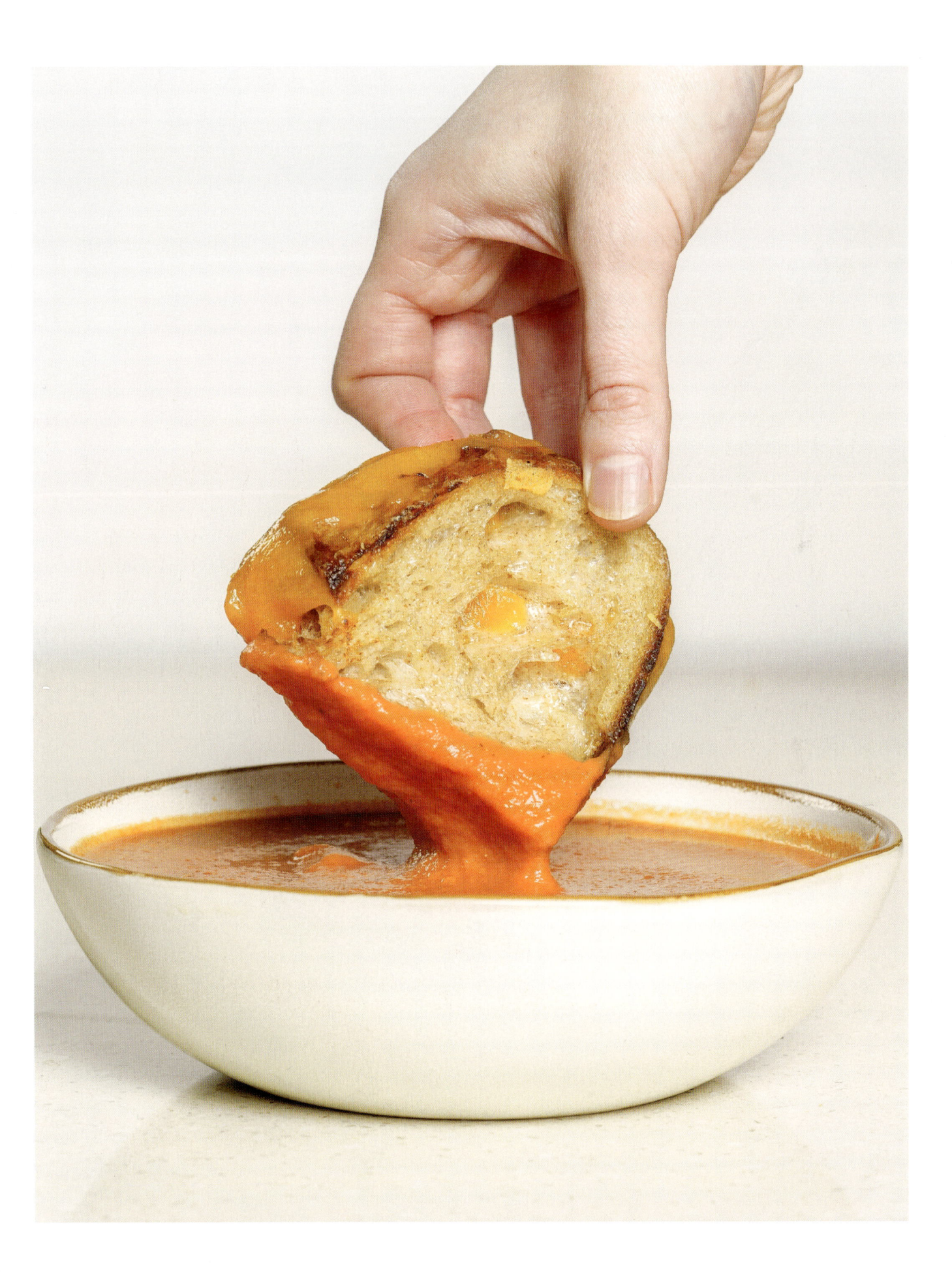

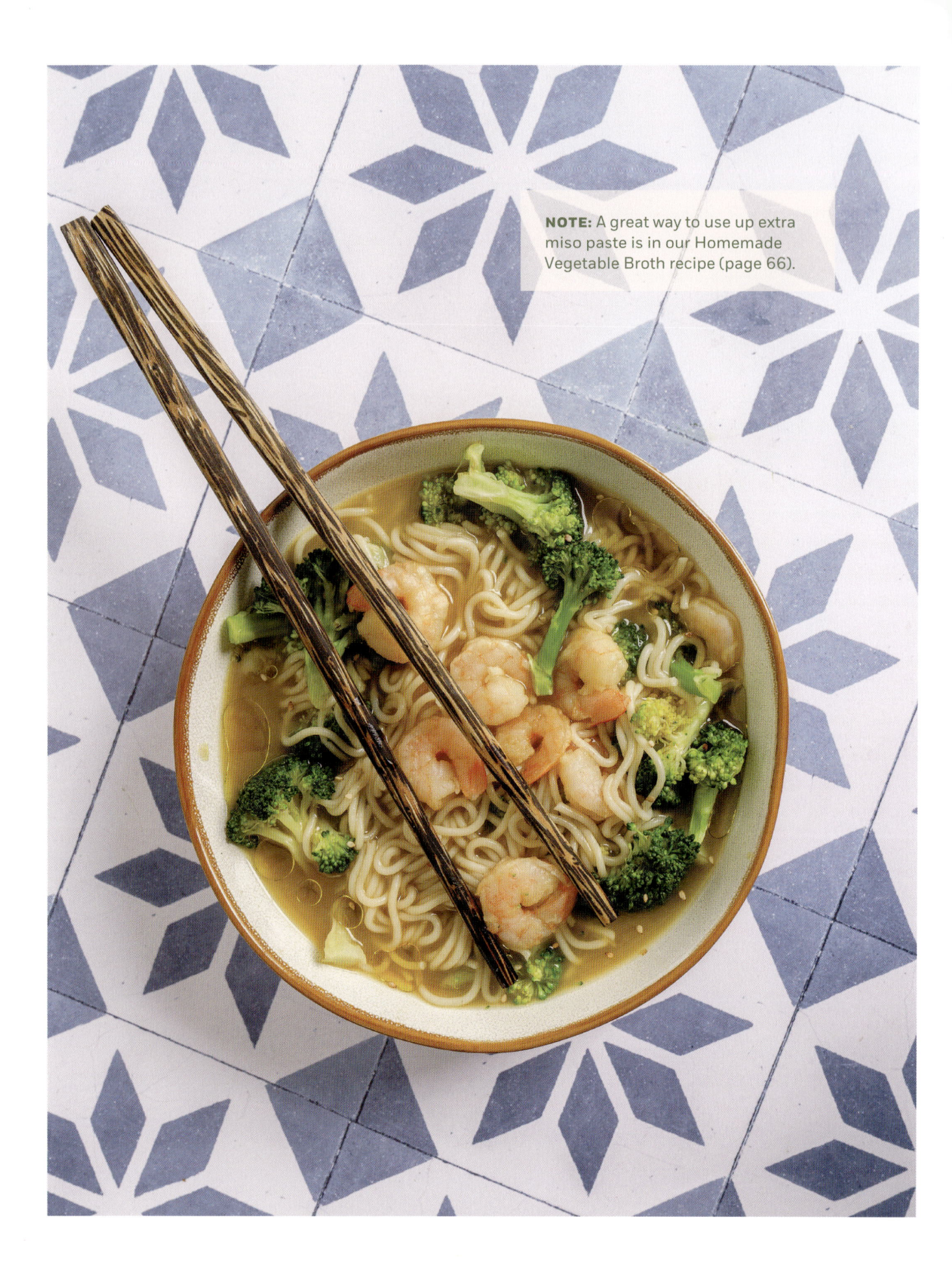

NOTE: A great way to use up extra miso paste is in our Homemade Vegetable Broth recipe (page 66).

Ramen Noodle Soup

SERVES 1
PREP TIME: 5 MINUTES
COOKING TIME: 10 MINUTES

1 ½ cups chicken or vegetable broth

1 (2-ounce) package brown rice ramen noodles

⅓ (15-ounce) block extra-firm tofu, drained and cubed, or 1 cup frozen shrimp

1 cup frozen broccoli

1 tablespoon miso paste, optional

1 teaspoon soy sauce, tamari, or coconut aminos

½ teaspoon fish sauce

Drizzle of sesame oil

½ teaspoon garlic powder

Per serving: Calories: 406
Fat: 9g | Carbohydrates: 53g
Fiber: 9g | Protein: 22g

Need dinner to be ready in less than 10 minutes with ingredients you probably have sitting around? Yes, please! This warm and comforting bowl of soup is a good source of protein and fiber that will help to keep you hydrated.

1. Place the broth in a saucepan over medium heat. Add the noodles and tofu, then the broccoli.

2. Bring broth up to a boil, then turn off the heat and let sit for about 3 minutes until the noodles are tender.

3. Add the miso paste, soy sauce, fish sauce, sesame oil, and garlic powder. Stir to combine.

Upgraded Boxed Mac and Cheese

SERVES 2
PREP TIME: 5 MINUTES
COOKING TIME: 10 MINUTES

1 (7.25-ounce) box of macaroni and cheese

2 frozen chicken sausage links (any flavor)

2 cups frozen broccoli

⅛ teaspoon black pepper

● **MAKE IT PLANT-BASED**

Use a plant-based mac and cheese box, and replace chicken sausage with veggie sausage.

Per serving: Calories: 559
Fat: 17g | Carbohydrates: 64g
Fiber: 6g | Protein: 28g

Not every night will be perfect. Improving easy and realistic options, such as boxed macaroni and cheese, can help you deal with a busy night and still meet your nutritional needs. The additions of chicken sausage and broccoli upgrade the nutrition profile of your mac and cheese with minimal effort.

1. In a large pot, boil the macaroni according to the package instructions (usually 8 minutes).

2. When there are 4 minutes left, add the whole frozen chicken sausages and bring the water back to a boil. Allow to cook for 2 minutes before adding the broccoli.

3. After 1–2 minutes more, test the macaroni for doneness. When done, drain into a colander and leave in the sink while you make the cheese sauce.

4. Make the cheese sauce in the pot according to the package instructions. Add the black pepper.

5. Slice the chicken sausage into bite-sized pieces.

6. Return the macaroni, chicken sausage, and broccoli to the pot with the sauce. Stir until combined.

Curry in a Hurry

SERVES 4
PREP TIME: 2 MINUTES
COOKING TIME: 10 MINUTES

1 (15-ounce) block firm tofu, drained and pressed

2 teaspoons olive oil

3 cups of frozen pepper-onion mix

1 (15.5-ounce) can chickpeas, drained and rinsed

1 (16-ounce) jar curry sauce

4 cups cooked brown rice

Per serving: Calories: 533
Fat: 14g | Carbohydrates: 65g
Fiber: 20g | Protein: 23g

This warm, comforting curry is bursting with flavor and potentially anti-inflammatory compounds, thanks to the spices found in curry, such as turmeric, coriander, and chili pepper. With minimal preparation, this recipe should become a staple in your kitchen for easy weeknight dinners.

1. Cut the tofu into 1-inch cubes.

2. Heat the olive oil in a medium-sized pan over medium heat. Add the pepper-onion mix and sauté until soft. Add the cubed tofu and chickpeas. Cook, stirring, for 4–5 minutes until the peppers are heated through. Pour the entire jar of curry into the pan, and stir and simmer for 5 minutes.

3. Serve over brown rice.

Butter Bean French Onion Soup

SERVES 3
PREP TIME: 5 MINUTES
COOKING TIME: 50 MINUTES

3 tablespoons unsalted butter or vegan butter, divided

2 tablespoons olive oil

2 white onions, sliced

1 teaspoon salt

2 tablespoons flour, white or whole-wheat

3 cups beef or vegetable broth

2 (15.5-ounce) cans butter or cannellini beans

½ teaspoon dried parsley

Black pepper, to taste

6 shakes Worcestershire sauce, optional

½ cup shredded Gruyère

● **MAKE IT GLUTEN-FREE**

Substitute flour with gluten-free or potato flour.

● **MAKE IT PLANT-BASED**

Replace Gruyère with plant-based cheese.

Per serving: Calories: 527
Fat: 26g | Carbohydrates: 42g
Fiber: 15g | Protein: 20g

Our take on warm and comforting French onion soup includes butter beans to enhance its creaminess while contributing protein. This soup is also packed with onions, which contain a large amount of quercetin, a flavonoid with antioxidant and anti-inflammatory properties.

1. Heat 2 tablespoons of the butter and the olive oil in a medium pot over medium heat.

2. Add the onions and salt. Let the onions cook slowly, turning or stirring so they cook evenly as they soften and brown, for about 40 minutes.

3. Once your onions are soft and brown, add the remaining 1 tablespoon of butter and the flour and stir. Let the flour cook for 2–3 minutes.

4. Add the broth, beans, dried parsley, black pepper, and Worcestershire (if using). Mix together and let simmer for at least 10 minutes.

5. Top with the cheese and allow it to melt before serving.

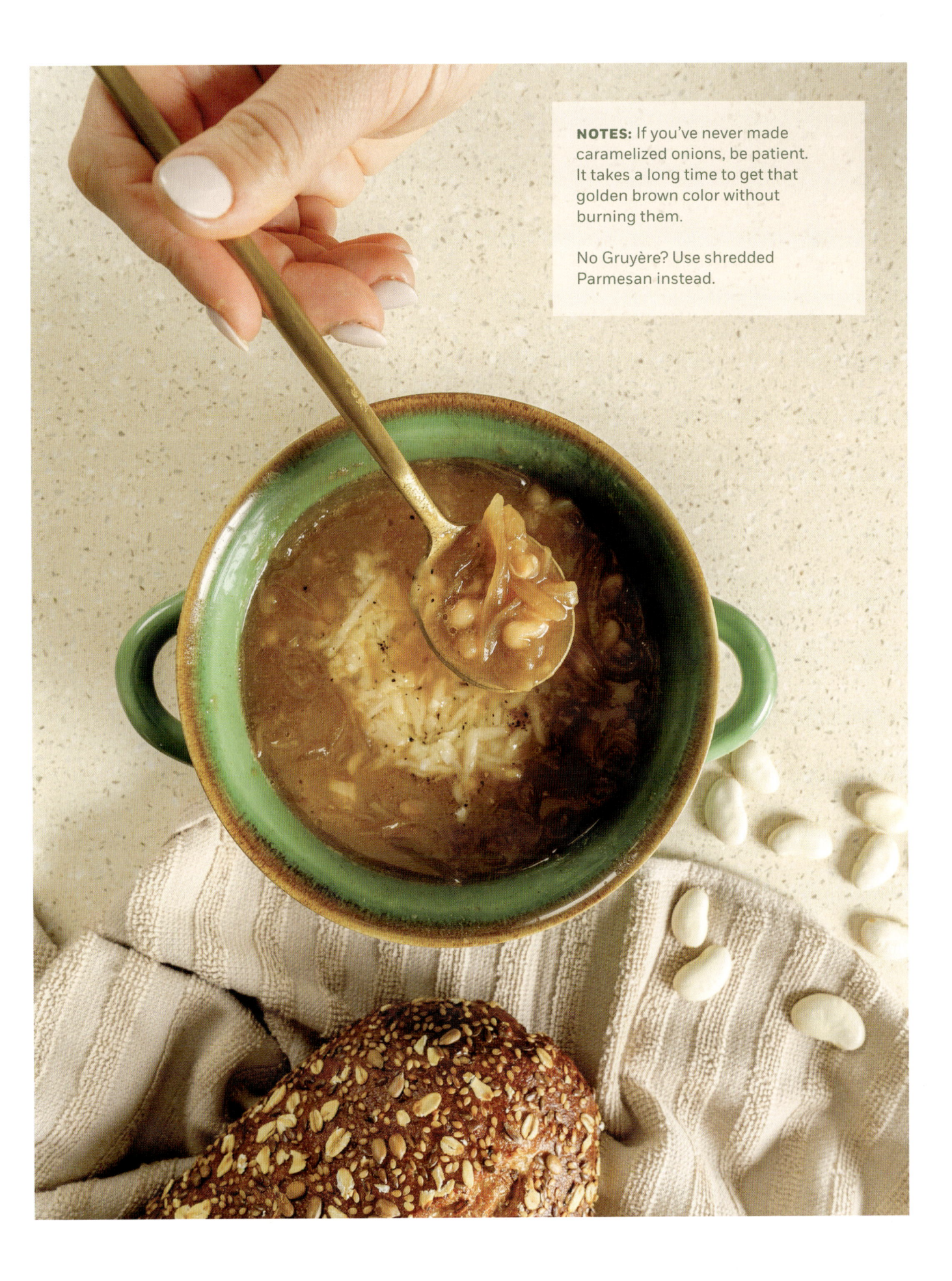

NOTES: If you've never made caramelized onions, be patient. It takes a long time to get that golden brown color without burning them.

No Gruyère? Use shredded Parmesan instead.

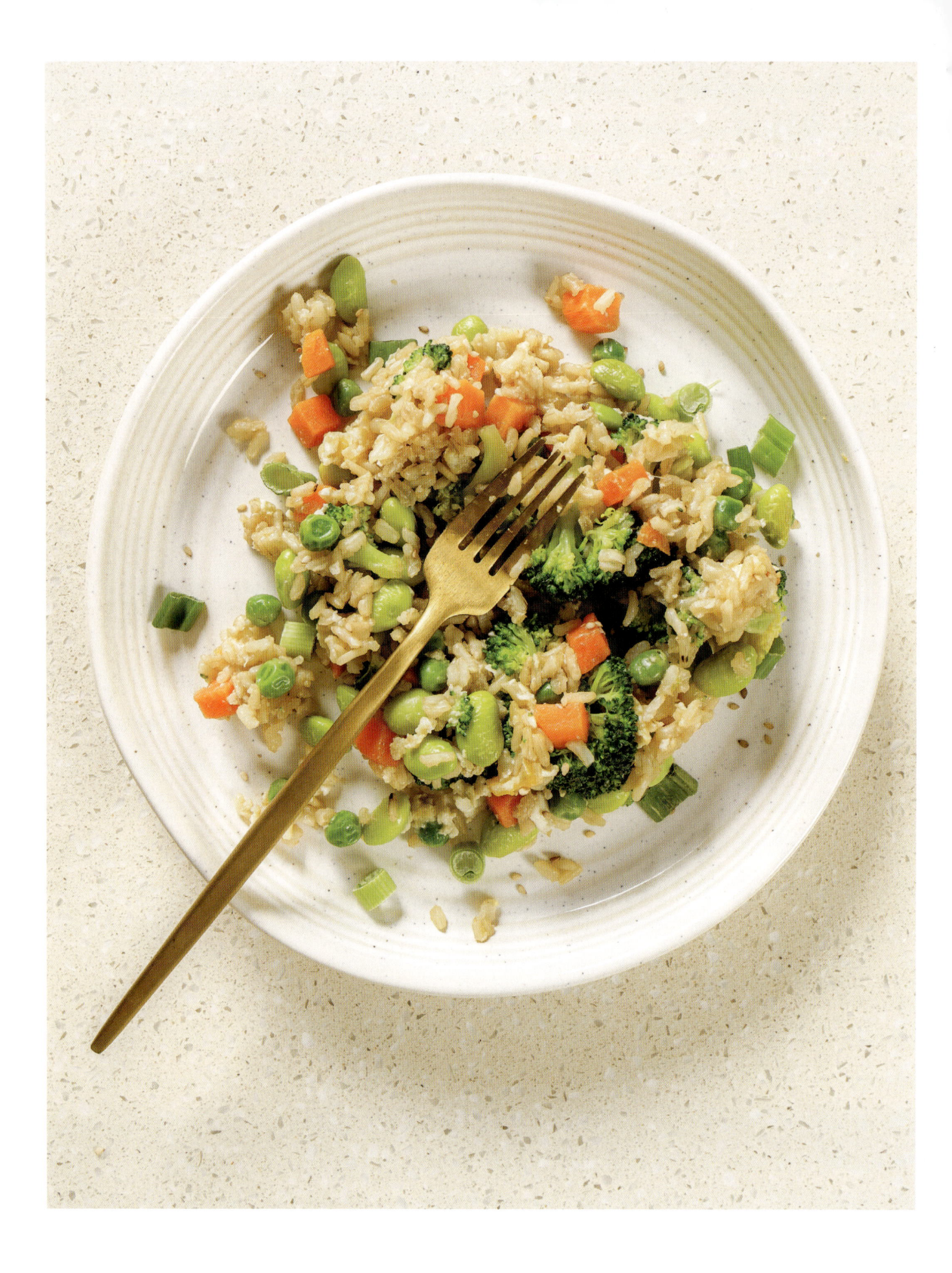

Veggie Fried Rice

SERVES 4
PREP TIME: 5 MINUTES
COOKING TIME: 20 MINUTES

1 tablespoon olive oil, divided

½ small white onion, finely chopped

2 cups frozen or fresh cooked brown rice

2 cups frozen edamame

2 cups frozen peas and carrots mix

2 cups frozen broccoli

2 garlic cloves, pressed or minced

2 eggs, beaten

2 tablespoons soy sauce, tamari, or coconut aminos

2 teaspoons sesame oil

Pinch of red pepper flakes

Chili-garlic sauce or sriracha for serving, optional

● PROTEIN ADD

Add ½ cup of shrimp (+12g), or add 1 (15-ounce) block of tofu, drained, pressed, and cubed (+8g per serving).

● MAKE IT PLANT-BASED

Omit the eggs.

Per serving: Calories: 346
Fat: 12g | Carbohydrates: 37g
Fiber: 9g | Protein: 17g

This veggie fried rice comes together in less than 30 minutes from start to finish. It's packed with tons of veggies that you can pull straight from the freezer to help you meet your fiber and vitamin C needs.

1. Add the olive oil to a large skillet and heat over medium heat. Sauté onions until tender (about 4 minutes).

2. Add in rice, edamame, peas and carrots, broccoli, and garlic. Sauté until they are heated through (roughly 6 minutes).

3. Make a small clearing in the skillet to add the beaten eggs. Allow them to cook until they become hard (about 3 minutes).

4. Scramble them with a spatula before incorporating the cooked eggs into the other ingredients.

5. Add in soy sauce, sesame oil, and red pepper flakes. Stir to combine and serve.

NOTE: This recipe is very customizable! Use any veggies in place of the peas, carrots, and broccoli.

Oven Black Bean Quesadillas

MAKES 3 QUESADILLAS
PREP TIME: 5 MINUTES
COOKING TIME: 15 MINUTES

1 tablespoon olive oil

2 cups frozen pepper-onion mix

1 (15.5-ounce) can black beans, drained and rinsed

1–2 teaspoons taco seasoning

1 garlic clove, minced

3 (10-inch) whole-wheat tortillas

¾ cup shredded cheese

● **MAKE IT GLUTEN-FREE**

Substitute tortillas for gluten-free or corn tortillas.

Per quesadilla: Calories: 448
Fat: 11g | Carbohydrates: 49g
Fiber: 19g | Protein: 24g

Using whole-wheat tortillas and plenty of veggies increases the fiber content in these healthy quesadillas, while black beans add both protein and fiber.

1. Heat the oil in a pan over medium heat. Once the oil is warm, add the frozen pepper-onion mix and cook, stirring until soft (5–7 minutes).

2. Add the black beans, taco seasoning, and garlic to the pan. Cook for an additional 5–7 minutes.

3. Preheat the broiler, or heat the oven to 450°F. Lay the tortillas out on a baking sheet. Add 2 tablespoons of cheese to one half of each tortilla, then top with ¾ cup of filling, then another 2 tablespoons of cheese.

4. Fold the tortillas closed and place under the broiler for 2 minutes on each side.

5. Slice into quarters to serve.

NOTE: No black beans? Use kidney, pinto, or red beans instead.

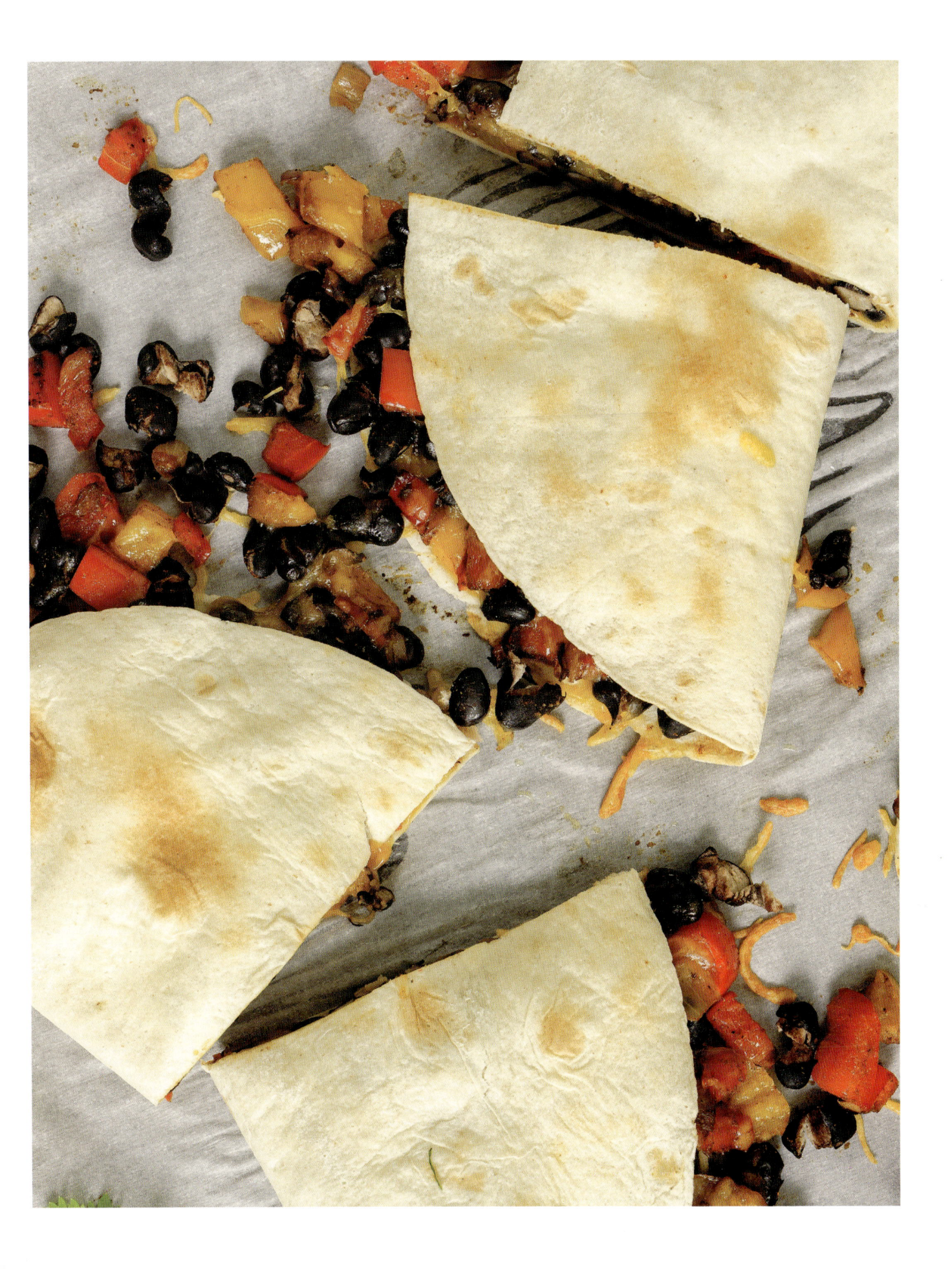

Teriyaki Salmon and Veggies

SERVES 2
PREP TIME: 2 MINUTES
COOKING TIME: 20 MINUTES

2 cups frozen brown rice

2 cups frozen green beans (or other sturdy vegetables such as broccoli, peas, Brussels sprouts)

2 teaspoons olive oil

2 (5-ounce) frozen salmon fillets

3–4 tablespoons teriyaki sauce

Per serving: Calories: 518
Fat: 15g | Carbohydrates: 51g
Fiber: 7g | Protein: 36g

Did you know you can cook fish straight from frozen? We didn't know either until we started experimenting for this book. This recipe is perfect for those days you forget to defrost your protein and need to make a complete meal straight from your freezer. Getting in your fish, and its omega-3s, has never been so easy.

1. Preheat the oven to 450°F. Line a baking sheet with parchment paper.

2. In a bowl, mix the brown rice, veggies, and oil. Toss until well combined.

3. Place the frozen salmon in the middle of the pan, and arrange the vegetables and rice around the salmon.

4. Bake for 10 minutes. Remove from the oven, stir the veggies and brown rice, and top the salmon with the teriyaki sauce.

5. Bake for 8–12 more minutes, depending on the size of your salmon, until the fish is cooked through and flaky.

Fancified Frozen Pizza

SERVES 1–2
PREP TIME: 5 MINUTES
COOKING TIME: 25 MINUTES

1 (11-inch) frozen pizza

½ cup frozen pepper-onion mix

½ cup frozen spinach

1–2 garlic cloves, sliced lengthwise

Olive oil, for drizzling

Red pepper flakes, optional

Italian seasoning, optional

● **PROTEIN ADD**

Add ½ cup shredded chicken (+26g total), or add 1 chopped tofurkey sausage link (+24g total).

Per pizza (will vary based on frozen pizza used):
Calories: 653 | Fat: 34g | Carbohydrates: 73g
Fiber: 5g | Protein: 27g

Sometimes a frozen pizza is just the reality of dinner. Use it as a canvas to create a more nutritious and balanced option by adding veggies, extra spices, and a protein source.

1. Preheat the oven according to the directions on the pizza box.

2. Top the frozen pizza with the pepper-onion mix, spinach, and garlic, and drizzle with a little olive oil.

3. Cook the pizza according to the instructions on the box. Add about 5 extra minutes to allow the frozen vegetables to cook all the way through, and check often to make sure the pizza doesn't burn.

4. Top with red pepper flakes and Italian seasoning, if desired.

NOTE: Frozen pizzas come in a lot of different sizes. Some may serve two, and the nutrition information likely varies.

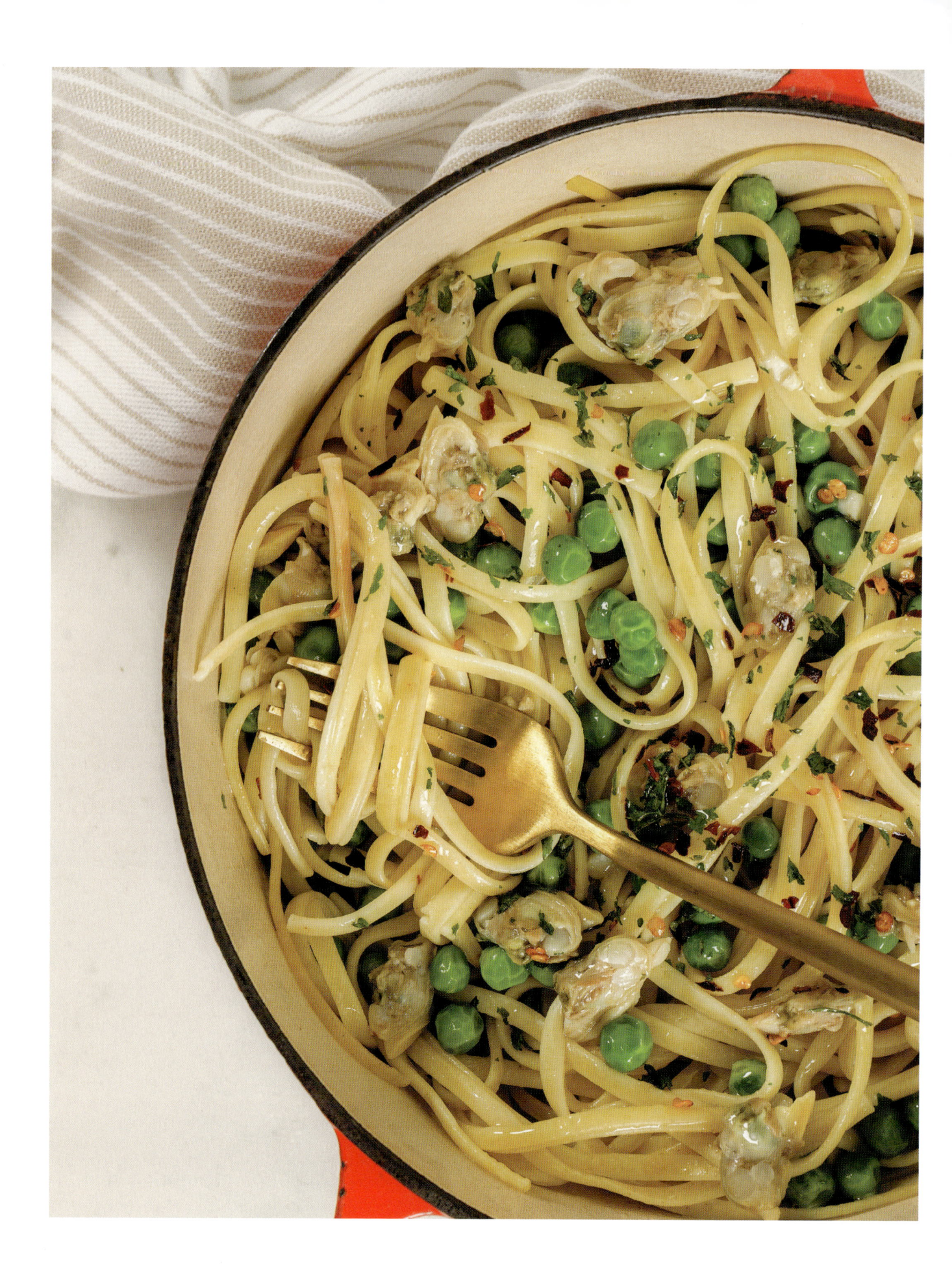

Linguine alla Vongole

SERVES 2
PREP TIME: 5 MINUTES
COOKING TIME: 15 MINUTES

¼ (16-ounce) box angel hair or linguine, whole-wheat or regular

2 cups frozen vegetables

1 tablespoon butter or vegan butter

1 tablespoon olive oil

2 garlic cloves, chopped

1 (10-ounce) can whole clams with liquid

¼ teaspoon dried parsley or thyme

Dash of black pepper

Salt, to taste

Red pepper flakes, optional

● **PROTEIN ADD**

Use a bean-based pasta (+13g), or add 1 tablespoon of hemp seeds per serving (+3g).

● **MAKE IT GLUTEN FREE**

Substitute pasta with gluten-free pasta.

Per serving: Calories: 473
Fat: 16g | Carbohydrates: 5g
Fiber: 9g | Protein: 17g

Clams and other mollusks such as mussels and oysters are great sources of iron, which is an important nutrient during the acute postpartum period to replenish any iron lost in delivery. Clams provide more iron per ounce than beef and can be conveniently stored in your pantry and eaten with minimal preparation.

1. Boil the pasta according to the package instructions. During the final minute of boiling, add the frozen vegetables and bring back up to a boil. Drain and set aside.

2. Set the pasta pot over medium-low heat and add the butter, olive oil and garlic. Sauté for 3–4 minutes until the garlic begins to soften and becomes fragrant.

3. Add the entire can of clams, including the liquid, the dried parsley or thyme, and a dash of black pepper. Cook for 3–4 minutes.

4. Add the pasta and vegetables back to the pot and cook for 2–3 minutes, stirring continuously. Remove from the pot and add salt and red pepper flakes to taste. How much salt you need will vary depending on the saltiness of your clams.

NOTE: If you can't find a 10-ounce can of clams, use 2 (6-ounce) cans.

Chickpea Toona Salad

SERVES 2
PREP TIME: 10 MINUTES
COOKING TIME: 0 MINUTES

1 (15.5-ounce) can chickpeas, drained and rinsed

¼ cup mayonnaise, vegan or regular

1 tablespoon capers, chopped

½ teaspoon caper brine

¼ teaspoon salt

¼ teaspoon black pepper

● **PROTEIN ADD**
Add 2 chopped hard-boiled eggs (+12g) or 3 tablespoons hemp seeds (+10g).

Per serving: Calories: 381
Fat: 22g | Carbohydrates: 23g
Fiber: 10g | Protein: 11g

This Chickpea Toona Salad brings the flavor of a traditional tuna salad without the fish. Capers add a nice saltiness to the dish, which you can whip up in 10 minutes or less. Plus, this recipe packs a ton of fiber, unlike regular tuna salad.

1. In a bowl, mash the chickpeas with the back of a fork, leaving a few chickpeas whole.

2. Add all the remaining ingredients and stir to combine.

3. Serve in a sandwich, with crackers, or with fresh vegetables such as carrot chips, cucumber boats, or celery.

NOTE: No chickpeas? Use white beans instead.

Sopa de Nopalitos

SERVES 4
PREP TIME: 3 MINUTES
COOKING TIME: 30 MINUTES

1 tablespoon olive oil

1 white onion, diced

8 garlic cloves, diced

1 (30-ounce) jar nopalitos, drained

1 (14.5-ounce) can diced tomatoes

1 (15.5-ounce) can black beans, drained and rinsed

2 cups chicken or vegetable broth

1 cup jarred tomatillo salsa

2 teaspoons dried oregano

1 teaspoon salt

½ teaspoon black pepper

● **PROTEIN ADD**

This dish is commonly served with 3 ounces of chicken (+21g per serving), or you can add 3.5-ounces of firm tofu (+9g per serving).

Per serving: Calories: 233
Fat: 8g | Carbohydrates: 32g
Fiber: 13g | Protein: 9g

Sopa de nopalitos is a traditional dish from Mexico recommended during the postpartum period. Nopales, or prickly pear cacti, are a good source of fiber, magnesium, vitamin C, and manganese. We've made this recipe even easier by using jarred nopalitos for a delicious pantry meal.

1. In a large pot, heat the olive oil over medium heat.

2. Add the onion and cook, stirring until tender (about 5 minutes).

3. Add the garlic and cook for 2–3 more minutes until fragrant.

4. Pour in the nopalitos, diced tomatoes, black beans, vegetable broth, tomatillo salsa, oregano, salt, and pepper. Bring to a simmer for 15 minutes.

NOTES: Traditionally, this recipe is made with fresh nopales. If you can find them, bring a large pot of water to a boil. Use a sharp knife to remove the spine around the outer rim of each nopal and the knobs that stick off the front and back. Rinse the nopal, then slice into 1-inch slices. Add 1 teaspoon of salt to the water, and boil the nopales for 15–20 minutes until tender. Add the cooked nopales in place of jarred nopalitos in the recipe.

Can't find jarred nopalitos? Substitute 2 (15-ounce) cans of chopped green beans.

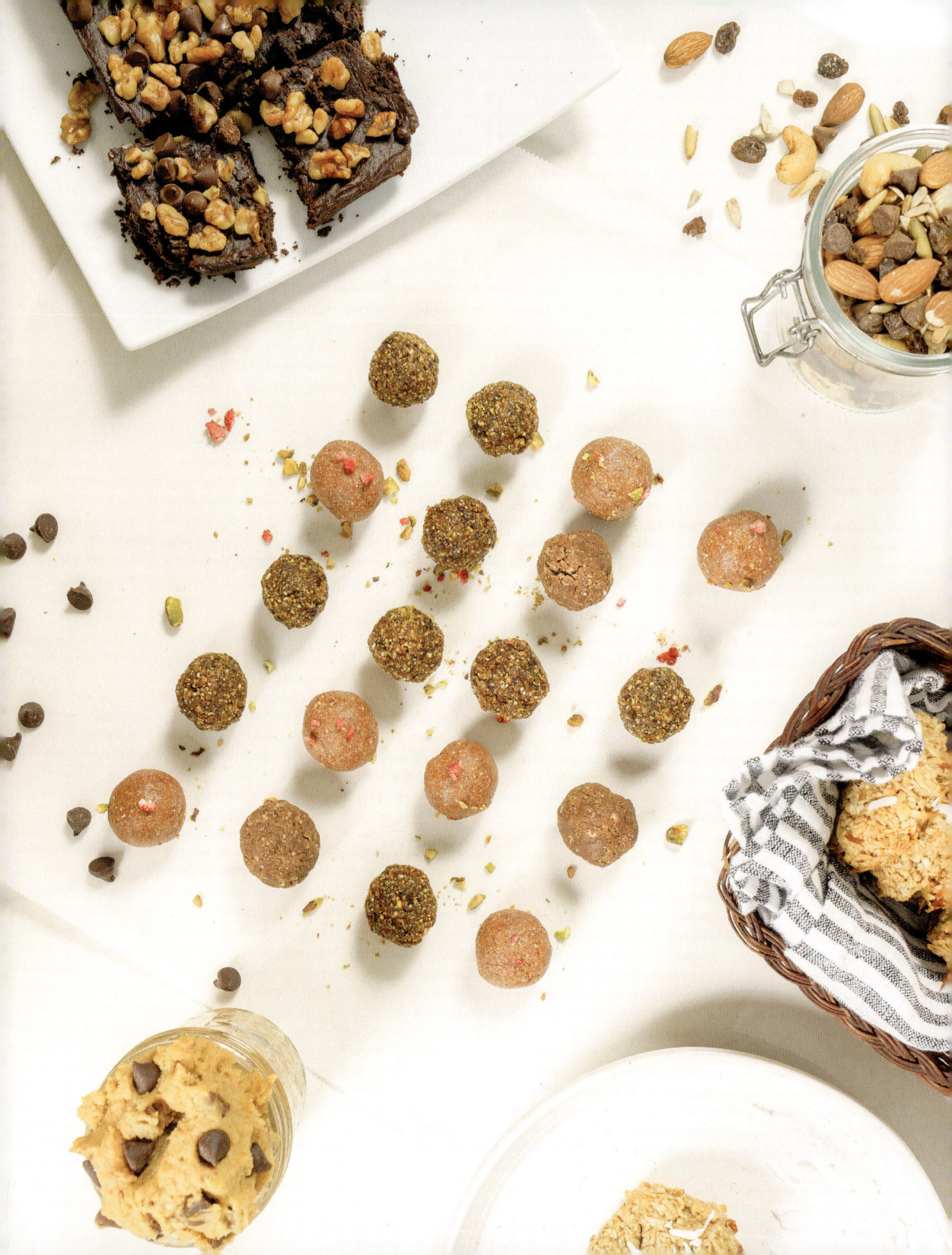

Snacks and Desserts

During the postpartum phase, you are likely to experience hunger like you've never experienced before. Having an arsenal of nutrient-dense, flavorful snacks and desserts can help to ensure you are satisfying your cravings while also meeting your nutrient needs. You deserve to enjoy and indulge in your favorite foods. We've included many of our favorite recipes, with ingredients intentionally chosen to maximize the nutrients your body needs without sacrificing tastiness. When you are so hungry that you will reach for anything, these are awesome options to have prepared!

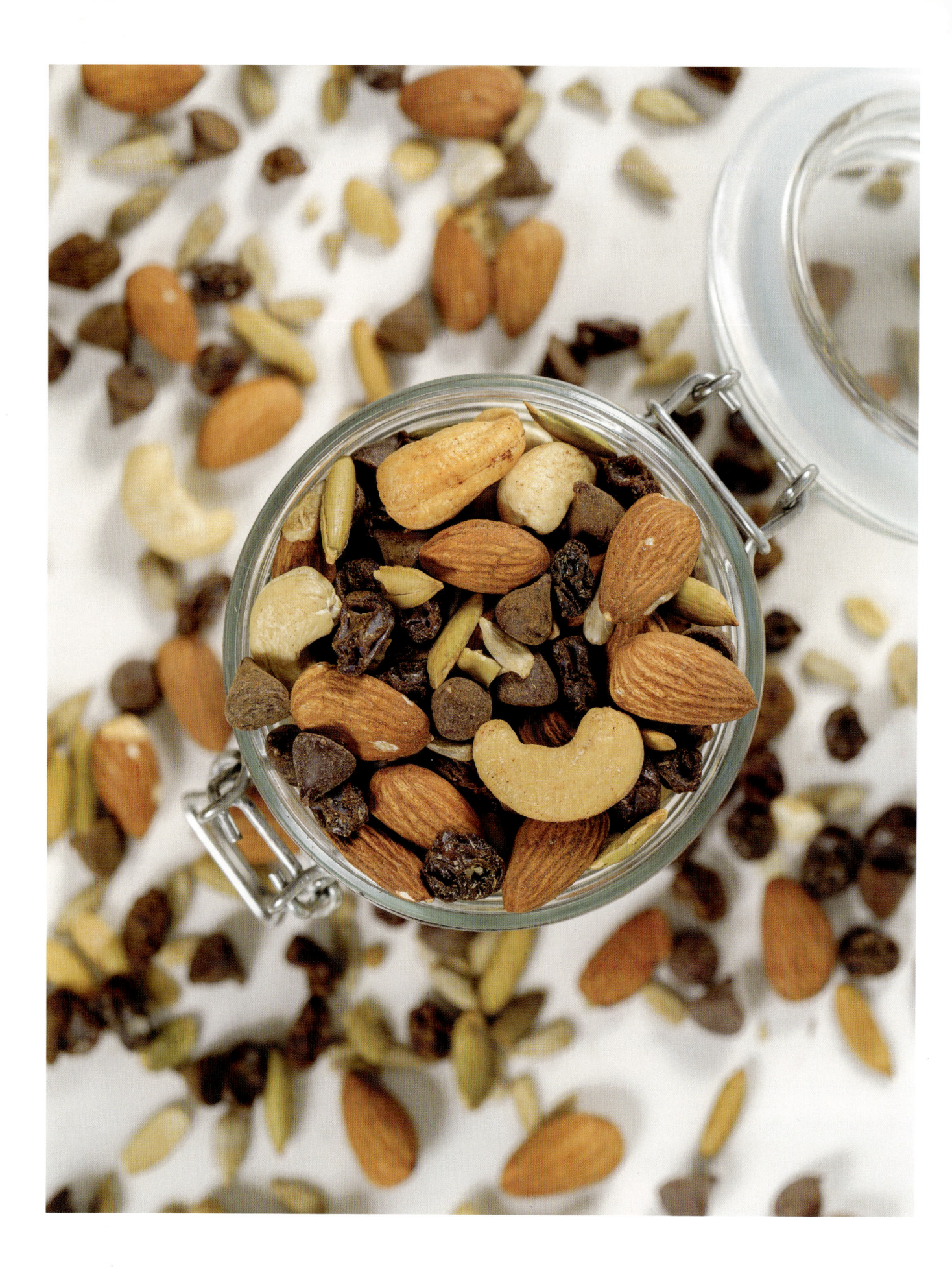

Midnight Trail Mix

MAKES 4 CUPS
PREP TIME: 5 MINUTES
COOKING TIME: 0 MINUTES

1 cup raisins

¾ cup almonds

¾ cup cashews

½ cup sunflower seeds

½ cup pumpkin seeds

½ cup chocolate chips or chopped dark chocolate

½ teaspoon ground cinnamon

¼ teaspoon salt (if using unsalted nuts and seeds)

● **MAKE IT NUT-FREE**

Omit the almonds and cashews, and increase the quantity of sunflower and pumpkin seeds.

Per 1/4 cup: Calories: 163
Fat: 11g | Carbohydrates: 13g
Fiber: 2g | Protein: 4g

This trail mix is a much better option than the bulk-size trail mix that we both devoured at 2 a.m. each night during our first weeks postpartum. We intentionally selected nuts and seeds for this recipe that are high in vitamin E, an essential antioxidant that helps your body recover. Vitamin E needs also increase by about 20% when breastfeeding. You will feel hunger like never before with round-the-clock feedings! Prepare for it by keeping this in a jar on your nightstand.

1. Combine all the ingredients in a large bowl and mix well.

2. Store in a ziplock bag or mason jar.

Pop's Rice Krispies Treats

SERVES 12
PREP TIME: 10 MINUTES
COOKING TIME: 5 MINUTES

⅔ cup creamy almond or peanut butter

⅓ cup maple syrup

½ cup white or dark chocolate chips

2-3 tablespoons unsweetened milk of choice

1 teaspoon vanilla extract

½ cup ground flaxseed

⅓ cup hemp seeds

½ teaspoon salt

½ teaspoon ground cinnamon

4 cups Rice Krispies

● **MAKE IT NUT-FREE**

Replace almond or peanut butter with sunflower seed butter.

Per serving: Calories: 229
Fat: 14g | Carbohydrates: 24g
Fiber: 3g | Protein: 7g

We've updated this classic snack with flaxseed and hemp seeds to boost the nutrient content without sacrificing flavor. Using either white or dark chocolate chips, you won't miss the marshmallows from the usual recipe. These are a great way to satisfy your breastfeeding hunger and sweet cravings.

1. In a large pot over low heat, melt the nut butter, maple syrup, and chocolate chips. Once melted, remove from the heat. Stir in the milk, vanilla extract, flaxseed, hemp seeds, salt, and cinnamon. The mixture should have enough liquid to mix with the cereal. Then add the Rice Krispies and thoroughly combine.

2. Pour into a parchment-lined 8 x 8-inch baking dish and gently push to flatten into a single layer. Allow to cool completely before cutting into squares.

3. These are best served immediately, or you can store them in an airtight container in the freezer.

NOTE: Try different flavor combinations by adding in dried fruit, nuts, spices, or extracts.

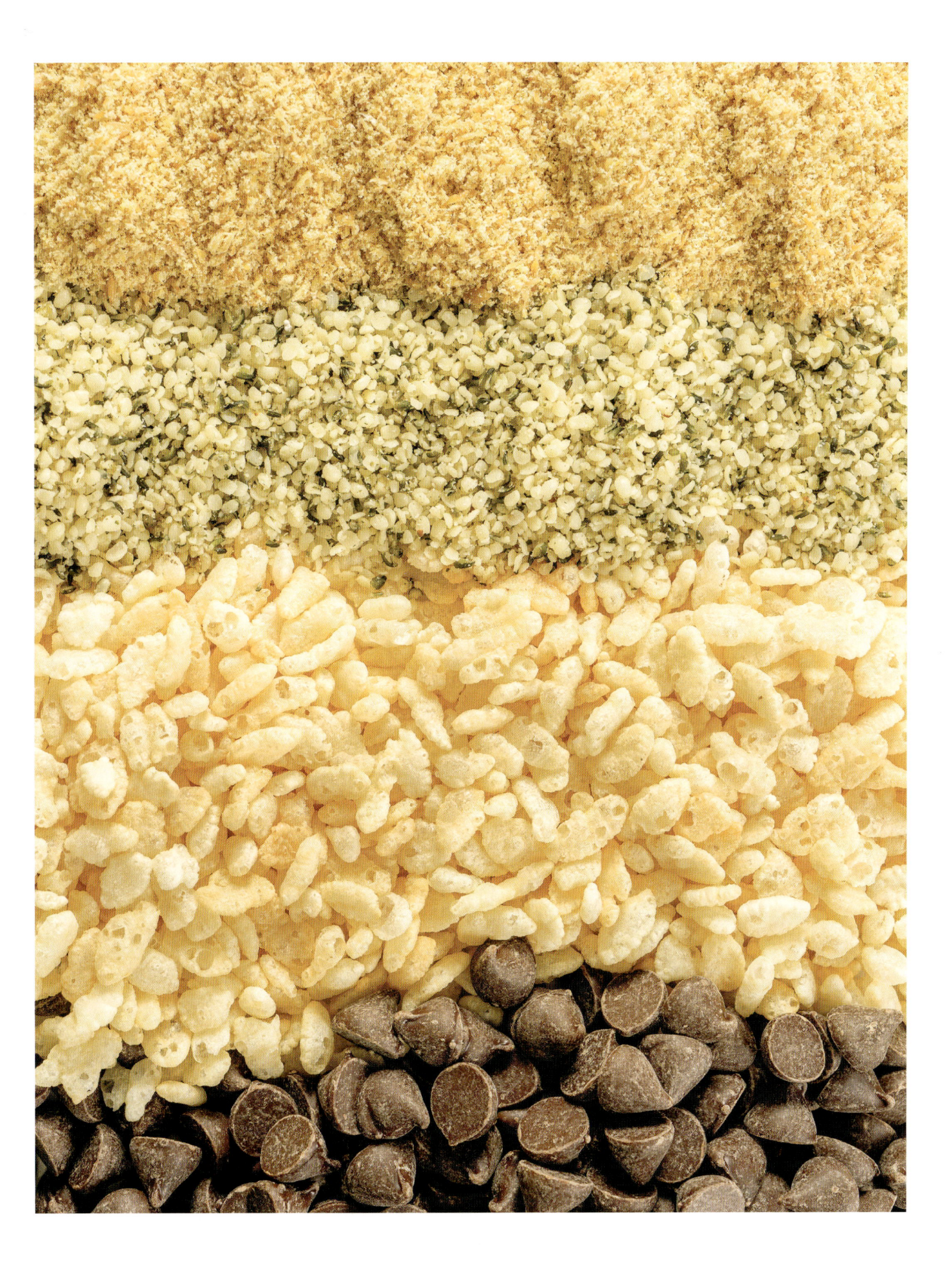

Gaia's Greek Yogurt Bowl

SERVES 1
PREP TIME: 5 MINUTES
COOKING TIME: 0 MINUTES

¾ cup unsweetened plain Greek yogurt

2 tablespoons vanilla protein powder

½ cup berries, fresh, or frozen and thawed

¼ cup shelled pistachios or walnuts

¼ cup granola

● **MAKE IT PLANT-BASED**

Use plant-based yogurt in place of the Greek yogurt.

Per serving: Calories: 467
Fat: 17g | Carbohydrates: 45g
Fiber: 9g | Protein: 36g

Turn your yogurt bowl into a power bowl with some intentional add-ins. These ingredients boost the protein, healthy fat, fiber, and antioxidant content, which are all important nutrients for you and your baby.

1. Combine the yogurt and protein powder in a bowl and stir until the protein powder is completely integrated.

2. Add the remaining ingredients and mix until well combined.

Iron-Filled Chocolate Mousse

SERVES 1
PREP TIME: 3 MINUTES
CHILLING TIME: 30 MINUTES

½ (15-ounce) package soft or silken tofu, drained

2 tablespoons cocoa powder

1–2 tablespoons maple syrup, depending on the desired level of sweetness

½ teaspoon vanilla extract

Per serving: Calories: 202
Fat: 8g | Carbohydrates: 25g
Fiber: 4g | Protein: 14g

Savor this chocolate mousse's rich, velvety goodness that will satisfy your sweet cravings while also providing a hearty serving of protein and a healthy 5-milligram dose of iron from the cocoa powder. Your iron needs may be elevated immediately following delivery to replenish blood loss. Once your monthly cycle returns, your iron needs will increase again.

1. In a blender or food processor, blend all the ingredients until creamy.

2. Pour the tofu-chocolate mixture into a bowl. Refrigerate for at least 2 hours, or place in the freezer for 30 minutes before eating.

NOTE: Use leftover silken tofu in our Creamy Pesto recipe on page 173.

Edible Chocolate Chip Cookie Dough

SERVES 4 (MAKES ABOUT 2 CUPS)
PREP TIME: 10 MINUTES
COOKING TIME: 0 MINUTES

1 (15.5-ounce) can chickpeas, drained and rinsed

⅓ cup smooth peanut butter

¼ cup maple syrup

1 teaspoon vanilla extract

3 tablespoons almond flour

⅛ teaspoon salt

½ cup chocolate chips

● **MAKE IT NUT-FREE**
Replace peanut butter with sunflower seed butter and almond flour with oat flour.

Per 1/2 cup: Calories: 422
Fat: 20g | Carbohydrates: 47g
Fiber: 6g | Protein: 11g

This edible chocolate chip cookie dough uses chickpeas as its base, providing a postpartum-friendly treat that combines nourishment with decadence. Chickpeas are a great source of vitamin B6, which plays an important role in postpartum recovery by replenishing blood loss from labor and after delivery. Your B6 needs also increase during breastfeeding.

1. In a food processor, process the chickpeas until smooth.

2. Add all the remaining ingredients except for the chocolate chips, and process until smooth.

3. Transfer the mixture to a bowl and fold in the chocolate chips.

NOTES: You can make this dough into cookies! Bake at 350°F for 15 minutes.

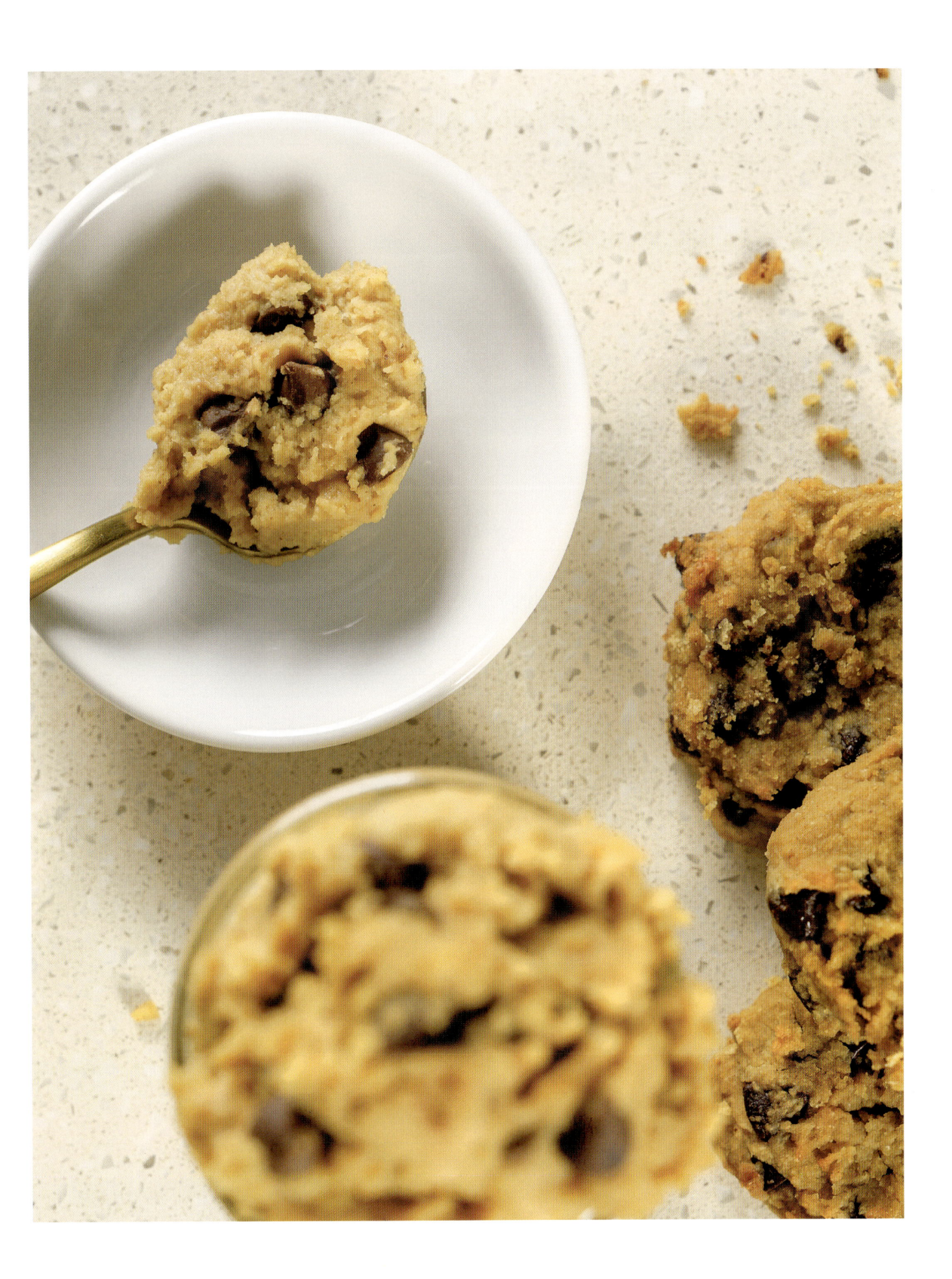

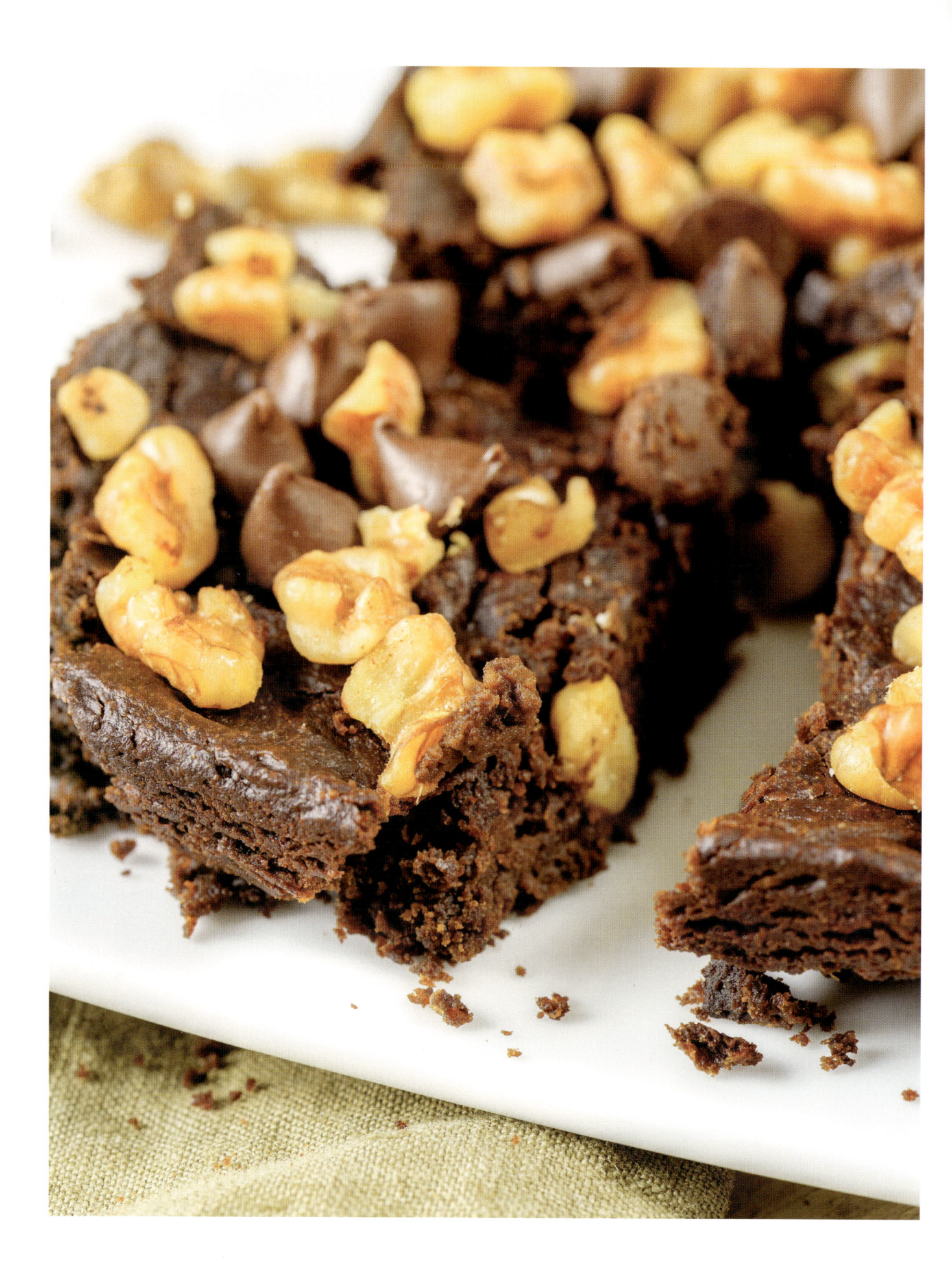

Beta-Carotene Brownies

SERVES 8
PREP TIME: 10 MINUTES
COOKING TIME: 1 HOUR

1 cup mashed cooked sweet potato

½ cup nut butter

3 tablespoons maple syrup

1 teaspoon vanilla extract

¼ cup cocoa powder

1 teaspoon baking powder

⅛ teaspoon salt

¼ cup chopped pecans or walnuts

2 tablespoons chocolate chips

● **MAKE IT NUT-FREE**

Replace peanut butter with sunflower seed butter. Omit pecans or walnuts.

Per brownie: Calories: 224
Fat: 14g | Carbohydrates: 20g
Fiber: 4g | Protein: 6g

Fudgier and healthier than a classic brownie, this version uses cocoa powder for its chocolate flavor and sweet potato in place of flour. Cocoa is rich in iron and polyphenols, compounds that help reduce inflammation. Sweet potato also provides a boost of beta-carotene, an important nutrient for postpartum wound-healing.

1. Preheat the oven to 350°F. Grease an 8 x 3-inch loaf pan and set it aside.

2. In a large bowl, thoroughly mash sweet potatoes with a fork until no large lumps remain. Combine with the nut butter, maple syrup, vanilla extract, cocoa powder, baking powder, and salt. Stir to combine. Pour into the baking pan and top with nuts and chocolate chips.

3. Bake for 50–60 minutes, or until a knife comes out clean. Remove from the oven and allow to cool completely before slicing and serving.

NOTES: You can freeze these sweet potato brownies. Wrap brownies individually in parchment paper and place them in a ziplock bag. Thaw brownies by setting them out at room temperature or in the fridge overnight.

No blender? No problem. You can also mix the batter vigorously in a bowl.

Sugar, Spice, and Everything Nice Cream (4 Ways)

SERVES 2
PREP TIME: 5 MINUTES
COOKING TIME: 0 MINUTES

BASE

2 ripe bananas, peeled, sliced, and frozen

¼ teaspoon ground cinnamon

CHOCOLATE

3 tablespoons cocoa powder

PEANUT BUTTER CHOCOLATE

3 tablespoons cocoa powder

2 tablespoons peanut butter

VANILLA CHOCOLATE CHIP

¼ cup chocolate chips, divided

1 teaspoon vanilla extract

CREAMY STRAWBERRY

1 cup frozen strawberries

¼ cup yogurt of choice

Did you know you can make "ice cream" from bananas? Our ice cream uses bananas as the base to boost potassium, as well as sweetness, without the need for added sugar. Experiment with different fruit and other add-ins to create your own favorite varieties.

1. Combine all the ingredients in a high-speed blender or food processor. (For the Vanilla Chocolate Chip, add only 2 tablespoons of chocolate chips to the blender.) Blend, occasionally scraping down the sides, until smooth (3–5 minutes). For the Vanilla Chocolate Chip, mix in the remaining 2 tablespoons of chocolate chips after blending.

2. Scoop into a bowl and enjoy immediately as soft serve, or for firmer ice cream, place in an airtight, freezer-safe container and freeze for at least 1 hour.

Per serving, Chocolate:
Calories: 123 | Fat: 2g
Carbohydrates: 26g
Fiber: 6g | Protein: 3g

Per serving, Peanut Butter Chocolate:
Calories: 219 | Fat: 10g
Carbohydrates: 28g
Fiber: 7g | Protein: 7g

Per serving, Vanilla Chocolate Chip:
Calories: 233 | Fat: 7g
Carbohydrates: 36g
Fiber: 4g | Protein: 3g

Per serving, Creamy Strawberry:
Calories: 143 | Fat: 1g
Carbohydrates: 29g
Fiber: 5g | Protein: 4g

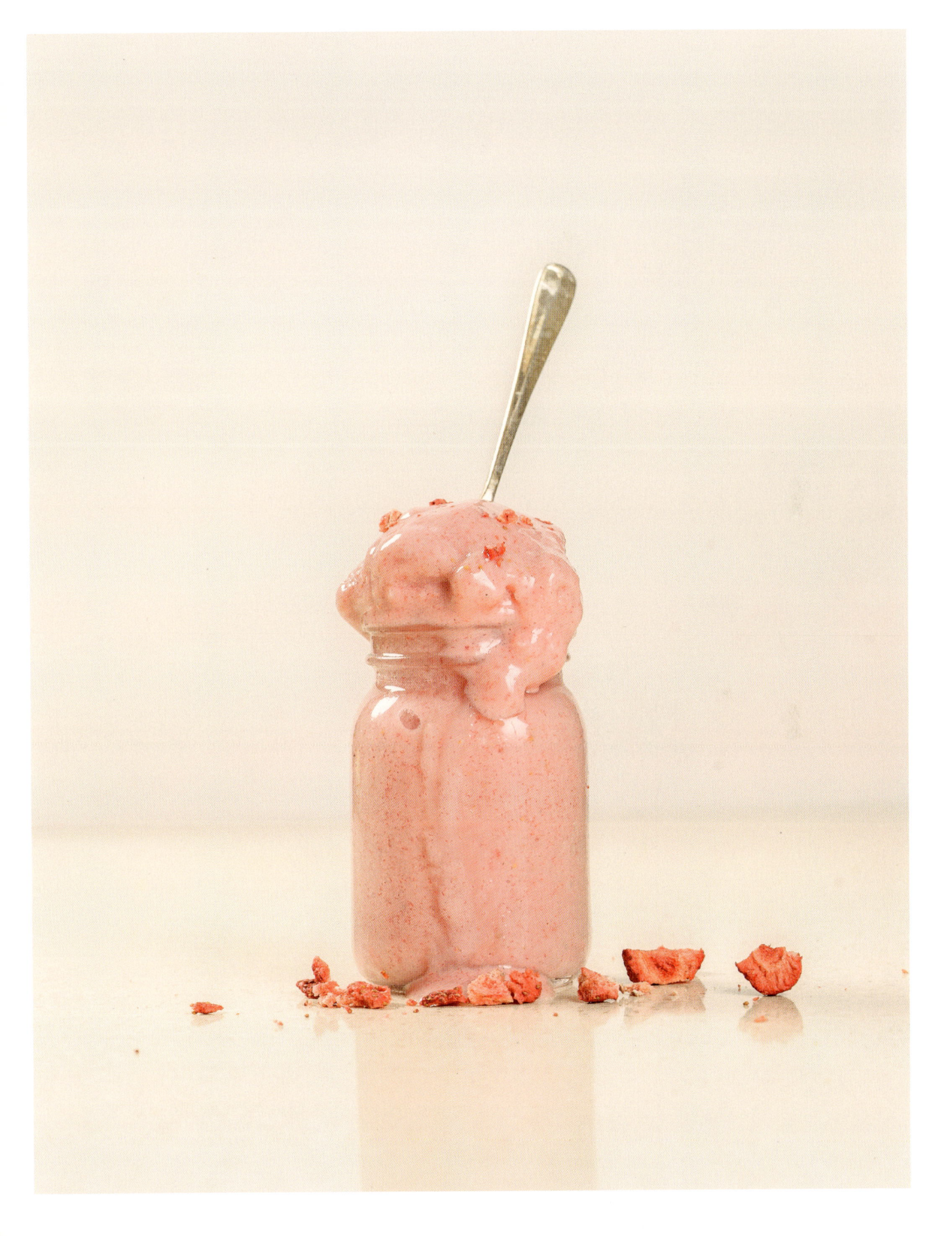

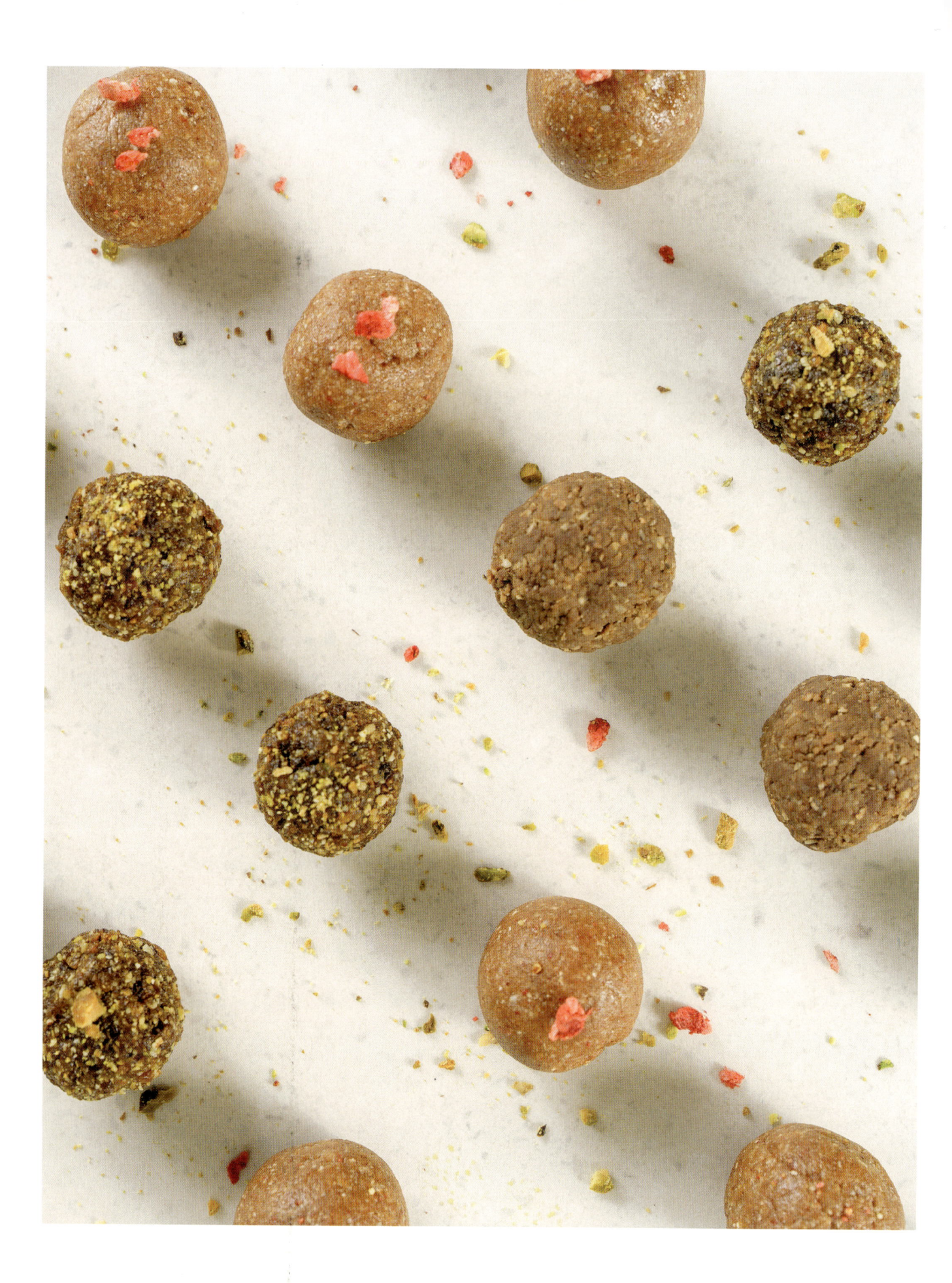

Energy Balls (3 Ways)

MAKES 24 BALLS
PREP TIME: 10 MINUTES
COOKING TIME: 0 MINUTES

PISTACHIO-APRICOT

2.5 cups dried apricots

1 cup roasted, unsalted almonds

1 cup roasted, unsalted pistachios

½ teaspoon ground cinnamon

¼ teaspoon ground ginger

PB&J

1 (1.2-ounce) package freeze-dried strawberries

2 cups roasted, unsalted peanuts

20 Medjool dates, pitted

½ cup rolled oats

CHOCOLATE PB

2 cups rolled oats

¾ cup chocolate protein powder

½ cup unsweetened peanut butter

½ cup honey

½ cup dark chocolate chips

Per ball, Pistachio Apricot:
Calories: 75 | Fat: 4g
Carbohydrates: 9g
Fiber: 2g | Protein: 2g

Per ball, PB&J:
Calories: 145 | Fat: 6g
Carbohydrates: 19g
Fiber: 3g | Protein: 4g

Per ball, Chocolate PB:
Calories: 127
Fat: 5g | Carbohydrates: 15g
Fiber: 2g | Protein: 7g

These poppable bites are awesome breastfeeding snacks. The Pistachio-Apricot balls are an excellent source of vitamin E, an important antioxidant during the acute postpartum period. The PB&J and Chocolate PB balls are delicious sweet treats that also provide filling fiber, healthy fats, and satisfying protein.

1. Combine all the ingredients in a food processor. Blend for 60–90 seconds until the ingredients form a paste. Scoop 2 tablespoons at a time into the palm of your hand and roll into balls.

2. These can be kept on the counter for 3 days, refrigerated for 2 weeks, or frozen for up to 1 year.

NOTE: The moisture content of dried fruit can alter the stickiness. If your balls aren't sticking together, add 1 teaspoon of honey at a time. After each addition, blend again and try to form a ball.

Lactation Cookies (3 Ways)

MAKES 12–14
PREP TIME: 10 MINUTES
COOKING TIME: 15 MINUTES

BASE

1 ⅔ cups oat flour (see Notes)

¾ cup rolled oats

1 teaspoon ground cinnamon

½ teaspoon baking powder

¼ teaspoon salt

⅓ cup coconut oil

⅓ cup maple syrup

1 teaspoon vanilla extract

1 flax egg (see Notes)

CHOCOLATE CHIP WALNUT

½ cup dark chocolate chips

¼ cup walnuts

BOOBIE BOOST

1 tablespoon unsweetened milk of choice

½ cup cranberries

¼ cup Brewer's yeast (we recommend the debittered kind, such as Solgars)

3 tablespoons orange zest

COCONUT ALMOND

½ cup shredded coconut

¼ cup chopped almonds

These lactation cookies are filled with nutrients from the oats, flaxseed, and even Brewer's yeast—all ingredients thought to help boost milk supply. While the research is still mixed on whether they actually improve breast milk production, these cookies still provide nutritional benefits such as fiber, omega-3s, and protein. They are the perfect breakfast carb, snack, or dessert.

1. Preheat the oven to 350°F, and line a baking pan with parchment paper.

2. In a bowl, mix the oat flour, oats, cinnamon, baking powder, and salt together until well combined.

3. In a separate bowl, whisk together the wet ingredients. For the Boobie Boost variation, add the milk.

4. Add the wet ingredients to the dry ingredients and mix until just combined.

5. Once combined, fold in any mix-ins for your preferred variation.

6. Evenly scoop out 12–14 cookies onto the baking sheet.

7. Bake for 10–15 minutes, or until a knife comes out clean.

Per cookie, Chocolate Chip Walnut:
Calories: 181 | Fat: 9g
Carbohydrates: 20g
Fiber: 3g | Protein: 3g

Per cookie, Boobie Boost:
Calories: 164 | Fat: 6g
Carbohydrates: 21g
Fiber: 3g | Protein: 5g

Per cookie, Coconut Almond:
Calories: 164 | Fat: 9g
Carbohydrates: 17g
Fiber: 3g | Protein: 3g

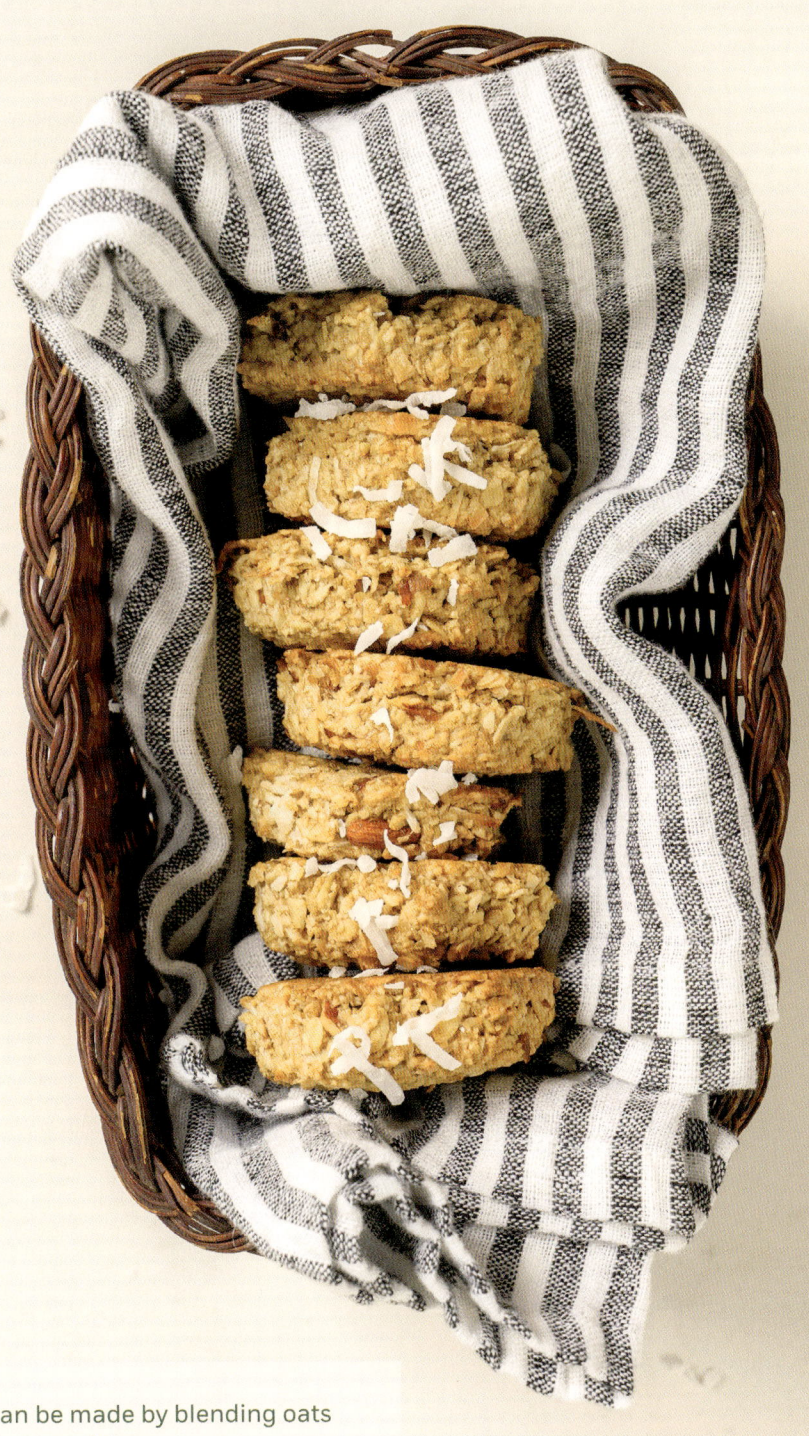

NOTES: Oat flour can be made by blending oats until you reach a fine consistency.

To make 1 flax egg, combine 1 tablespoon ground flaxseed and 2 ½ tablespoons water. Stir and let sit for at least 5 minutes.

Mix-and-Match Savory Snacks

SERVES 1
PREP TIME: 5–10 MINUTES
COOKING TIME: 0 MINUTES

VEGGIE OPTIONS

1 cup sliced bell peppers

1 cup baby carrots

1 cup sliced cucumbers

15 snap peas

4 celery sticks

12 cherry tomatoes

CARB OPTIONS

8 seed crackers

1 slice whole-wheat toast

2 rice cakes

3 cups popcorn

PROTEIN/FAT OPTIONS

2 string cheeses

¼ cup hummus

2 tablespoons nut butter

¼ cup nuts (such as almonds, pistachios, walnuts)

2 hard-boiled eggs

½ cup yogurt or cottage cheese

½ cup shelled edamame (fresh or dried)

10 olives

We know you won't always be craving sweet snacks, so we wanted to include some ideas for creating a balanced salty snack. These mix-and-match categories provide a customizable array of protein-rich and nutrient-dense options for you to combine.

- Pick one food from the veggie category and pair it with one food from the carb category and one to two foods from the protein/fat category.

Chocolate Truffle Bites

MAKES 24
PREP TIME: 15 MINUTES
COOKING TIME: 0 MINUTES

1 cup pitted Medjool dates (8–10 dates)

¼ cup walnuts or pecans

¼ cup cashews

2 tablespoons cocoa powder, plus more for dusting

1 tablespoon nut butter or tahini

1 ½ teaspoons unsweetened non-dairy milk

¼ teaspoon vanilla extract

Pinch of salt

Per ball: Calories: 37
Fat: 2g | Carbohydrates: 5g
Fiber: 1g | Protein: 1g

These bites are not only a naturally sweetened and indulgent treat, they also contribute to the nourishment and energy you need during the postpartum period. They are high in fiber, healthy fats, and antioxidants.

1. Combine all the ingredients in a food processor and blend until smooth and combined.

2. Roll the mixture into small balls and dust with cocoa powder. Store in an airtight container on the counter for 1 week, or freeze for up to 3 months.

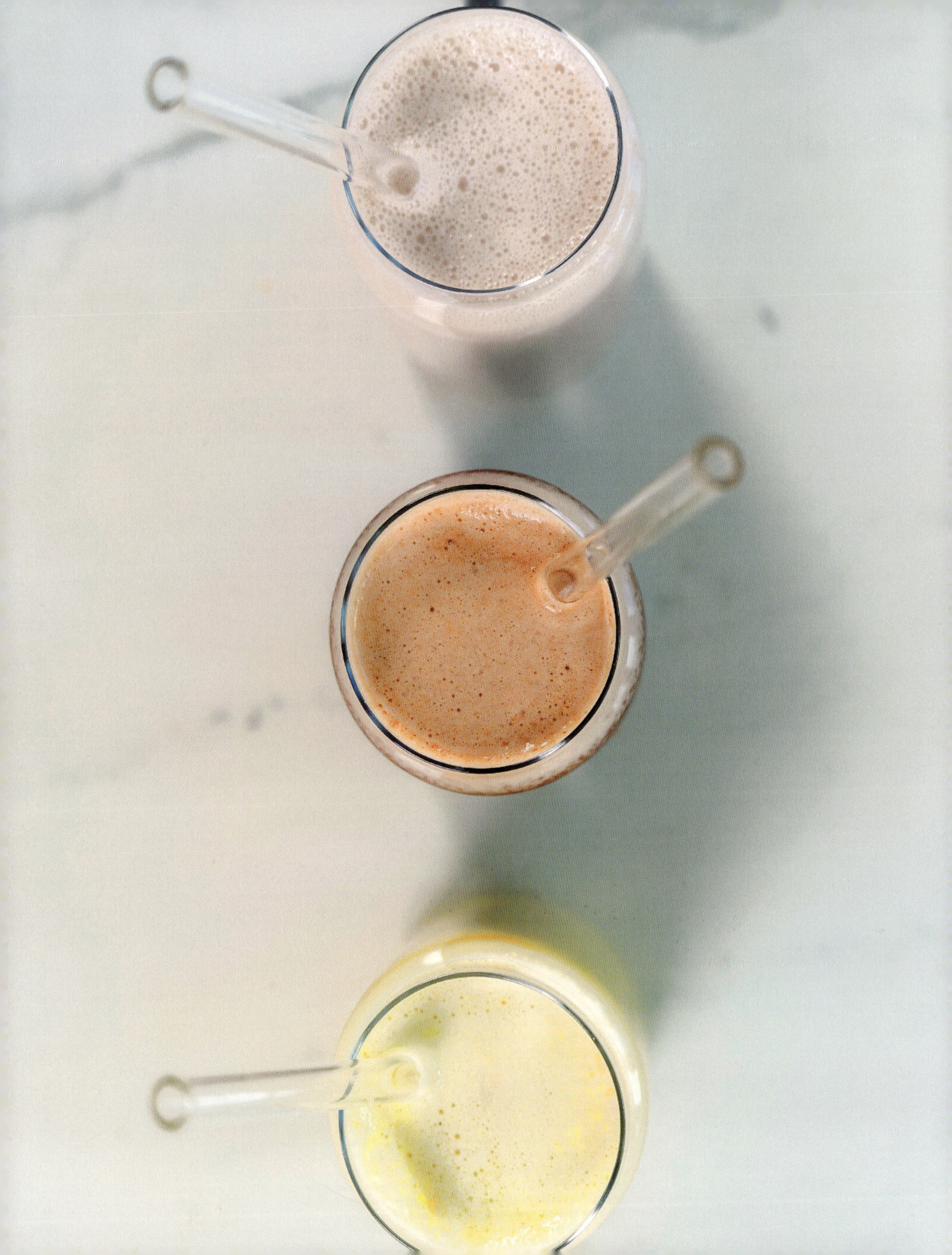

Smoothies

We wanted to include a whole chapter on smoothies because they are an easy option for a full meal or a quick snack and a great way to boost the antioxidant content in your day. You'll find a variety of meal-sized smoothies here, as well as a few lighter ones—some are great before a walk outside, while others are a perfect dessert before bed. Unlike most of our other recipes, we haven't included protein additions for all of these smoothies, because some just taste better without it. We recommend either pairing our lower-protein smoothies with a protein-containing meal or snack or having them before you are physically active.

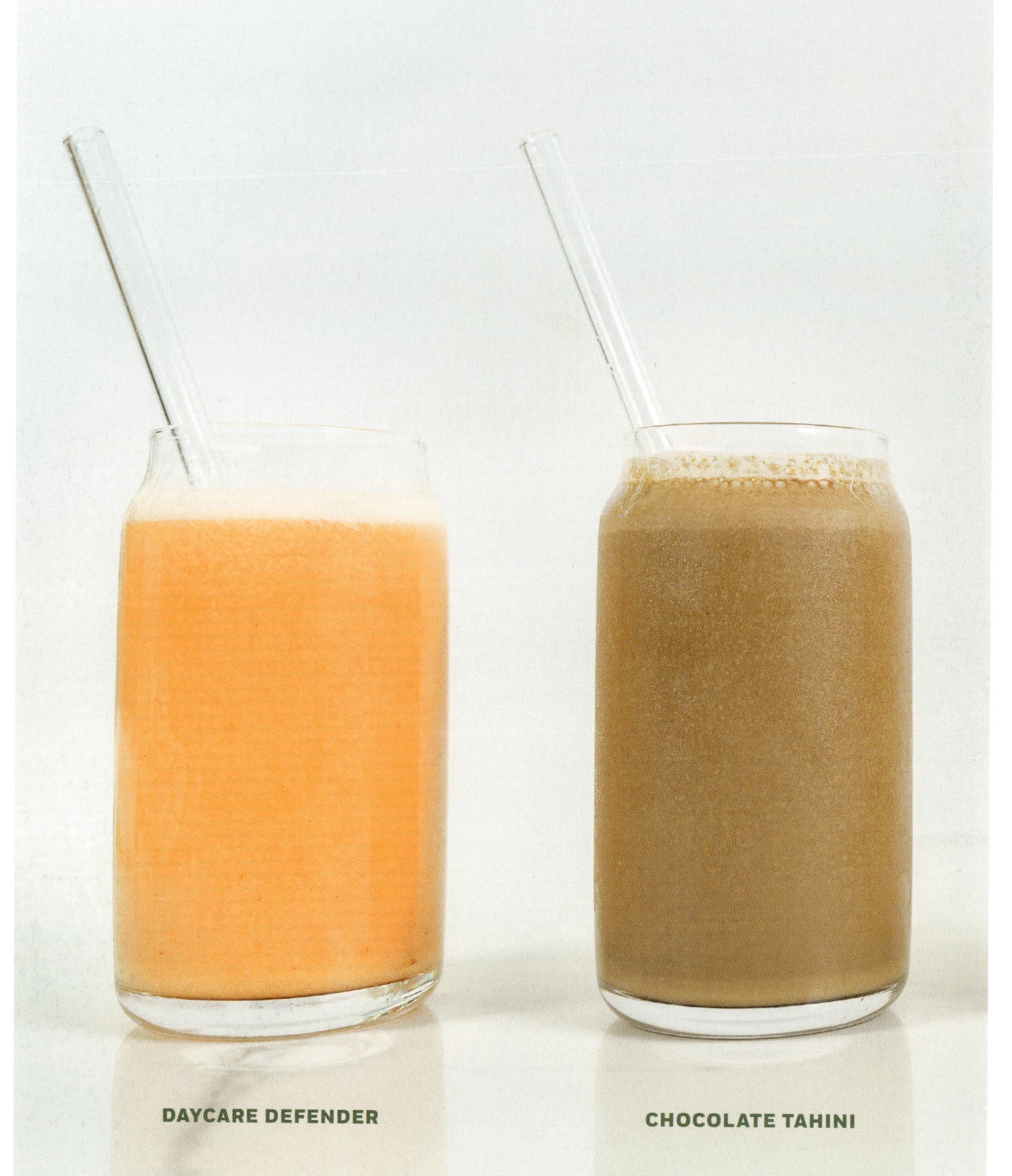

DAYCARE DEFENDER **CHOCOLATE TAHINI**

Daycare Defender Smoothie

SERVES 1
PREP TIME: 5 MINUTES
COOKING TIME: 0 MINUTES

½ cup frozen strawberries

½ cup frozen mango

½ cup frozen pineapple

2 clementines

½ cup water

Per serving: Calories: 196
Fat: 2g | Carbohydrates: 50g
Fiber: 3g | Protein: 3g

Holy daycare germs! While this recipe won't keep coughs and snot out of your face, it can help to make sure that your body has all it needs when those daycare illnesses just keep coming. This tasty drink has 200% of your daily recommended amount of vitamin C and 300% of the daily recommended amount of beta-carotene.

- Place all the ingredients in a blender, and blend until smooth.

NOTE: This is a perfect recipe to turn into ice pops for you and your little ones.

Chocolate Tahini Milkshake

SERVES 1
PREP TIME: 5 MINUTES
COOKING TIME: 0 MINUTES

¾ cup unsweetened milk of choice, plus more as needed

½ cup ice

1 frozen ripe banana

2 tablespoons cocoa powder

1 ½ tablespoons tahini

Per serving: Calories: 323
Fat: 17g | Carbohydrates: 32g
Fiber: 9g | Protein: 13g

This creamy smoothie is perfect if you're craving something chocolatey and sweet. The milk and tahini provide a boost of calcium, which is essential for postpartum bone health.

- Place all the ingredients in a blender, and blend until smooth.

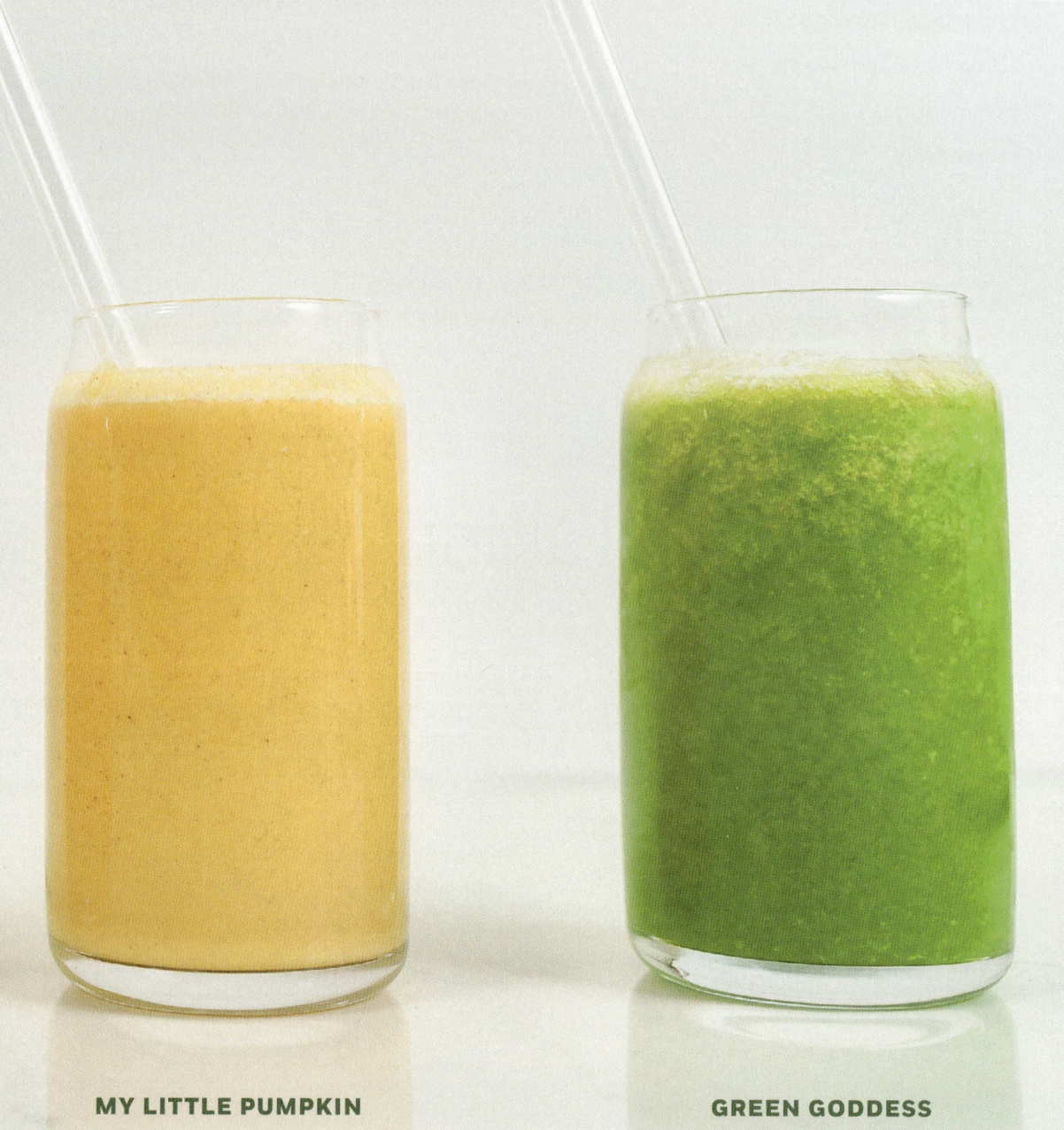

MY LITTLE PUMPKIN

GREEN GODDESS

My Little Pumpkin Smoothie

SERVES 1
PREP TIME: 5 MINUTES
COOKING TIME: 0 MINUTES

1 cup unsweetened milk of choice

½–1 cup water, depending on desired consistency

½ (15-ounce) can pureed pumpkin

¼ cup rolled oats

1 tablespoon chia seeds

1 tablespoon peanut, almond, or sunflower seed butter

2–3 teaspoons maple syrup or molasses

2–3 dates

¼ teaspoon pumpkin spice seasoning (cinnamon, nutmeg, and cloves)

1 cup ice

2 tablespoons vanilla protein powder

This festive fall smoothie is packed with not only delicious pumpkin flavor but protein, fiber, and beta-carotene, too. It's an awesome smoothie to enjoy during the acute recovery phase to meet your nutrient needs and help you regain normal digestion.

- Combine all the ingredients except the ice and protein powder in a blender. Blend on high until the ingredients are smooth. Add the ice and protein powder, and blend again until combine

NOTE: Enjoy immediately! The oats and chia seeds will thicken the smoothie if it's allowed to sit for a long period. You can also use 2–3 dates for this recipe in place of the maple syrup.

Per serving: Calories: 510
Fat: 21g | Carbohydrates: 58g
Fiber: 11g | Protein: 28g

Green Goddess Smoothie

SERVES 1
PREP TIME: 5 MINUTES
COOKING TIME: 0 MINUTES

1 handful of spinach or baby kale

1 celery stalk

½ green apple, cored

½ cup frozen mango

½ teaspoon grated fresh ginger

1–1 ½ cups water, depending on desired consistency

1 tablespoon fresh lemon juice

This Green Goddess Smoothie is packed with leafy greens, fruit, and zesty flavors designed to nourish and energize you on those mornings when you feel like you can't get out of bed.

- Place all the ingredients in a blender, and blend until smooth.

Per serving: Calories: 194
Fat: 5g | Carbohydrates: 27g
Fiber: 6g | Protein: 9g

Iron Infuser

SERVES 1
PREP TIME: 5 MINUTES
COOKING TIME: 0 MINUTES

1 cup frozen mango

1 cup frozen spinach or kale

½–1 cup water, depending on desired consistency

½ cup orange juice

2 tablespoons hemp seeds

2 tablespoons chia seeds

Per serving: Calories: 452
Fat: 22g | Carbohydrates: 38g
Fiber: 13g | Protein: 18g

It's crucial to replenish iron lost through blood loss, which begins during labor and delivery and continues weeks after delivery through lochia. This Iron Infuser smoothie provides 6 milligrams of iron (about 75% of the daily value), and the vitamin C found in the mango and orange juice helps enhance its absorption.

- Place all the ingredients in a blender, and blend until smooth.

NOTE: Calcium tends to inhibit iron absorption, so try to avoid having any dairy or other calcium-containing foods with this smoothie.

Mocha Mama Smoothie

SERVES 1
PREP TIME: 5 MINUTES
COOKING TIME: 0 MINUTES

1 cup ice

1 cup chilled black coffee

1 cup unsweetened milk of choice

¼ cup chocolate protein powder

1 tablespoon cocoa powder

Per serving: Calories: 266
Fat: 9g | Carbohydrates: 20g
Fiber: 2g | Protein: 28g

Some mornings (okay, maybe most mornings), your need for a strong cup of coffee may feel more important than eating. On those days, opt for this smoothie instead. It's high in protein to start your day on a well-nourished foot while also providing your much-needed caffeine.

- Place all the ingredients in a blender, and blend until smooth.

It's a Girl! Smoothie

SERVES 1
PREP TIME: 5 MINUTES
COOKING TIME: 0 MINUTES

1 cup unsweetened milk of choice, plus more as needed

½ cup unsweetened plain Greek yogurt

½ cup frozen cauliflower, optional

½ cup frozen strawberries

1 frozen ripe banana

½ teaspoon vanilla extract

¼ teaspoon ground cinnamon

● **MAKE IT PLANT-BASED**
Use plant-based yogurt in place of the Greek yogurt.

Meeting your nutrition needs during the postpartum period can be challenging at times. With this pretty pink smoothie, you'll not only get plenty of protein, you'll also get a whole serving of vegetables if you choose to add the cauliflower. We promise you won't even taste it!

- Place all the ingredients in a blender, and blend until smooth.

Per serving: Calories: 288
Fat: 5g | Carbohydrates: 36g
Fiber: 7g | Protein: 20g

Midwife Mix-Up

SERVES 1
PREP TIME: 5 MINUTES
COOKING TIME: 0 MINUTES

1 cup frozen berries

½ cup frozen mango

½ cup plain unsweetened Greek yogurt

2 tablespoons peanut butter

2 tablespoons vanilla protein powder

Dash of ground cinnamon

Per serving: Calories: 437
Fat: 18g | Carbohydrates: 42g
Fiber: 8g | Protein: 30g

Take advantage of this meal-sized smoothie to easily get in all the nutrients you need. This PB&J-flavored smoothie was inspired by the one Ashley's midwife created when she was too nauseous to eat during her first trimester. It remains a staple portable meal to this day!

- Combine all the ingredients in a blender. Fill the blender with enough water to cover the ingredients. Blend until smooth.

● **MAKE IT NUT-FREE**
Replace peanut butter with sunflower seed butter.

● **MAKE IT PLANT-BASED**
Use plant-based yogurt in place of the Greek yogurt.

IT'S A GIRL!

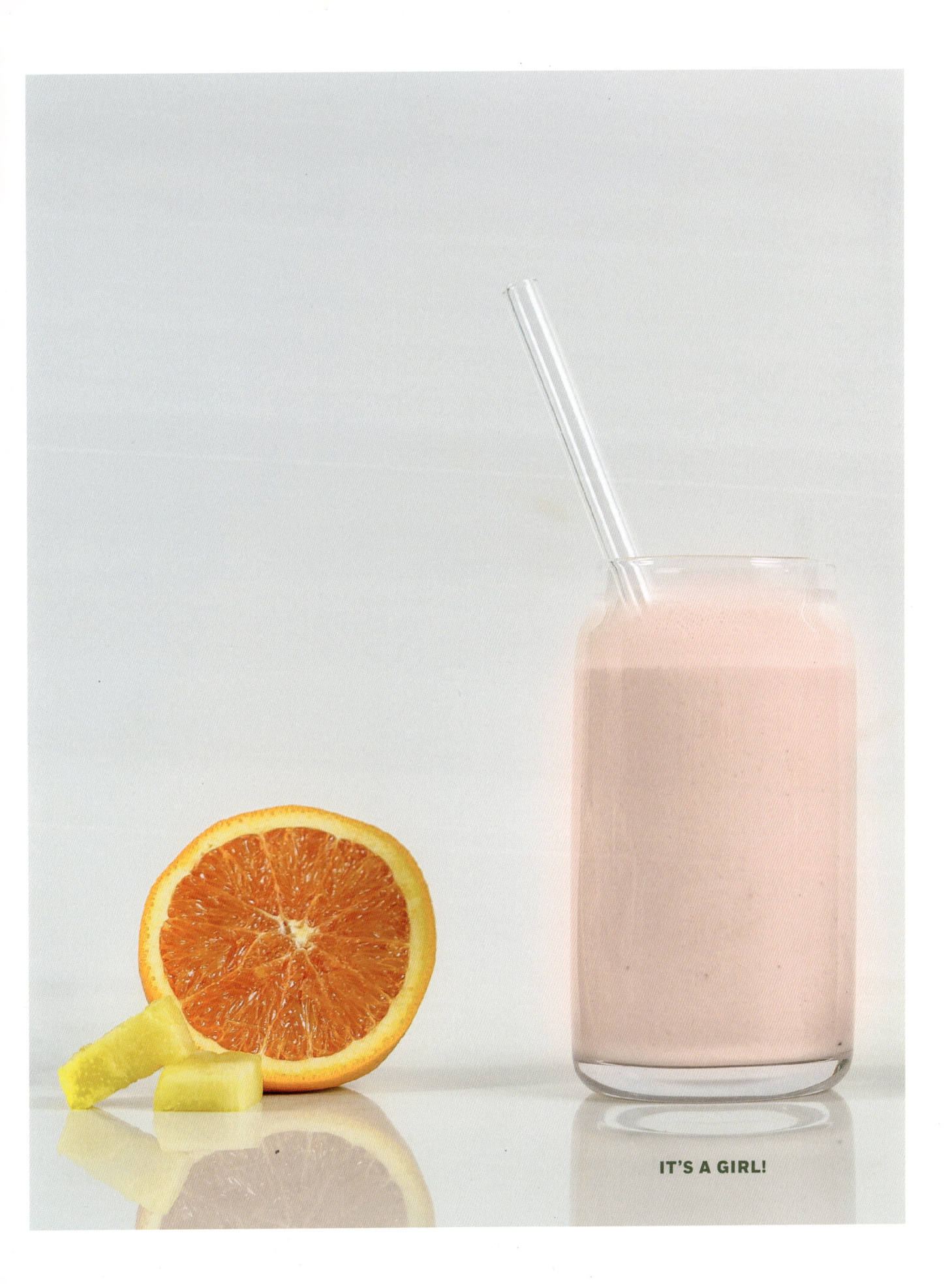

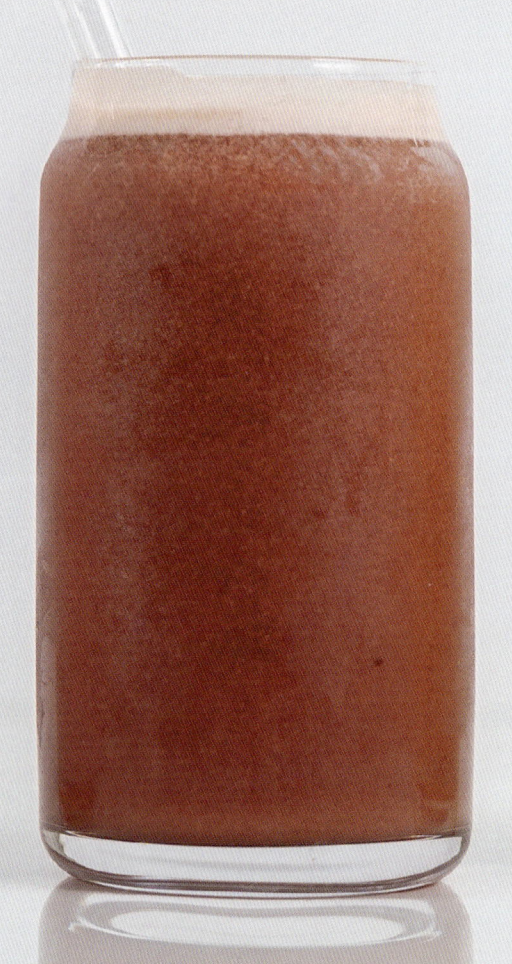

CHERRY ANTIOXIDANT   **TATA'S MORIR SOÑANDO**

Cherry Antioxidant Smoothie

SERVES 1
PREP TIME: 5 MINUTES
COOKING TIME: 0 MINUTES

¾ cup coconut water

½ cup frozen cherries

½ cup frozen pineapple

1 ½ teaspoons lime juice

½ teaspoon grated fresh ginger

Per serving: Calories: 122
Fat: 1g | Carbohydrates: 25g
Fiber: 5g | Protein: 3g

Right after giving birth, inflammation is generally at its peak as the body begins to heal in the acute recovery phase. Incorporating foods that have antioxidants and anti-inflammatory properties can aid in the recovery process. This hydrating smoothie is high in vitamin C, an antioxidant that plays a critical role during the inflammatory phase of healing. Ginger and cherries both contain other antioxidants as well.

- Place all the ingredients in a blender, and blend until smooth.

Tata's Morir Soñando

SERVES 1
PREP TIME: 5 MINUTES
COOKING TIME: 0 MINUTES

½ (12-ounce) can evaporated milk

Juice of 2 large oranges

½ cup ice

½ teaspoon agave

½ teaspoon vanilla extract

● **MAKE IT PLANT-BASED**

Use soy milk in place of the evaporated milk.

Per serving: Calories: 294
Fat: 13g | Carbohydrates: 31g
Fiber: 0g | Protein: 12g

Tata, a family friend from the Dominican Republic, introduced Diana's family to this postpartum drink. Literally translated, its name means "to die dreaming" because of its "to-die-for" flavors. It's a delicious drink often given to Dominican mothers to help boost milk production. Evaporated milk is also a great source of calcium.

- Combine all the ingredients in a blender, and blend until smooth.

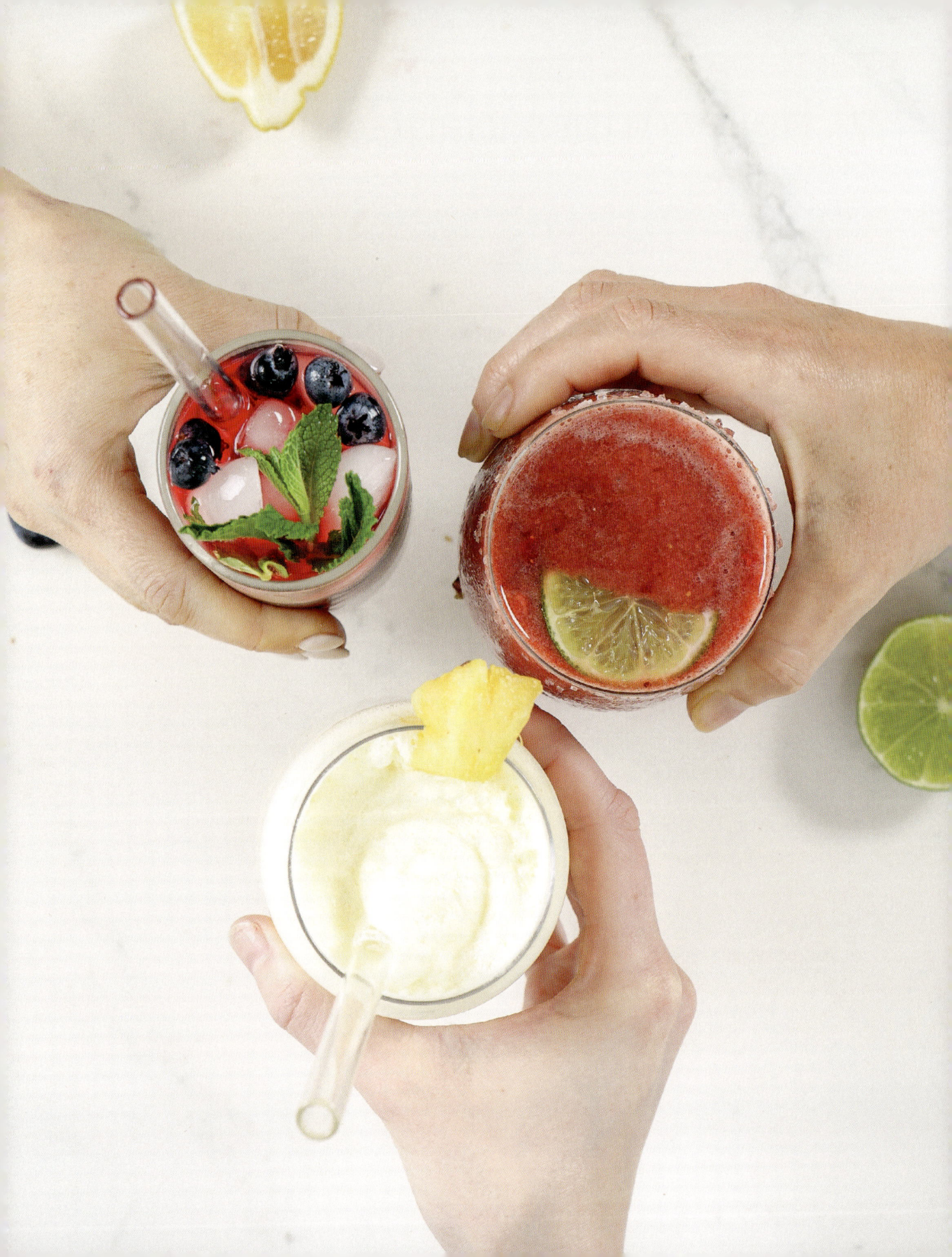

Mocktails and More

No need to just drink water while everyone else is sipping cocktails—no alcohol does not mean no enjoyment or relaxation! Shake one of these mocktails up, pour it into your favorite glass, add a straw, and sip slowly. Our mocktails are not only delicious, they also include ingredients that can be helpful during the postpartum phase. And this chapter includes more than just mocktails: we've got you covered with teas, electrolyte drinks, and other options for sipping, too.

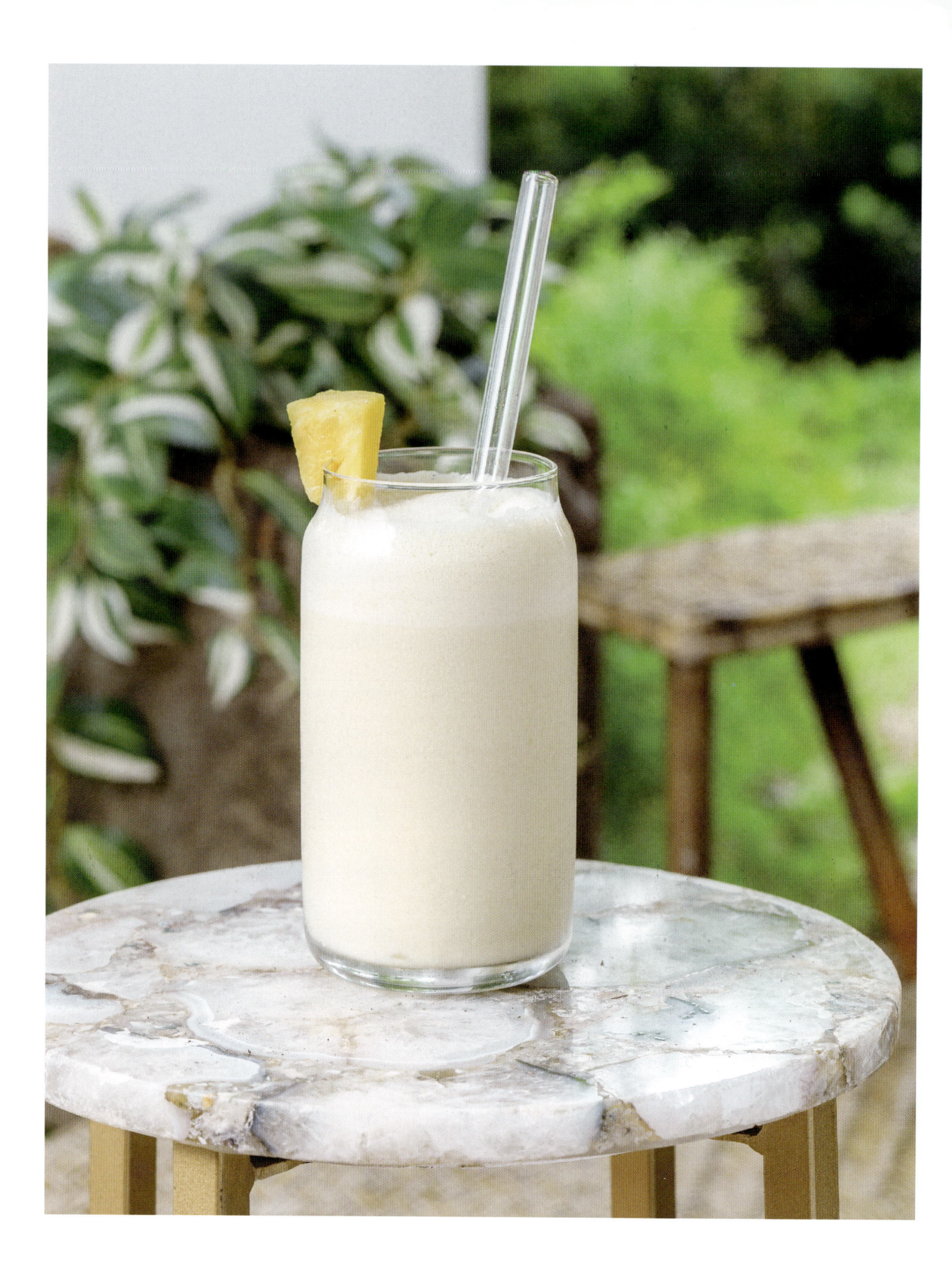

(She Ain't a) Virgin Piña Colada

SERVES 1
PREP TIME: 5 MINUTES
COOKING TIME: 0 MINUTES

1 ½ cups frozen pineapple

½ cup canned light coconut milk

1 ½ teaspoons agave

Per serving: Calories: 240
Fat: 7g | Carbohydrates: 40g
Fiber: 4g | Protein: 1g

This piña colada mocktail will make you feel like you are in the tropics and tastes much better without the rum (in our opinion). Treat yourself to a mini vacation that also provides fiber without all the added sugar of a regular piña colada.

1. Allow the pineapple to thaw for 2–3 minutes.
2. Combine all the ingredients in a blender, and blend until smooth.

NOTE: Make sure to pick the most yellow pieces of pineapple from the bag! Pale pineapple lacks flavor and sweetness.

Watermelon Lime Cooler

SERVES 1–2
PREP TIME: 5 MINUTES
COOKING TIME: 0 MINUTES

1 ½ cups frozen watermelon

1 cup seltzer

1 teaspoon lime juice

3 fresh mint leaves or 2 fresh basil leaves

Pinch of salt

Per 1-cup serving: Calories: 70
Fat: 0g | Carbohydrates: 18g
Fiber: 1g | Protein: 1g

This mocktail is incredibly refreshing and a great way to use up extra watermelon. Watermelon provides more than just water: it's also a good source of vitamin C and potassium. Potassium, along with the sodium found in salt, is one of the two main electrolytes that help to keep us hydrated.

- Combine all the ingredients in a blender, and blend until smooth.

Mama's Mule

SERVES 1
PREP TIME: 3 MINUTES
COOKING TIME: 0 MINUTES

1 cup seltzer

1 tablespoon agave

1 tablespoon fresh lime juice

1 ½ teaspoons freshly grated ginger

1 cup ice

Lime wedges for garnish, optional

Per serving: Calories: 72
Fat: 0g | Carbohydrates: 18g
Fiber: 0g | Protein: 0g

Packed with freshly grated ginger, a root known for its anti-inflammatory properties, this alcohol-free version of a Moscow mule will not only satisfy your taste buds but also support postpartum health and hydration.

1. In a cup, combine the seltzer, agave, lime juice, and ginger, and stir.

2. Strain the mixture through a fine-mesh strainer into a highball glass to remove the ginger bits.

3. Add the ice and stir again.

4. Garnish with lime wedges, if using.

Pomegranate Fizz

SERVES 1
PREP TIME: 3 MINUTES
COOKING TIME: 0 MINUTES

½ cup pomegranate juice

½ cup seltzer

3 tablespoons orange juice

1 cup ice

Per serving: Calories: 68
Fat: 0g | Carbohydrates: 16g
Fiber: 0g | Protein: 0g

This mocktail combines the antioxidant-rich goodness of pomegranate juice with the citrusy zing of orange juice for a nourishing postpartum option. Pomegranate juice is one of the most nutrient-dense juices available, providing a significant amount of potassium, vitamin C, and many antioxidants.

1. Combine the pomegranate juice, seltzer, and orange juice in a highball glass and stir.
2. Add the ice and stir again.

NOTES: If you like a tangier drink, add 1 teaspoon of apple cider vinegar.

We love the brand POM for pomegranate juice.

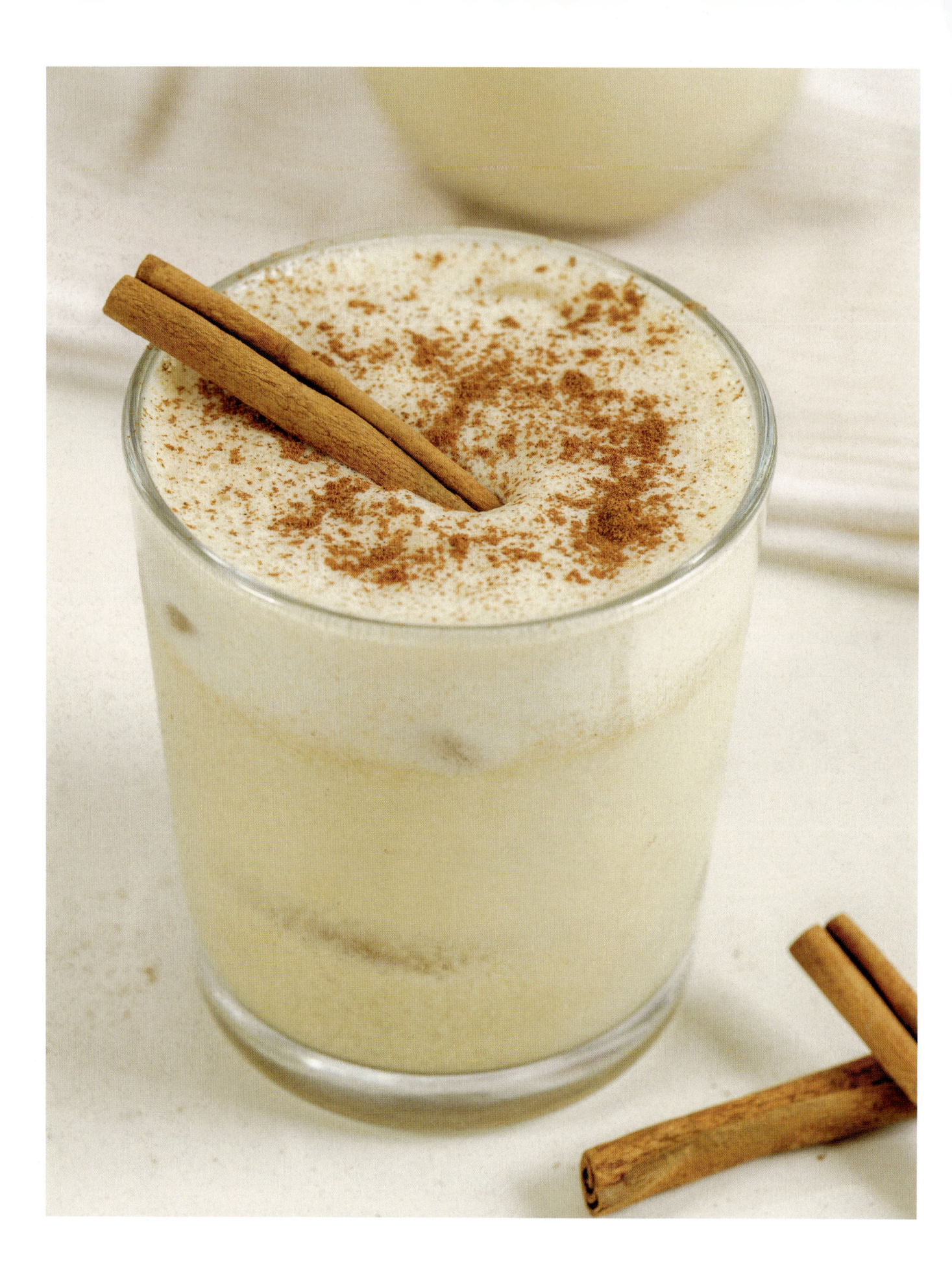

Titi Rita's Horchata

SERVES 4
PREP TIME: 5 MINUTES
COOKING TIME: 5 MINUTES

1 cup sesame seeds

4 cups unsweetened milk of choice

1 tablespoon maple syrup

½ teaspoon vanilla extract

1 teaspoon ground cinnamon

Per serving: Calories: 97
Fat: 4g | Carbohydrates: 7g
Fiber: 2g | Protein: 7g

Diana had her son in Puerto Rico, where her family is from. Her aunt always brought her horchata de ajonjli (sesame seed milk), which is commonly served to breastfeeding mothers in Puerto Rico. It's thought to promote milk production because of its high amounts of calcium, lecithin, and healthy fats.

1. Heat a large skillet over medium heat. Add the sesame seeds and toast, stirring almost constantly, for about 5 minutes.

2. Transfer the seeds to a blender or food processor and blend into a fine powder.

3. Add the milk and blend until smooth. Strain the blended sesame mixture into a pitcher using a fine-mesh strainer. Use the back of a spoon to press the liquid through the strainer.

4. Stir in the remaining ingredients and chill in the refrigerator until ready to serve.

NOTES: The contents of this recipe may separate, so shake well before using.

This goes great in coffee!

Frozen Strawberry-Lime Mock-a-Rita

SERVES 1
PREP TIME: 3 MINUTES
COOKING TIME: 0 MINUTES

1 cup frozen strawberries

½ cup water

Juice of 1 lime

1 tablespoon agave

⅛ teaspoon salt

Per serving: Calories: 119
Fat: 1g | Carbohydrates: 27g
Fiber: 3g | Protein: 1g

We improved the nutrient profile found in traditional frozen margaritas with this healthier, alcohol-free version. The strawberries and lime provide fiber and a healthy dose of vitamin C—both important postpartum nutrients.

- Combine all the ingredients in a blender, and blend until smooth.

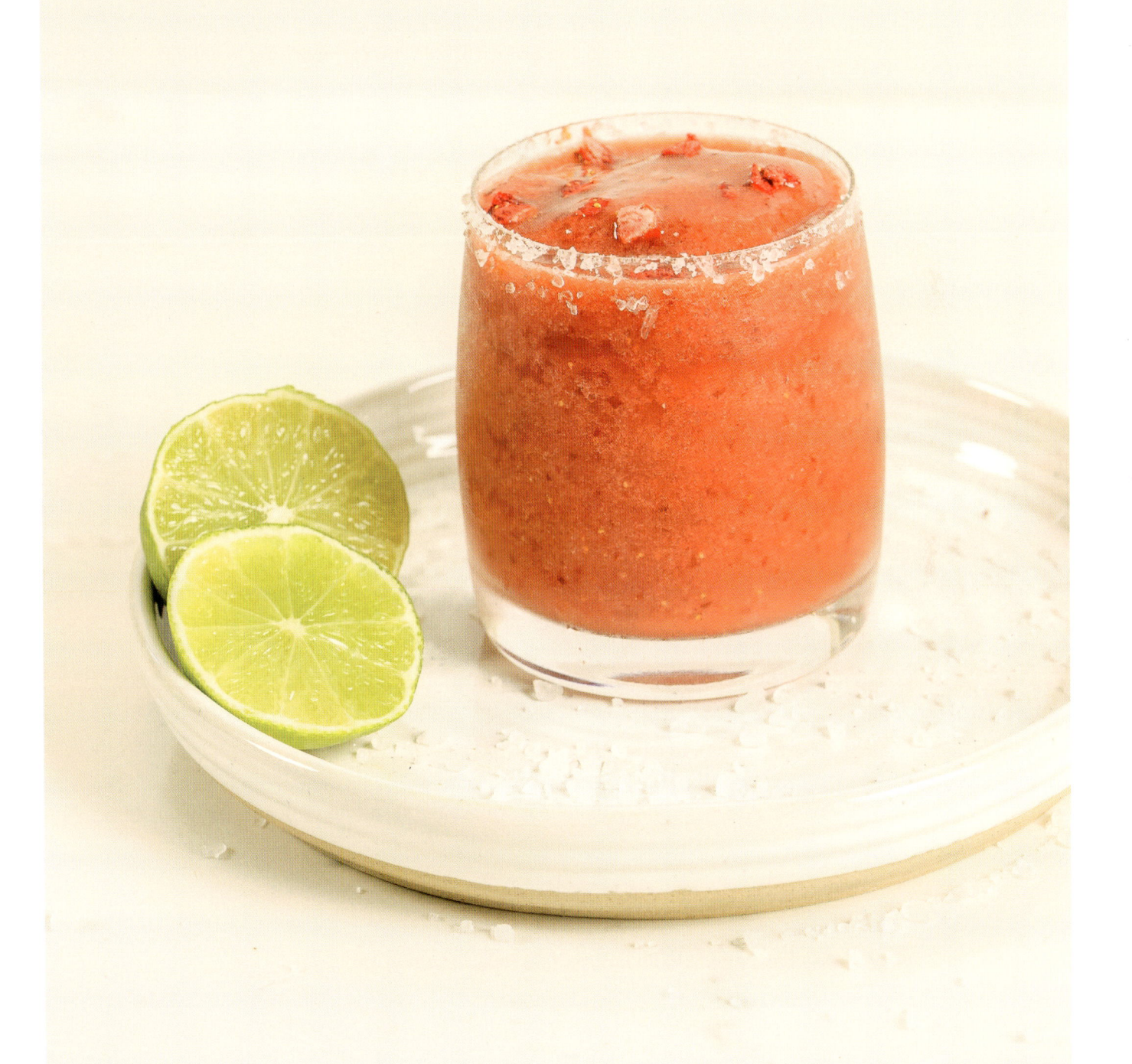

Electrolyte Replenisher

SERVES 1
PREP TIME: 5 MINUTES
COOKING TIME: 0 MINUTES

½ cup coconut water

¼ cup potassium-rich juice (such as pomegranate, orange, or pineapple juice)

1 ½ teaspoons lemon juice

⅛ teaspoon salt

½ cup seltzer

Per serving: Calories: 58
Fat: 0g | Carbohydrates: 12g
Fiber: 1g | Protein: 1g

Electrolytes are minerals such as sodium, potassium, and magnesium that help regulate bodily functions, including balancing the amount of water in the body. Skip the Gatorade and make your own nutritious electrolyte drink instead. By combining coconut water, a potassium-rich juice, and a pinch of salt, you can easily get in enough electrolytes with this drink.

1. In a shaker full of ice, combine the coconut water, juice, lemon juice, and salt. Shake.

2. Pour into a highball glass full of ice. Top with the seltzer. Stir.

Brewed Fennel Tea

SERVES 1
PREP TIME: 0 MINUTES
COOKING TIME: 10 MINUTES

1 cup boiling water

2 tablespoons fennel seed

Per serving: Calories: 0
Fat: 0 | Carbs: 0
Fiber: 0 | Protein: 0

Diana's son's nanny from Colombia recommended this drink after Mateo was born, as drinking fennel tea is encouraged to increase milk supply in many cultures. A compound found in fennel, anethol, may increase the level of prolactin, the hormone responsible for milk production.

- Combine the ingredients and allow to steep for 10 minutes. Remove the seeds. Serve hot or cold.

Sassy Spritzer

SERVES 1
PREP TIME: 3 MINUTES
COOKING TIME: 0 MINUTES

⅔ cup seltzer, flavor of choice

½ cup kombucha, flavor of choice

1 teaspoon lemon juice

Fresh mint leaves for garnish, optional

Per serving: Calories: 13
Fat: 0g | Carbohydrates: 3g
Fiber: 0g | Protein: 0g

This refreshing beverage was inspired by our friend Laura at The Sassy Dietitian. This simple but "sassy" mocktail combines the benefits of probiotic-rich kombucha with seltzer water to offer a hydrating option that supports digestive health during the postpartum phase.

1. Fill a wineglass with ice. Combine all the ingredients in the ice-filled glass.

2. Stir and garnish with mint leaves, if desired.

Summer Shandy

SERVES 1
PREP TIME: 3 MINUTES
COOKING TIME: 0 MINUTES

1 handful of ice

½ cup coconut water

2 tablespoons lemon juice

1 ½ teaspoons agave

½ (12-ounce) can nonalcoholic beer

Lemon slices for garnish, optional

Per serving: Calories: 97
Fat: 0g | Carbohydrates: 21g
Fiber: 1g | Protein: 1g

The combination of nonalcoholic beer, coconut water, fresh lemon juice, and a touch of agave nectar delivers the taste of a summer shandy without the booze. This mocktail is a refreshing and hydrating option, especially during those hot summer days.

1. Combine all the ingredients except the beer in a cocktail shaker.

2. Shake well and strain into a highball glass.

3. Top with the beer and stir.

4. Garnish with lemon slices, if using.

NOTE: We love the brand Athletic Brewing for nonalcoholic beers.

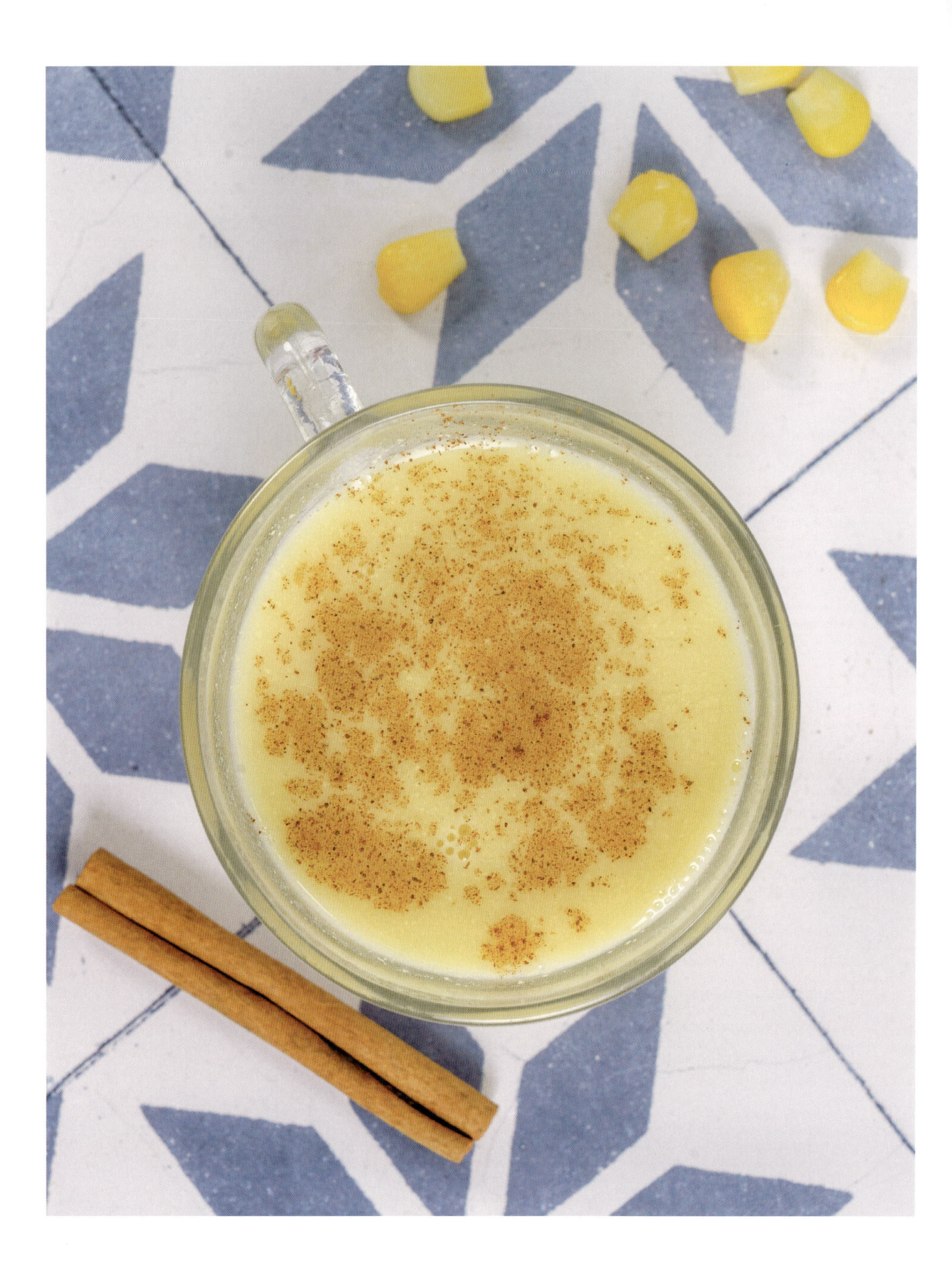

Mexican Atole

SERVES 3
PREP TIME: 5 MINUTES
COOKING TIME: 25 MINUTES

1 cup frozen or fresh corn

2 cups unsweetened milk of choice, divided

1 cup water

1 cinnamon stick

2 tablespoons agave

1 teaspoon vanilla extract

1 tablespoon cornstarch

Ground cinnamon, for garnish

Per serving: Calories: 148
Fat: 4g | Carbohydrates: 18g
Fiber: 2g | Protein: 7g

Atole is a common beverage in Mexican cuisine made from corn. Postpartum Mexican moms have traditionally turned to atole as a way to support their milk supply, since this creamy drink is energy- and nutrient-dense.

1. Combine the corn and 1 cup of milk in a blender, and blend until smooth.

2. In a medium pot or saucepan, bring the water to a simmer over medium-low heat. Add the cinnamon stick and simmer for 3 minutes. Add the agave and stir until fully dissolved.

3. Strain the corn mixture into the pot through a fine-mesh strainer. Stir in ½ cup of milk and the vanilla extract. Continue to gently simmer the atole mixture for 5 minutes, stirring continuously.

4. Make a cornstarch slurry by whisking together the cornstarch with the remaining ½ cup milk until fully combined. Slowly pour it into the pot while whisking.

5. Gently simmer the atole for 10–15 minutes to allow the mixture to thicken.

6. Remove the cinnamon stick before serving.

7. Top with ground cinnamon, if desired.

NOTE: This is also often made with oats for extra potential milk-boosting benefits! Just swap the corn for an equal amount of oats.

Smooth Move Mocktail

SERVES 1
PREP TIME: 3 MINUTES
COOKING TIME: 0 MINUTES

4 ounces apple juice

1 tablespoon chia seeds

1 tablespoon lemon juice

4–8 ounces flavored seltzer of choice

Per serving: Calories: 114
Fat: 4g | Carbohydrates: 15g
Fiber: 4g | Protein: 2g

Sorbitol, a natural sugar alcohol found in apple juice, acts as a gentle laxative, promoting digestive regularity, while the soluble fiber content in chia seeds contributes to overall digestive health. This mocktail is perfect to combat constipation—a common issue during those early postpartum days.

1. In a highball glass, combine the apple juice, chia seeds, and lemon juice. Mix well and let sit for at least 15 minutes, or until the seeds have formed a gel-like consistency.

2. Add the seltzer and stir.

NOTE: You can make a big batch of the juice-chia base and let it sit in the fridge. When you're ready to drink it, top it with the seltzer.

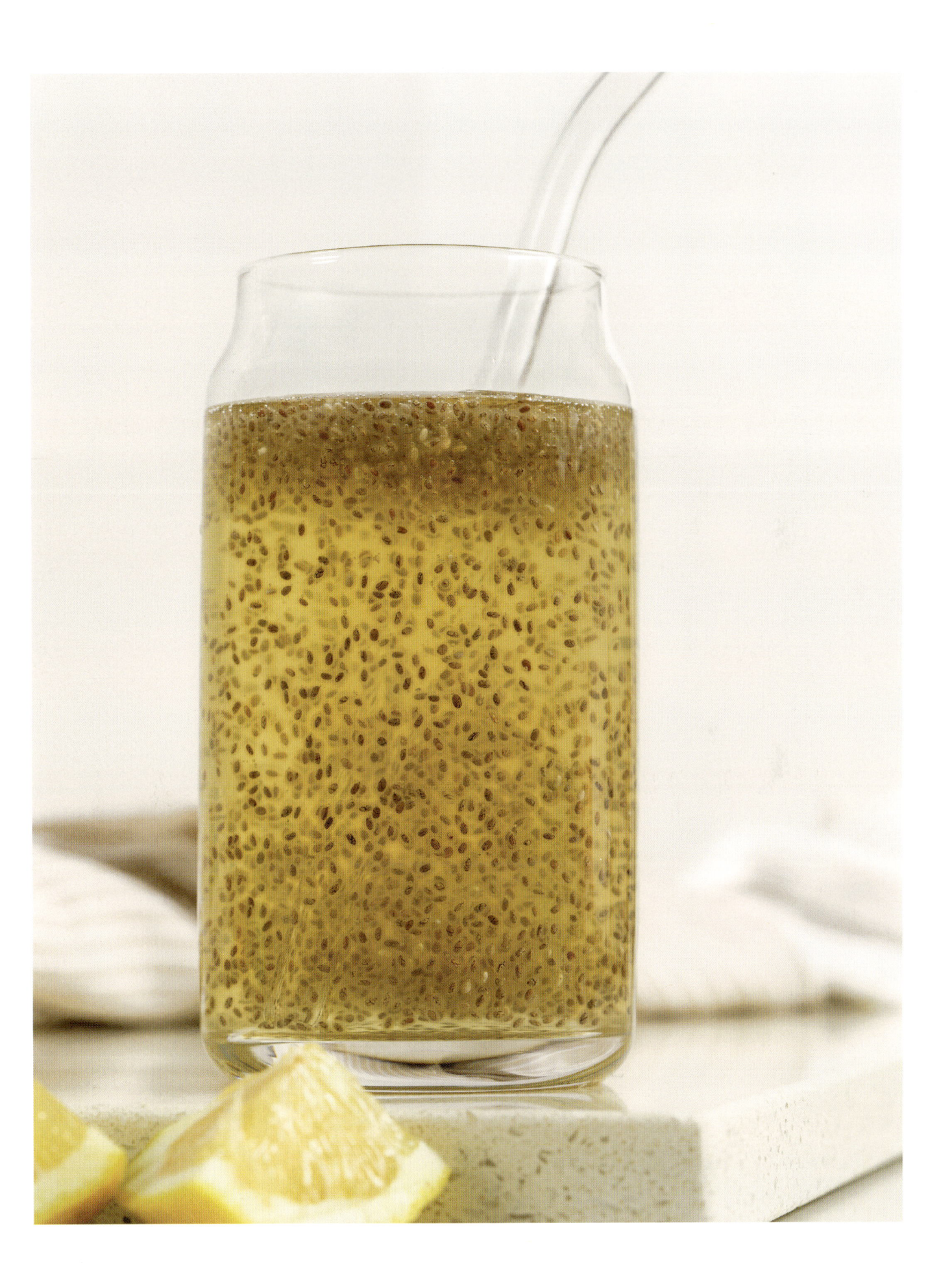

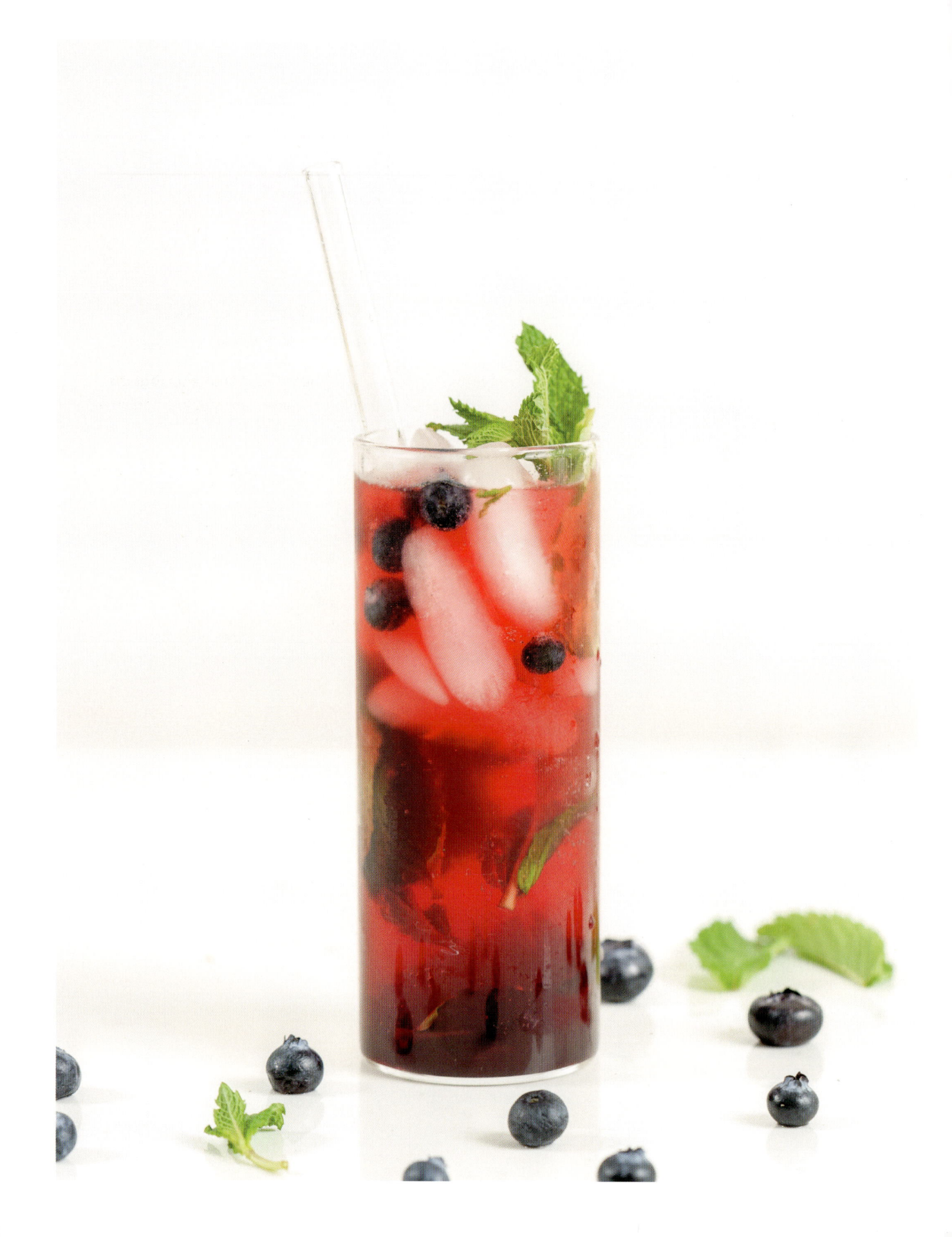

Berry Nojito

SERVES 1
PREP TIME: 3 MINUTES
COOKING TIME: 0 MINUTES

¼ cup blueberries, fresh or frozen (see Notes)

5 large fresh mint leaves

1 teaspoon agave

1 teaspoon lime juice

½–1 cup ice

½ (6-ounce) can lime or regular seltzer

Per serving: Calories: 30
Fat: 0g | Carbohydrates: 8g
Fiber: 1g | Protein: 0g

Enjoy this berry mojito-inspired mocktail on the couch after your baby goes to bed, or sip it while getting some time outdoors. It's the perfect opportunity to meet your hydration needs while taking a few minutes for yourself.

1. In the bottom of a highball glass, combine the blueberries, mint leaves, agave, and lime juice.

2. With a fork or muddler, mash the ingredients together until the berries begin to break down and you can smell the aroma of the mint.

3. Fill the glass with ice and pour seltzer over the top. Stir.

NOTES: For a tangier drink, add ¼ teaspoon of apple cider vinegar.

If using frozen blueberries, let the blueberries thaw in the cup that you intend to use (to capture the juices).

Nana's Aynar Spiced Tea

SERVES 4
PREP TIME: 2 MINUTES
COOKING TIME: 45 MINUTES

6 cups water

2 cinnamon sticks

1 tablespoon anise seeds

1 teaspoon caraway seeds

⅛ teaspoon ground nutmeg

¼ cup honey

½ cup assorted nuts (such as pine nuts, chopped walnuts, and slivered almonds)

Per serving: Calories: 160
Fat: 10g | Carbohydrates: 18g
Fiber: 1g | Protein: 2g

This recipe was inspired by Diana's mother-in-law, who has Lebanese roots. Aynar spiced tea is often referred to as "post-pregnancy tea" in Lebanon and is drunk in celebration of the baby. Assorted spices, honey, and nuts give the tea a sweet kick, while the anise seed is supposed to soothe moms and help their bodies recover.

1. In a medium saucepan, heat the water over high heat. Add the cinnamon sticks, anise seeds, caraway seeds, and nutmeg, and bring to a boil.

2. Cover and simmer for at least 45 minutes, or until it's flavored strongly enough.

3. Whisk in the honey and simmer until it's dissolved. Remove from the heat and strain through a fine-mesh sieve. Discard the spices.

4. Place one-quarter of the chopped nuts in the bottom of each teacup. Pour in the hot tea and serve.

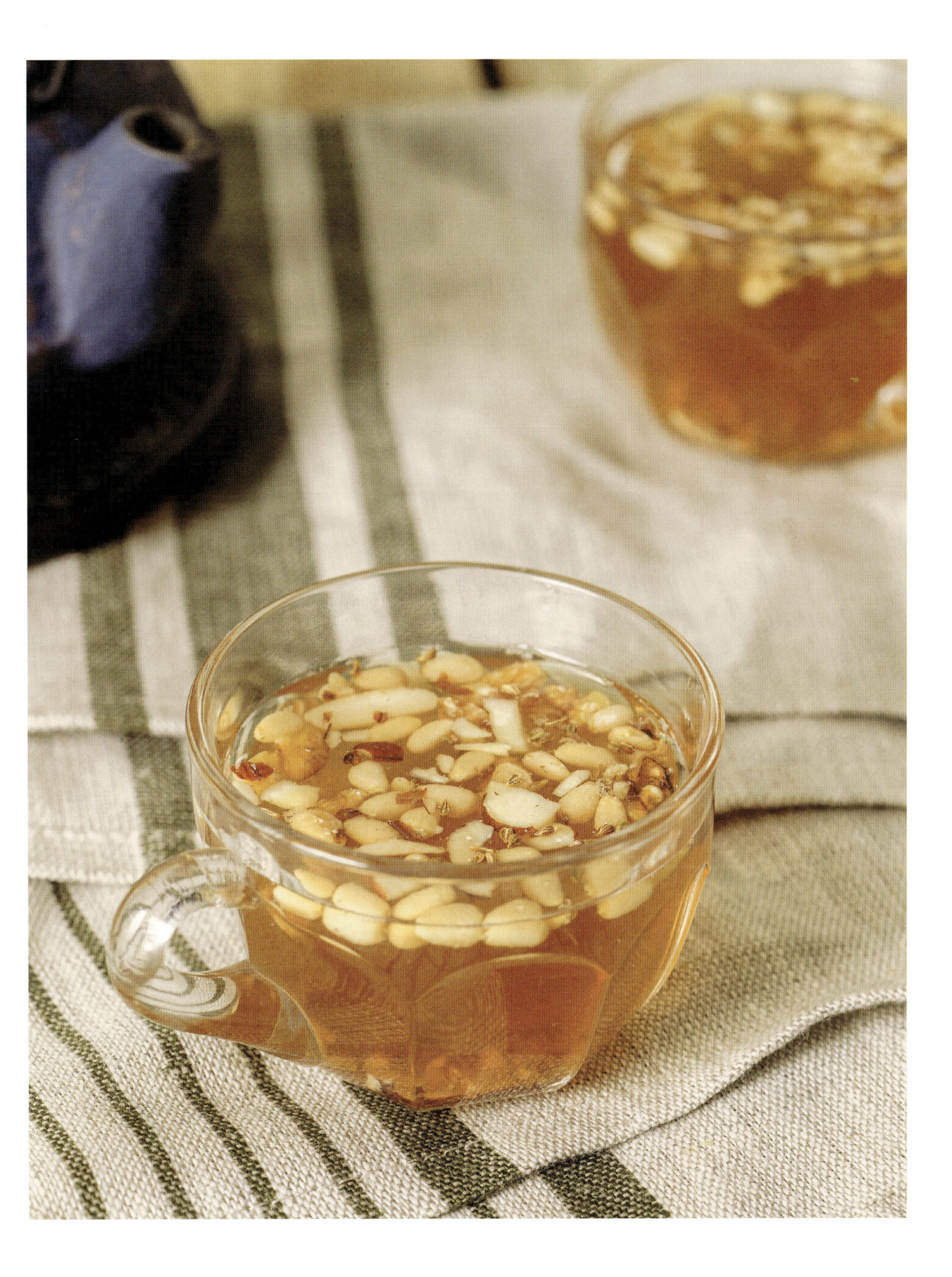

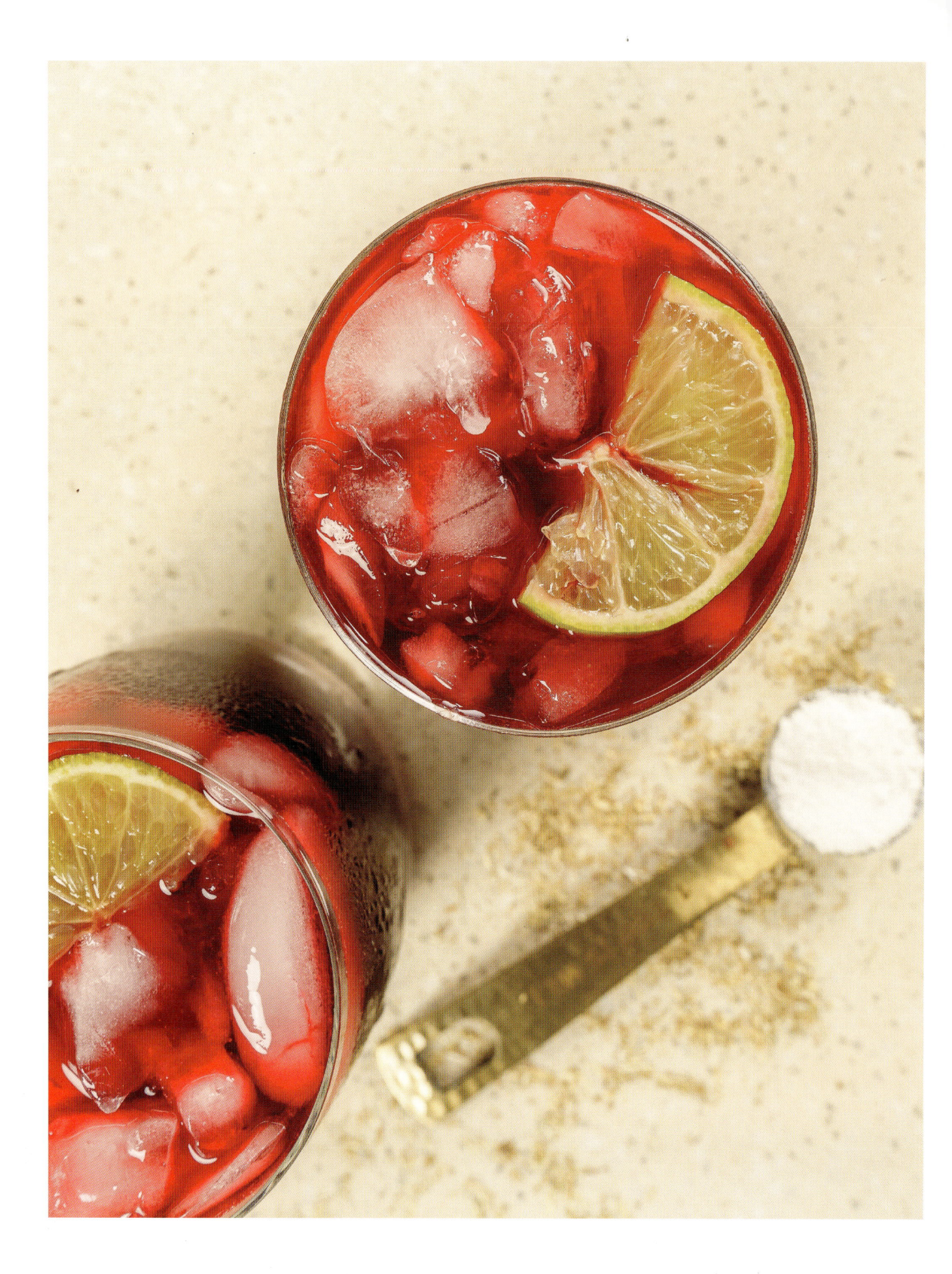

Abu's Sleepy Time Mocktail

SERVES 1
PREP TIME: 3 MINUTES
COOKING TIME: 0 MINUTES

1 cup brewed and cooled chamomile tea

½ cup pure tart cherry juice

Squeeze of lime juice

1 teaspoon magnesium powder

Per serving: Calories: 66
Fat: 0g | Carbohydrates: 16g
Fiber: 0g | Protein: 1g

Chamomile has a mild sedative effect believed to be caused by a compound called apigenin. Coupled with tart cherry juice, which may elevate melatonin levels, and magnesium, a mineral linked to relaxation of the muscles, this tea will have you sleep like a baby... until yours wakes up, anyway.

- Fill a highball glass with ice. Add all the ingredients and stir well.

NOTE: Hibiscus tea would also work well in place of the chamomile but should not be consumed during pregnancy.

APPENDIX I

Prepping Your Postpartum Freezer

We hope this resource helps you feel like you *can* stock your freezer to fuel your recovery. This guide includes a three-day cooking breakdown to help you make up to nineteen freezer meals, complete with grocery lists, needed equipment, and step-by-step instructions. We've included two separate plans: one for omnivore moms and one for plant-based moms.

You can execute either of these cooking plans over three consecutive days or space your cooking days out with one per week during the weeks leading up to your due date. Even better, recruit friends or family members to cook through these plans with you. The hands-on work should take no more than three hours each day.

These meals will last in the freezer for up to six months, but we recommend having them within three months of preparation, so don't get started on cooking too early. Once you've prepared them, you can use these freezer meals as part of our First-Week-Home Meal Plan (page 260).

Omnivore Cooking Plan

DAY 1	DAY 2	DAY 3
STOVE: Mom's Spaghetti Sauce (page 60) Egg Breakfast Burritos (page 84) **OVEN:** BeaBea's Lasagna (page 62) Ma! The Meatloaf! (page 67) **INSTANT POT:** Shredded Chicken (page 79) Ironclad Beef Stew (page 74)	**STOVE:** Mushroom Black Bean Burgers (page 81) Creamy Enchilada Casserole (page 69) Mediterranean Turkey Burgers (page 82) **OVEN:** Mighty Miles's Meatballs: Beef (page 77) Mighty Miles's Meatballs: Chicken (page 77) Mighty Miles's Meatballs: Pork (page 77) **INSTANT POT:** Shredded Beef (page 79)	**STOVE:** Life-Giving Lentil Soup (page 73) White Bean Chicken Chili (page 70) **OVEN:** Apple Cider Oatmeal Bread (page 92) Maple Pistachio Oatmeal Muffins (page 89) **INSTANT POT:** Shredded Pork (page 79) Homemade Chicken Broth (page 65)

Day 1

SHOPPING LIST

Meat and Dairy

12 eggs

4 pounds ground beef or ancestral blend

2 pounds beef stew meat, chuck roast, or round roast

2 pounds boneless, skinless chicken thighs

2 (6-ounce) bags shredded mozzarella cheese

1 (64-ounce) carton unsweetened milk of choice

Produce

3 large onions

4 celery stalks

5 large carrots

3 large russet potatoes

1 head garlic

2 bell peppers

8 ounces mushrooms

4 cups fresh spinach

Dried Herbs and Spices

Bay leaves

Black pepper

Dried thyme

Garlic powder

Salt

Condiments and Baking Needs

Spreadable sauce (our favorites: Bitchin' sauce, guacamole crema, chimichurri)

BBQ sauce

Cornstarch

Olive oil

Beans and Other Canned Goods

1 (28-ounce) can diced tomatoes

1 (28-ounce) jar marinara sauce

2 (15-ounce) cans black beans

1 (16-ounce) jar salsa

1 cup chicken, beef, or vegetable broth

Whole Grains and Pastas

Bread

Tortillas, flour or whole-wheat (10-inch)

1 (16-ounce) box lasagna noodles

COOKING PLAN

Cut all the vegetables:

- Dice 3 onions
- Dice 2 bell peppers
- Dice 4 celery stalks
- Peel and cut 5 carrots into half-moons
- Slice 8 ounces mushrooms
- Dice 3 russet potatoes into cubes
- Finely dice 8 cloves garlic

Make **Mom's Spaghetti Sauce** on the stovetop.

While the sauce is simmering, bring a separate pot of water up to a boil and cook the lasagna noodles.

While the pasta is cooking, add the chicken thighs to an Instant Pot for **Shredded Chicken**. Following the recipe, cook for 10 minutes with a 5-minute natural release.

Preheat the oven to 350°F.

Mix together the **Ma! The Meatloaf!** ingredients and assemble into pans. When the lasagna noodles are finished boiling, assemble **BeaBea's Lasagna**. Place the lasagna and meatloaf pans on baking sheets and bake for 45–50 minutes. Remove from the oven and let them completely cool before freezing.

Remove the chicken from the Instant Pot and shred. Allow to completely cool before storing and freezing.

Rinse the Instant Pot and assemble the **Ironclad Beef Stew**. Cook for 45 minutes under high pressure and allow a 15–20 minute natural release.

While the beef stew is cooking, scramble the eggs for **Egg Breakfast Burritos**. Allow the eggs to cool completely before assembling the burritos according to the recipe. Wrap them in foil and store in a labeled bag.

When the beef stew is finished cooking, stir in the cornstarch mixture and allow to sit for 5–10 minutes. Transfer to a storage container and allow to completely cool before freezing.

Celebrate! You've just prepped 6 recipes and 48 servings of food! Go put your feet up, knowing you have enough food to at least get you through the first week home.

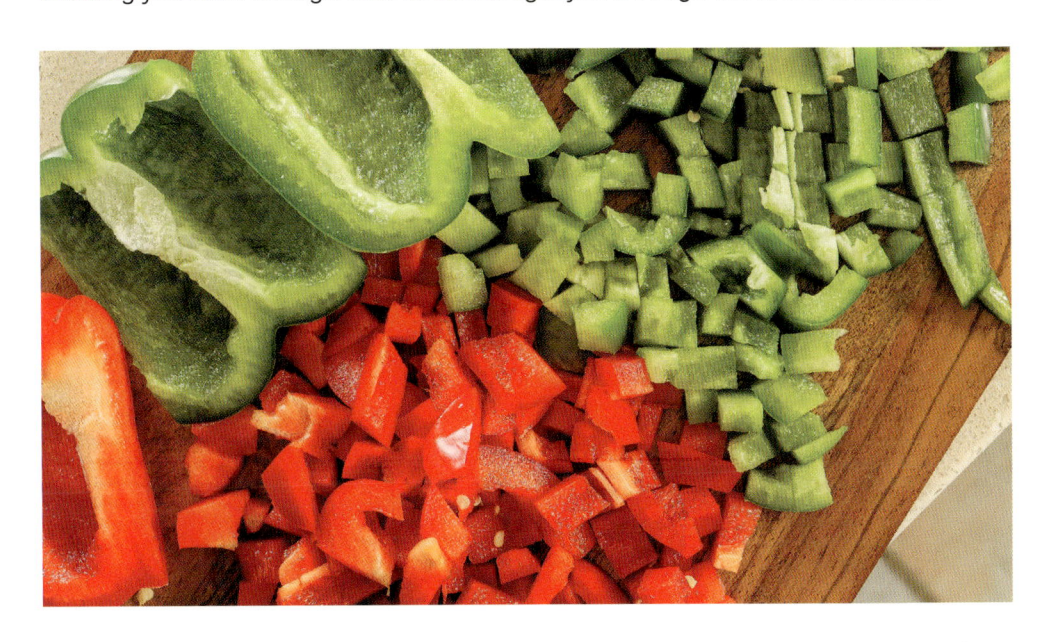

Day 2

SHOPPING LIST

Meat and Dairy

2 eggs

2 pounds ground pork

2 pounds ground chicken

2 pounds ground beef or ancestral blend

2 pounds ground turkey

1 (16-ounce) container cottage cheese

1 (6-ounce) package cheddar or Monterey Jack shredded cheese

4 ounces feta cheese

3 cups unsweetened milk of choice

Produce

4 onions

2 heads garlic

8 ounces mushrooms

1 bell pepper

4 cups any dark leafy greens

2 limes

1 bunch cilantro

Dried Herbs and Spices

Ground cumin

Garlic powder

Olive oil

Onion powder

Pepper

Red pepper flakes

Salt

Condiments and Baking Needs

Ketchup or mayonnaise

Beans and Other Canned Goods

2 (15-ounce) cans black beans

2 (15.5-ounce) cans pinto, black, or kidney beans

1 small jar sun-dried tomatoes

1 (15-ounce) jar enchilada sauce

Nuts and Seeds

Ground flaxseed

Whole Grains and Pastas

White bread

Corn tortillas (6-inch)

Frozen

Frozen spinach

COOKING PLAN

Prepare the **Shredded Beef** recipe in an Instant Pot. Cook under high pressure for 45 minutes and allow a 20-minute natural release.

While the beef cooks, prepare the vegetables for **Mushroom Black Bean Burgers**, **Mediterranean Turkey Burgers**, and **Creamy Enchilada Casserole**:

- Dice 2 onions
- Roughly chop 2 onions
- Dice 1 bell pepper
- Chop 8 ounces mushrooms
- Chop 12 sun-dried tomatoes
- Separate and remove skins from 2 heads garlic

Preheat the oven to 375°F.

On the stovetop, prepare the filling for the **Creamy Enchilada Casserole**. Assemble and bake for 20 minutes.

Prepare the **Mushroom Black Bean Burgers** and arrange on a baking sheet. Prepare the **Mediterranean Turkey Burgers** and arrange on another baking sheet. Add both burgers to the oven when the **Creamy Enchilada Casserole** is finished cooking.

To prepare all three **Mighty Miles's Meatballs** recipes: Combine 6 slices of torn white bread, 3 cups of milk, 1 ½ diced onions, 18 cloves of garlic, 3 teaspoons of salt, and 3 teaspoons of pepper in a blender. Blend until pureed.

Divide the mixture evenly among 3 bowls. Add the meat and specific seasonings for the beef, chicken, and pork variations to each bowl. Mix the meatballs and roll into 32 balls for each variation. Place on two to three lined baking sheets.

When the burgers are finished cooking, reduce the oven temperature to 350°F. Bake the meatballs for 25 minutes, or until the internal temperature reaches 165°F. If making in the air fryer, fry in small batches until all the meatballs have been cooked.

Allow all the recipes to cool before freezing in airtight containers.

Another day is done, and you have at least 50 more servings ready for the freezer! Mix up a mocktail and relax.

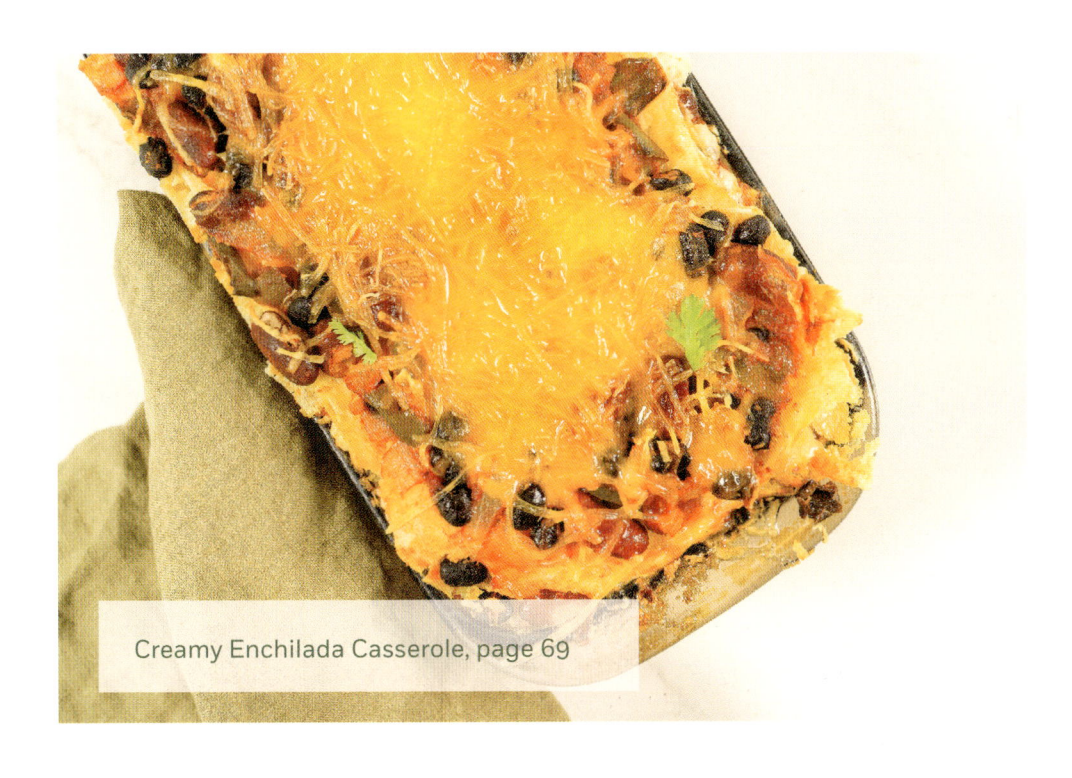

Creamy Enchilada Casserole, page 69

Day 3

SHOPPING LIST

Meat and Dairy

5 eggs

4 chicken backs or 1 turkey back

2 pounds pork butt or shoulder roast

1 pound boneless, skinless chicken thighs

1 (64-ounce) carton unsweetened milk of choice

Produce

1 apple

7 carrots

6 celery stalks

2 large onions

1 head garlic

1 medium yellow onion

1 large red onion

3 cups spinach

1 lemon

1 lime

1 cup apple cider

Dried Herbs and Spices

Bay leaves

Black pepper

Ground cinnamon

Chili powder

Cumin

Dried thyme

Ground ginger

Nutmeg

Paprika

Condiments and Baking Needs

Baking soda

Baking powder

Maple syrup

Olive or vegetable oil

Vanilla extract

Beans and Other Canned Goods

1 (14-ounce) can fire-roasted crushed tomatoes

1 (4-ounce) can green chiles

2 (32-ounce) cartons chicken or vegetable broth

2 (15.5-ounce) cans white beans

Dried brown or black lentils

Nuts and Seeds

Chia seeds

Pistachios

Chopped pecans

Whole Grains and Pastas

Rolled oats

Whole-wheat flour

Frozen

Frozen corn

COOKING PLAN

Make the **Maple Pistachio Oatmeal Muffins,** following the recipe. While it is soaking, prepare the oatmeal for the **Apple Cider Oatmeal Bread**. Allow the oatmeal to cool completely (about 10 minutes) before mixing with the remainder of the ingredients. While waiting, dice the apples into small pieces.

Preheat the oven to 350°F. Assemble the **Apple Cider Oatmeal Bread** in a baking dish. After the **Maple Pistachio Oatmeal Muffin** mixture has soaked for 25 minutes, pour it into a muffin tin. Bake the oatmeal cups for 20 minutes and the bread for 50 minutes. Set an alarm and be mindful of their baking times!

Cut the pork into 2-inch cubes for **Shredded Pork**. Place in an Instant Pot with 1 teaspoon salt and ½ cup water. Cook under high pressure for 28 minutes and allow a 15-minute natural release.

While the pork is cooking, chop the vegetables for **Life-Giving Lentil Soup** and **White Bean Chicken Chili**:

- Dice 1 large red onion
- Dice 1 medium yellow onion
- Mince 5 garlic cloves
- Chop 1 large carrot
- Chop 2 celery stalks

In a large pot, begin the **Life-Giving Lentil Soup** recipe. While it is simmering, dice the chicken thighs into 1-inch pieces and begin making the **White Bean Chicken Chili** recipe.

Once cooked, allow the soups to cool completely before freezing in airtight containers such as silicone soup cubes, ziplock or reusable silicone bags, or freezer-safe glass jars.

When the pork has finished its natural release, shred and remove it from the Instant Pot. Allow to cool completely before freezing.

Roughly chop the vegetables for the **Homemade Chicken Broth**. Rinse the Instant Pot and assemble the chicken broth ingredients in it. Select the slow cooker function and cook for 20 hours.

Once the oatmeal cups have completely cooled, store in an airtight container and freeze. The apple bread can either be frozen whole or cut into individual servings. Store in an airtight container and freeze.

When the broth has finished cooking the next day, allow it to cool slightly so it can be handled. Place a colander over a large bowl. Pour the broth into the colander to catch large pieces and discard. Allow the broth to cool completely before portioning it into containers for the freezer. Be sure to leave space at the top of the containers, as the broth will expand by roughly 10% when frozen.

CONGRATS! You have now fully stocked your freezer for your postpartum recovery! You've made over 125 servings of food to help ensure your body has the fuel it needs to heal and breastfeed.

Plant-Based Cooking Plan

DAY 1	DAY 2	DAY 3
STOVE: Lentil Spaghetti Sauce (page 61) Vegan Breakfast Burritos (page 87) White Bean Chicken Chili (page 70) **OVEN:** BeaBea's Lasagna (page 62) Butternut Squash Soup (page 161) **INSTANT POT:** Homemade Vegetable Broth (page 66)	**STOVE:** Life-Giving Lentil Soup (page 73) Sopa de Nopalitos (page 191) **OVEN:** Mushroom Black Bean Burgers (page 81) Eggless "Egg" Cups (page 96) Creamy Enchilada Casserole (page 69) **INSTANT POT:** 3-Bean Chili (page 150)	**STOVE:** Mateo's Minestrone (page 146) **OVEN:** Maple Pistachio Oatmeal Muffins (page 89) Baked Blueberry Oatmeal (page 107) Apple Cider Oatmeal Bread (page 92)

Day 1

SHOPPING LIST

Soy and Non-Dairy

2 (6-ounce) bags shredded vegan mozzarella cheese

1 (15-ounce) block extra-firm tofu

Produce

12 medium carrots

4 medium tomatoes

5 large yellow onions

6 celery stalks

2 red bell peppers

2 heads garlic

4 cups kale or spinach

1 large red onion

1 butternut, acorn, or kabocha squash or one (12-ounce) container peeled and cut squash

1 lime

1 cup mushrooms

1-inch fresh ginger

1-inch fresh turmeric

Dried Herbs and Spices

Black pepper

Chili powder

Cumin

Nutritional yeast

Red pepper flakes

Salt

1 cup dried shiitake mushrooms

Condiments and Baking Needs

Olive oil

Beans and Other Canned Goods

3 (32-ounce) cartons vegetable broth

3 (15.5-ounce) cans white beans

1 (15.5-ounce) can black beans

1 (15.5-ounce) can cannellini beans

1 (6-ounce) can tomato paste

1 (4-ounce) can green chiles

1 pound dried red lentils

1 jar salsa

Miso paste

Nuts and Seeds

Hemp seeds

Whole Grains and Pastas

Tortillas, flour or whole-wheat (10-inch)

1 (16-ounce) box lasagna noodles

Frozen

Frozen corn

COOKING PLAN

Cut all the vegetables:

- Mince or chop 10 garlic cloves
- Dice 2 ½ onions
- Peel and halve 1 onion
- Finely dice 1 ½ cups carrots
- Peel 4 carrots and remove tops
- Dice 4 medium tomatoes, reserving juices
- Dice 1 cup mushrooms
- Halve 1 butternut, acorn, or kabocha squash and remove seeds
- Cut off entire top of 1 head of garlic
- Halve 2 red bell peppers

Follow the instructions for the **Homemade Vegetable Broth** recipe and set in an Instant Pot for 20 hours.

Preheat the oven to 350°F.

Make **Lentil Spaghetti Sauce** on the stovetop.

While the sauce is simmering, bring a separate pot of water up to a boil and cook the lasagna noodles.

When the lasagna noodles are finished boiling, assemble **BeaBea's Lasagna** and set aside.

Follow the instructions for the **Butternut Squash Soup** by placing all the ingredients onto a sheet pan.

Place the lasagna and squash soup ingredients in the oven and bake for 40–45 minutes. Remove from the oven and let both completely cool.

While the lasagna and soup ingredients are cooking, drain and press the tofu for the **Vegan Breakfast Burritos**. Follow the recipe, then wrap the burritos in foil and store in a labeled bag.

Follow the recipe for the **White Bean Chicken Chili**, but replace the chicken with an extra can of white beans. Allow to cool before pouring into containers and freezing.

Once the lasagna has cooled completely, wrap in foil and freeze. Once the squash soup ingredients have cooled, transfer to a blender, and blend until creamy. Transfer to storage containers and freeze.

Celebrate! You've just prepped 6 recipes and 30 servings of food! Go put your feet up, knowing you've got enough food to at least get you through the first week home.

Day 2

SHOPPING LIST

Soy and Non-Dairy

1 (6-ounce) bag vegan shredded cheese

1 (15-ounce) block extra-firm tofu, drained and pressed

Produce

5 medium yellow onions

1 large white onion

3 heads garlic

1 large carrot

2 celery stalks

3 cups spinach

8 ounces mushrooms

1 lemon

2 limes

1 bunch cilantro

1 jalapeño

3 red bell peppers

½ cup chopped baby spinach

4 cups any dark leafy greens

Dried Herbs and Spices

Bay leaves

Black pepper

Chili powder

Cumin

Garlic powder

Nutritional yeast

Onion powder

Oregano

Paprika

Red pepper flakes

Salt

Turmeric

Condiments and Baking Needs

Ketchup or mayonnaise

Olive oil

Nuts and Seeds

Ground flaxseed

Beans and Other Canned Goods

1 (30-ounce) jar nopalitos

2 (32-ounce) cartons vegetable broth

1 (16-ounce) jar tomatillo salsa

5 (15.5-ounce) cans black beans

1 (15.5-ounce) can pinto beans

1 (15.5-ounce) can chickpeas

1 (15.5-ounce) can kidney beans

1 (15-ounce) jar enchilada sauce

1 (14-ounce) can fire-roasted crushed tomatoes

3 (14.5-ounce) cans diced tomatoes

1 (6-ounce) can tomato paste

1 pound dried brown or black lentils

Whole Grains and Pastas

Corn tortillas (6-inch)

Frozen

Frozen corn

COOKING PLAN

Cut all the vegetables:

- Dice 8 garlic cloves
- Mince 8 garlic cloves
- Chop 2 celery stalks
- Chop 1 ½ cups mushrooms
- Dice 4 yellow onions
- Dice 1 yellow onion
- Chop 1 large carrot
- Chop ½ cup fresh cilantro
- Chop ½ cup baby spinach
- Seed and dice 1 jalapeño
- Finely dice ½ red bell pepper
- Dice 2 red bell peppers

Preheat the oven to 375°F.

Assemble the **Mushroom Black Bean Burgers** by following the recipe instructions and freezing.

Assemble the **Creamy Enchilada Casserole** and set aside. Prepare the **Eggless "Egg" Cups**. Place both in the oven and bake for 30–35 minutes.

While they cook, follow the instructions for the **Life-Giving Lentil Soup** recipe. While that is simmering, follow the recipe for the **3-Bean Chili** using your Instant Pot. Once the two recipes are done, allow to cool.

While they cool, follow the **Sopa de Nopalitos** recipe, then allow to cool. Transfer the three soups to storage containers and freeze. Allow the casserole to cool completely, wrap tightly in foil, and freeze. Place the egg cups in an airtight container or bag and freeze.

Another day is done, and you have at least 30 more servings ready for the freezer! Mix up a mocktail and relax.

APPENDIX II

First-Week-Home Meal Plan

This First-Week-Home Meal Plan offers a sample meal plan, including a grocery list, for what to eat the first week after your baby is born. This grocery list can even be ordered on your way home from the hospital! Many of the meals listed below will (hopefully) come from your already-stocked freezer, while also incorporating a few fresh ingredients to support your healing. We've also included plant-based options for every recipe.

Here's why we chose these particular recipes for our sample meal plan:

- **Breakfast:** Oats are a fiber-filled breakfast option to make those post-delivery bowel movements a little smoother. They may also help to support your developing milk supply. Make your overnight oats in one large batch, and divide it into four containers for a grab-and-go breakfast option. Egg or vegan burritos can be heated straight from the freezer for a protein-packed and savory start to your morning.

- **Lunch:** We want to focus on filling you up and keeping you full with high-protein and high-fiber lunches. Beef and beans are also good sources of iron, which can help replenish your iron stores that may have been lost during delivery.

- **Dinner:** Soup! Comforting, warm, and relaxing. . . need we say more?

- **Snack 1:** These snacks will help you reach your increased calorie needs during the acute recovery phase. We've planned a smoothie for each of your days during this first week to ensure you're taking in a high amount of the antioxidant vitamin C to support the healing process.

- **Snack 2:** This trail mix is a healthier option than most store-bought varieties and an easy way to satisfy the nonstop hunger you'll feel as you deal with round-the-clock feedings! We intentionally selected nuts and seeds that are high in vitamin E, which you need about 20% more of when breastfeeding and is an essential antioxidant to help your body recover.

- **Sipping:** Choose either a sweet or savory option (or both!) to help you reach your increased hydration needs. Either option will provide water, sodium, and potassium.

MEALS FROM THE FREEZER:
- Egg or Vegan Breakfast Burritos (pages 84 and 87)
- Ironclad Beef Stew or Life-Giving Lentil Soup (pages 74 and 73)
- Mediterranean Turkey or Mushroom Black Bean Burgers (pages 82 and 81)
- White Bean Chicken Chili (page 70)
- Homemade Chicken or Vegetable Broth (pages 65 and 66)

QUICK MEALS TO MAKE WHEN YOU GET HOME:
- Mateo's Minestrone (page 146)
- Cherry Cheesecake Overnight Oats (page 104)
- Tuna and Chickpea or Chickpea Toona Salad (pages 119 and 190)
- Electrolyte Replenisher (page 234)
- Midnight Trail Mix (page 195)

MAKE EACH DAY:
- Green Goddess Smoothie (page 217)
- Cherry Antioxidant Smoothie (page 223)

	DAY 1	DAY 2	DAY 3	DAY 4	DAY 5	DAY 6	DAY 7
BREAKFAST	Cherry Cheesecake Overnight Oats	Egg or Vegan Breakfast Burritos	Cherry Cheesecake Overnight Oats	Egg or Vegan Breakfast Burritos	Cherry Cheesecake Overnight Oats	Egg or Vegan Breakfast Burritos	Cherry Cheesecake Overnight Oats
LUNCH	Ironclad Beef Stew or Life-Giving Lentil Soup + bagged salad	Mediterranean Turkey or Mushroom Black Bean Burgers + bagged salad	Ironclad Beef Stew or Life-Giving Lentil Soup + bagged salad	Mediterranean Turkey or Mushroom Black Bean Burgers + bagged salad	White Bean Chicken Chili	Tuna and Chickpea Salad or Chickpea Toona Salad	Takeout
DINNER	White Bean Chicken Chili	Mateo's Minestrone	White Bean Chicken Chili	Mateo's Minestrone	Takeout	Mateo's Minestrone	Tuna and Chickpea Salad or Chickpea Toona Salad
SNACK 1	Cherry Antioxidant Smoothie	Iron Infuser	Cherry Antioxidant Smoothie	Iron Infuser	Cherry Antioxidant Smoothie	Iron Infuser	Cherry Antioxidant Smoothie
SNACK 2	Midnight Trail Mix	Midnight Trail Mix	Midnight Trail Mix	Midnight Trail Mix	Midnight Trail Mix	Midnight Trail Mix	Midnight Trail Mix
SIPPING	Electrolyte Replenisher or Homemade Chicken or Vegetable Broth	Electrolyte Replenisher or Homemade Chicken or Vegetable Broth	Electrolyte Replenisher or Homemade Chicken or Vegetable Broth	Electrolyte Replenisher or Homemade Chicken or Vegetable Broth	Electrolyte Replenisher or Homemade Chicken or Vegetable Broth	Electrolyte Replenisher or Homemade Chicken or Vegetable Broth	Electrolyte Replenisher or Homemade Chicken or Vegetable Broth

Shopping List (Omnivore)

If you've already stocked your freezer using the plan on page 59, just pick up the items listed here, and you'll have everything you need to get through the week!

Meat and Dairy

1 carton unsweetened milk of choice

1 pint Greek yogurt

Produce

4 bagged salads

3 garlic cloves

2 medium carrots

2 celery stalks

1 medium onion

1 green onion

1 small lemon

½ teaspoon grated fresh ginger

2 tablespoons lime juice

1 lemon

1 quart potassium-rich juice (such as pomegranate, orange, or pineapple juice)

1 pint orange juice

Dried Herbs and Spices

Bay leaves

Dried parsley

Italian seasoning

Condiments and Baking Needs

Maple syrup

Vanilla extract

Beans and Other Canned Goods

2 quarts coconut water

4 cups seltzer

1 (32-ounce) carton vegetable broth

1 (28-ounce) diced or crushed tomatoes

1 (15-ounce) can chickpeas

1 (15-ounce) can kidney beans

1 (15-ounce) can chickpeas

1 (5-ounce) can tuna

Nuts and Seeds

Hemp seeds

Chia seeds

Raisins

Almonds

Cashews

Sunflower seeds

Pumpkin seeds

Chocolate chips or chopped dark chocolate

Whole Grains and Pastas

Whole-wheat bread or tortillas

1 canister rolled oats

Frozen

1 bag frozen cherries

1 bag frozen mango

1 bag frozen spinach or kale

1 bag frozen corn

1 bag frozen pineapple

1 bag frozen green beans

Shopping List (Plant-Based)

If you've already stocked your freezer using the plan on page 59, just pick up the items listed here, and you'll have everything you need to get through the week!

Soy and Non-Dairy

1 (64-ounce) carton unsweetened milk of choice

1 pint plant-based Greek yogurt

Produce

4 bagged salads

Fresh ginger

1 medium onion

1 lemon

1 lime

1 quart potassium-rich juice (such as pomegranate, orange, or pineapple juice)

1 pint orange juice

Condiments and Baking Needs

Maple syrup

Vegan mayonnaise

Vanilla extract

Beans and Other Canned Goods

2 quarts coconut water

4 cups seltzer

1 (2-ounce) jar capers

Nuts and Seeds

Hemp seeds

Chia seeds

Raisins

Almonds

Cashews

Sunflower seeds

Pumpkin seeds

Chocolate chips or chopped dark chocolate

Whole Grains and Pastas

1 canister rolled oats

Frozen

1 bag frozen cherries

1 bag frozen mango

1 small container dark leafy greens (such as spinach or kale), fresh or frozen

1 bag frozen pineapple

1 bag frozen green beans

APPENDIX III

Sample Weekly Meal Plan

This sample meal plan works for any week. It includes a mixture of recipes from all of our chapters, including both frozen meals and freshly prepared recipes. As in the other appendices, we've included plant-based options for every recipe and grocery lists for both the plant-based and omnivore options. To simplify feeding yourself and your family, use the meal plan we've created:

- One breakfast freezer meal (Apple Cider Oatmeal Bread, page 92)
- One to two make-ahead breakfasts (Green Eggs and Ham Cups or Eggless "Egg" Cups, pages 95 and 96; Banana Bread Baked Pancakes, page 100)
- Two lunch/dinner freezer meals (BeaBea's Lasagna, page 62; Creamy Enchilada Casserole, page 69)
- Two pantry meals (Grandma's Tomato Soup and Grilled Cheese, page 174; Fancified Frozen Pizza, page 187)
- Two freshly made recipes (Thai Peanut Chicken Salad, page 132; Sheet-Pan Steak Fajitas, page 156)
- Two takeout options

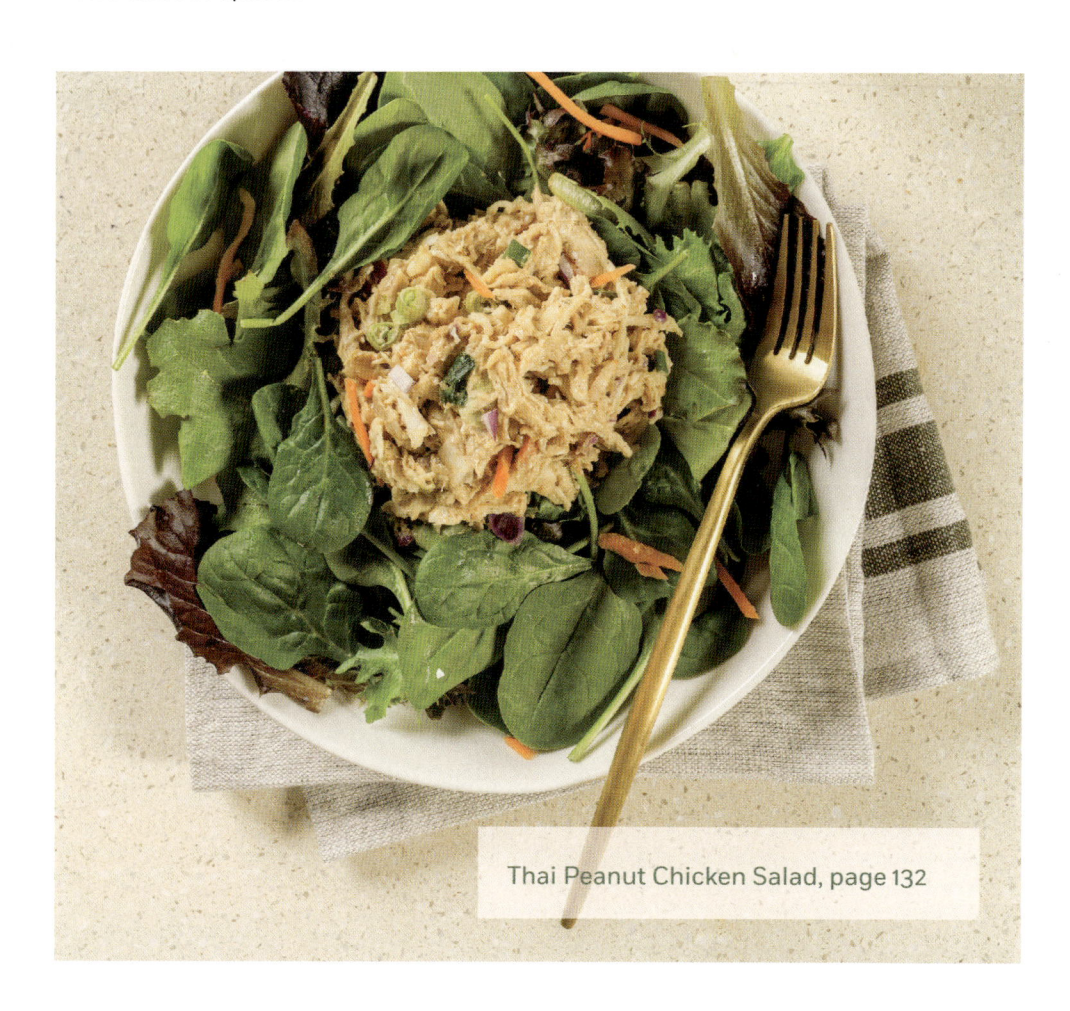

Thai Peanut Chicken Salad, page 132

	MONDAY	TUESDAY	WEDNESDAY	THURSDAY	FRIDAY	SATURDAY	SUNDAY
BREAKFAST	Apple Cider Oatmeal Bread **and** Green Eggs and Ham Cups or Eggless "Egg" Cups	Banana Bread Baked Pancakes	Apple Cider Oatmeal Bread **and** Green Eggs and Ham Cups or Eggless "Egg" Cups	Banana Bread Baked Pancakes	Apple Cider Oatmeal Bread **and** Green Eggs and Ham Cups or Eggless "Egg" Cups	Banana Bread Baked Pancakes	Apple Cider Oatmeal Bread **and** Green Eggs and Ham Cups or Eggless "Egg" Cups
LUNCH	Thai Peanut Chicken Salad	Creamy Enchilada Casserole	Sheet-Pan Steak Fajitas	Creamy Enchilada Casserole	Thai Peanut Chicken Salad	Creamy Enchilada Casserole	Takeout
DINNER	BeaBea's Lasagna	Sheet-Pan Steak Fajitas	Thai Peanut Chicken Salad	BeaBea's Lasagna	Grandma's Tomato Soup and Grilled Cheese	Takeout	Fancified Frozen Pizza

APPENDIX III: SAMPLE WEEKLY MEAL PLAN

Shopping List (Omnivore)

If you've already stocked your freezer using the plan on page 59, just pick up the items listed here, and you'll have everything you need to get through the week!

Meat and Dairy

4 ounces ham steak, deli ham, or pancetta

2 (1-ounce) slices white cheddar cheese

2 large chicken breasts (or 3 cups frozen shredded chicken)

1 pound skirt or flank steak

12 eggs

1 carton unsweetened milk of choice

Produce

4 green onions

3 bananas

3 cups fresh spinach

2 green bell peppers

2 red bell peppers

1–2 garlic cloves

1 large onion

1 bunch cilantro

1 small shallot

1 (12-ounce) bag coleslaw mix

Dried Herbs and Spices

Black pepper

Cinnamon

Chili powder

Coriander

Cumin

Garlic powder

Italian seasoning

Nutmeg

Onion powder

Salt

Condiments and Baking Needs

Baking powder

Creamy peanut butter

Maple syrup

Nonstick cooking spray

Olive oil

Rice wine vinegar

Sesame oil

Soy sauce, tamari, or coconut aminos

Beans and Other Canned Goods

1 (32-ounce) carton chicken or vegetable broth

1 (15.5-ounce) can cannellini or Great Northern beans

1 (14.5-ounce) can pureed or diced tomatoes

1 (4.6-ounce) tube or 1 (6-ounce) can tomato paste

Nuts and Seeds

Hemp seeds

Walnuts

Whole Grains and Pastas

8 (6-inch) flour or corn tortillas

1 canister rolled oats

2 slices whole-wheat bread

Frozen

1 (11-inch) frozen pizza

Frozen pepper-onion mix

1 bag frozen spinach

Shopping List (Plant-Based)

If you've already stocked your freezer using the plan on page 59, just pick up the items listed here, and you'll have everything you need to get through the week!

Soy and Non-Dairy

2 (1-ounce) slices vegan white cheddar cheese

3 (15-ounce) blocks extra-firm tofu

Produce

4 green onions

3 green bell peppers

3 bananas

2 red bell peppers

2 large onions

1 bunch cilantro

1 (12-ounce) bag coleslaw mix

1–2 garlic cloves

1 small container baby spinach

Dried Herbs and Spices

Black pepper

Chili powder

Cinnamon

Cumin

Coriander

Garlic powder

Italian seasoning

Nutmeg

Nutritional yeast

Onion powder

Salt

Turmeric

Condiments and Baking Needs

Baking powder

Creamy peanut butter

Maple syrup

Nonstick cooking spray

Olive oil

Rice wine vinegar

Sesame oil

Soy sauce, tamari, or coconut aminos

Beans and Other Canned Goods

1 (14.5-ounce) can pureed or diced tomatoes

1 (15.5-ounce) can cannellini or Great Northern beans

1 (32-ounce) carton vegetable broth

1 (4.6-ounce) tube or 1 (6-ounce) can tomato paste

Nuts and Seeds

Walnuts

Hemp seeds

Flaxseed

Whole Grains and Pasta

2 slices whole-wheat bread

8 (6-inch) flour or corn tortillas

1 canister rolled oats

Frozen

1 (11-inch) frozen pizza

1 bag frozen pepper-onion mix

1 bag frozen spinach

Index

Page numbers appearing in *italic* type contain images. The letter *t* following a page number denotes a table.

A

Abu's Sleepy Time Mocktail, *244–245*
air fryer recipes, *76–77*, *84–85*, 143
alcohol, 32
American College of Obstetrics and Gynecology, 7, 32
American Gastroenterological Association, 16
amino acids, *10–11*, 18
anti-inflammatory recipes
  breakfast, 96
  dessert, *202–203*
  drinks, *222–223*, 228
  soup, *180–181*
  tofu, 179
antioxidant defense network, 20, 22–23
antioxidant-rich recipes
  breakfast, 96, *98–99*, *106–107*, 198
  dinner, chicken, *152–153*
  drinks, *222–223*, 229
  sandwich, *128–129*
  snacks and desserts, *194–195*, 198, *206–207*, 211
  soup, *180–181*
Apple Cider Oatmeal Bread, *92–93*
appliances, kitchen, 41, 45

B

Baby Caesar Salad Wrap, 123
Baked Blueberry Oatmeal, *106–107*
Baked French Toast, *110–111*
Baked Sweet Potato Hash, 113
Banana Bread Baked Pancakes, *100–101*
BeaBea's Lasagna, *62–63*
Beef Stew, Ironclad, *74–75*
Berry Nojito, *240–241*
beta-carotene, 9, 20
Beta-Carotene Brownies, *202–203*
beta-carotene-rich recipes
  breakfast, *98–99*, 113
  brownies, *202–203*
  drinks, *214–217*
  lasagna, *62–63*
Blender Blueberry Muffins, 97
Bread, Apple Cider Oatmeal, *92–93*

breakfast
  bread and baked goods, *92–93*, *100–101*, *110*–112
  burritos, 84–87
  chia seed pudding, 105
  egg-based, *84–85*, *94–95*, *102–103*
  hash, 113
  muffins, *88–89*, 97–99
  oats-based, 104, *106–107*
  savory, 96, *108–109*, 112, *114–115*
breastfeeding
  galactagogues, 26
  and hydration, 31–32
  lactation process, 10–11
  nutrient needs for, 14t
  recipes (drinks) that may support, *222–223*, *230*–231, 234, *236–237*
  recipes (food) that may support, *88–89*, *110*–111, *208–209*
breast tissue, 4–5
Brewed Fennel Tea, 234
Broth, Homemade Chicken, *64–65*
Broth, Homemade Vegetable, 66
Brownies, Beta-Carotene, *202–203*
BTLT: BBQ Tempeh, Lettuce, and Tomato, *130*–131
Buffalo Tofu Wrap, *136–137*
Burgers, Mediterranean Turkey, *82–83*
Burgers, Mushroom Black Bean, *80–81*
burritos
  breakfast, 84–87
  shredded beef, 170
Butter Bean French Onion Soup, *180–181*
Butternut Squash Soup, *160–161*
B vitamins. *See* vitamin B complex

C

caffeine, 32
calcium
  as an electrolyte, 31
  increased need for during pregnancy, 4, 6
  overview, 24–25
  for postpartum recovery, 36–37t
  in various types of milk, 57
  Vitamin D role in absorption of, 23–24
calcium-rich recipes
  drinks and smoothies, *214–215*, *222–223*, *230*–231
  pasta, *162–163*

tofu, *154–155*
calories, 9, 14t, 15–16, 36–37t
carbohydrate-rich recipes, *62–63*, *114–115*, 126
carbohydrates, 11, 14t, 15–16, 36–37t
cardiovascular system, 3–4, 5
Cherry Antioxidant Smoothie, *222–223*
Chia Seed Pudding, Creamy, 105
Chicken, Pressure Cooker Cashew, 158
Chicken and Rice, Spanish, 159
Chicken Barley Stew, 151
Chicken Broth, Homemade, *64–65*
Chicken Drumsticks with Crispy Polenta, 143
Chicken or the Egg Salad, 127
Chicken Quinoa Bake, Creamy, 142
Chicken Salad, Pesto, 122
Chicken Salad, Thai Peanut, *132–133*
Chickpea Toona Salad, 190
Chili, 3-Bean, 150
Chili, White Bean Chicken, *70–71*
Chocolate Chip Cookie Dough, Edible, *200–201*
Chocolate Mousse, Iron-Filled, 199
Chocolate Tahini Milkshake, *214–215*
Chocolate Truffle Bites, 211
cholesterol, 33
choline, 14t, 25, 36–37t
choline-rich recipes
  breakfast, *84–85*, *94–95*, *102*–103
  salad, *118*–119
  turkey burgers, *82–83*
cold foods, 34
collagen
  overview, 17–18
  for postpartum recovery, 9, 47
  recipes supporting production of, *74–75*, *80–81*, *100–101*, *148–149*
  supplements, 18
  and vitamin C, 22, 47
  and zinc, 29
community support for meal planning, 51–52
Congee Bowl, Savory, *114–115*
cookies and bars, *196–197*, *200–203*, *208–209*
Creamy Chia Seed Pudding, 105
Creamy Chicken Quinoa Bake, 142
Creamy Enchilada Casserole, *68*–69
Creamy Pesto Pasta, *172–173*
Creamy Tomato-Feta Pasta Bake, *162–163*
Curried Lentils with Kale and Cauliflower, *148–149*
Curry in a Hurry, 179
Customizable Tofu Wrap, 126

D
Daycare Defender Smoothie, *214–215*
desserts, 199, *204–205*, 211
Dietary Guidelines for Americans, 16, 24
digestive system, 4–5
drink recipes
  atole, *236–237*
  electrolyte replenisher, 234
  horchata, *230–231*
  mocktails, *226–229*, *232–233*, 235, *238–241*, *244–245*
  smoothies, *214–223*
  tea, 234, *242–243*

E
Edible Chocolate Chip Cookie Dough, *200–201*
Egg Breakfast Burritos, *84–85*
Eggless "Egg" Cups, 96
Eggs, Pizza, *102–103*
Eggs and Ham Cups, Green, *94–95*
Electrolyte Replenisher, 234
electrolyte-rich foods, *64–65*, 150, 228, 234
electrolytes, 31
Elevated PB&J Sandwich, *124–125*
emotional impacts of pregnancy and childbirth, 6, 7–8, 10
Enchilada Casserole, Creamy, *68*–69
endocrine system, 5–6
Energy Balls (3 Ways), *206–207*

F
fact or fiction
  biotin supplements, 21
  caffeine and alcohol, 32
  cold foods, 34
  collagen supplements, 18
  galactagogues, 26
  placentophagia, 28
family involvement in meal planning, 50–51
Fancified Frozen Pizza, 187
fat, 10–11, 18–20, 23–24. *See also* omega-3s
fiber, 16, 33, 36–37t
fiber-rich recipes
  bread and muffins, *88–89*, *92–93*, *98–99*
  breakfast, *84–85*, *105–107*, *113–115*
  chili, *70–71*, 150
  dinner, 142, *148–149*, *152–155*
  drinks and smoothies, *216–217*, *226–227*, *232–233*, *238–239*
  freezer meals, *68–69*, *80–81*, *84–85*, *88–89*
  pantry meals, *168–169*, *172–173*, *182–185*

271

salads, *118–121*, 190
sandwiches, *124–126*
snacks and desserts, 198, *206–209*, 211
soup, *176–177*, 191
stew, 151
Fish and Chips, Sheet-Pan, *140–141*
flax egg, recipes using, *88–89*, *92–93*, *98–101*, *106–107*, *208–209*
folate, 21–22, 36–37t. *See also* vitamin B complex
food storage supplies, 41
fourth trimester, *8–10*
freezer meals
  preparation and storage, 45–48
  recipes, breakfast, 84–89
  recipes, broth, *64–66*
  recipes, casserole, *62–63*, *68–69*
  recipes, dinner, *67–68*, *70–75*, *80–83*
  recipes, meat, *76–79*
  recipes, sauce, *60–61*
  vitamin C boost, 56
French Toast, Baked, *110–111*
French Toast, Savory Baked, 112
Frito-less Taco Salad, *120–121*
Frozen Strawberry-Lime Mock-a-Rita, *232–233*

G

Gaia's Greek Yogurt Bowl, 198
galactagogues, 26. *See also* breastfeeding
gestational diabetes mellitus, 32–33
glucose, 10–11, 15, 32–33
gluten-free option, 56
  breakfast, 84–87, *92–93*, *98–99*
  freezer meals, *62–63*, *67–68*, *76–78*
  pantry meals, *184–185*, *188–189*
  sandwiches and wraps, *123–126*, *130–131*, *136–137*, 171, *174–175*
  soup, *146–147*, *174–175*, *180–181*
  stew, 151
Grandma's Tomato Soup and Grilled Cheese, *174–175*
Greek Yogurt Bowl, Gaia's, 198
Green Eggs and Ham Cups, *94–95*
Green Goddess Smoothie, *216–217*

H

hair loss, 9
heart, 3–4
heart-healthy recipes, 151, *168–169*
Homemade Chicken Broth, *64–65*
Homemade Vegetable Broth, 66
Horchata, Titi Rita's, *230–231*

hormones
  and the endocrine system, 6
  insulin, 15, 32–33
  and placentophagia, 28
  during postpartum recovery, 8–9
  prolactin, 234
  protein role in, 17
  thyroid, 26
hydrating recipes
  broth, *64–66*
  chili, 150
  drinks and smoothies, *222–223*, 228, 235, *240–241*
  soup, *176–177*
hydration, 30–31

I

ice cream alternative, *204–205*
inflammation, 8–9, 20, 22. *See also* anti-inflammatory recipes
Instant Pot recipes
  breakfast, *114–115*
  broth, *64–66*
  chili, 150
  meat-based, 79, *158–159*, *170–171*
  stew, *74–75*, 151
insulin, 15, 32–33
iodine, 14t, 26–27, 36–37t
iodine-rich stew recipe, *164–165*
iron
  calcium role in absorption of, 218
  increased need for during pregnancy, 3–4
  overview, 27, 29
  and placentophagia, 28
  for postpartum recovery, 14t, 36–37t
  vitamin C role in absorption of, 22, 29
Ironclad Beef Stew, *74–75*
Iron-Filled Chocolate Mousse, 199
Iron Infuser, 218
iron-rich recipes
  breakfast, *86–87*
  freezer meals, *62–63*, *67–68*, *76–78*
  pantry meals, 170, *188–189*
  plant-based, *72–73*, *148–149*, *154–155*
  smoothie, 218
  snacks and desserts, 199, *202–203*
  spaghetti sauce, *60–61*
  stew, *74–75*
It's a Girl! Smoothie, *220–221*

K
kitchen tools and appliances, 41, 45

L
labor and delivery, impacts of, 6–7
lactation. See breastfeeding
Lactation Cookies (3 Ways), 40, 208–209
Lasagna, BeaBea's, 62–63
Lentil Soup, Life-Giving, 72–73
Lentil Spaghetti Sauce, 61
Lentils with Kale and Cauliflower, Curried, 148–149
Linguine alla Vongole, 188–189

M
Mac and Cheese, Upgraded Boxed, 178
magnesium, 31, 36–37t
magnesium-rich recipes, 191, 234, 244–245
make it gluten-free. See gluten-free option
make it nut-free. See nut-free option
make it plant-based. See plant-based option
Mama's Mule, 228
Maple Pistachio Oatmeal Muffins, 88–89
Mateo's Minestrone, 146–147
Ma! The Meatloaf!, 67
meal planning, 45–48, 49t, 50–52
Meat, Shredded (3 Ways), 79
Meatballs, Mighty Miles's (3 Ways), 76–78
Meatloaf!, Ma! The, 67
Mediterranean Turkey Burgers, 82–83
mental and emotional impacts of childbirth, 6–10
Mexican Atole, 236–237
Midnight Trail Mix, 194–195
Midwife Mix-Up, 220
Mighty Miles's Meatballs (3 Ways), 76–78
Milkshake, Chocolate Tahini, 214–215
milk supply. See breastfeeding
milk varieties, 57
Minestrone, Mateo's, 146–147
Mix-and-Match Savory Snacks, 210
Mocha Mama Smoothie, 219
Mock-a-Rita, Frozen Strawberry-Lime, 232–233
mocktail recipes, 226–229, 232–233, 235, 238–241, 244–245
Mom's Spaghetti Sauce, 60
Moroccan Chicken, Chickpeas, and Sweet Potatoes, 152–153
Muffins, Blender Blueberry, 97
Muffins, Pumpkin Chocolate Chip, 98–99
Mule, Mama's, 228, 244–245

musculoskeletal system, 5–6
Mushroom Black Bean Burgers, 80–81
My Little Pumpkin Smoothie, 216–217

N
Nana's Aynar Spiced Tea, 242–243
nesting party, 52
Nice Cream (4 Ways), Sugar, Spice, and Everything, 204–205
nut-free option, 56
  breakfast, 92–93, 100–101, 104, 106–107
  muffins, 88–89
  sandwich, 124–125
  smoothie, 220
  snacks and desserts, 194–197, 200–203
  tofu, 154–155
nutrient needs for postpartum recovery, 14t, 36–37t

O
oats, recipes using, 88–89, 92–93, 106–107
omega-3s
  overview, 18–20
  for postpartum recovery, 10, 14t, 36–37t
omega-3s, recipes rich in
  breakfast, 88–89, 105, 108–109
  cookies, 208–209
  salad, 118–119, 134–135
  salmon, 108–109, 186
  shrimp, 144–145
Omega-Boosting Salmon Salad, 134–135
One-Pan Shrimp Boil, 144–145
Oven Black Bean Quesadillas, 184–185
Overnight Oats (3 Ways), 104

P
pantry essentials, 42–43
pasta
  meals using, 62–63, 162–163, 168–169, 172–173, 188–189
  sauce recipes for, 60–61
  in soup, 146–147
Pasta, Spinach Artichoke, 168–169
Pasta Bake, Creamy Tomato-Feta, 162–163
Peanut BBT (Broccoli, Brussels, and Tofu), 154–155
Pesto Chicken Salad, 122
Piña Colada, (She Ain't a) Virgin, 226–227
Pizza, Fancified Frozen, 187
Pizza Eggs, 102–103

placenta
  as an endocrine gland, 6
  delivery of, 7–8
  development in pregnancy, 3
  placentophagia, 28
plant-based option, 56
  cheese alternative, 62–63, 162–163, 168–169, 174–175, 178, 180–181
  egg alternative, 106–107
  meat alternative, 70–71, 114–115, 120–121, 132–133, 142, 144–145, 151, 164–165, 170, 178
  milk alternative, 222–223
  yogurt alternative, 105, 198, 220–221
plant-based recipes
  black bean burgers, 80–81
  breakfast, 86–87
  broth, 66
  chili, 150
  lentils, 61, 72–73, 148–149
  salad, 190
  sandwiches and wraps, 128–131, 136–137
  soup, 72–73
Pomegranate Fizz, 229
Pop's Rice Krispies Treats, 196–197
postpartum depression, 9–10, 19, 24
postpartum recovery, 7–10, 14t, 36–37t
potassium, 31
potassium-rich recipes
  chili, 150
  drinks, 228–229, 234
  snacks and desserts, 204–205
  tofu, 154–155
preeclampsia, 25, 33
pregnancy impacts on body, 3–6
Pressure Cooker Cashew Chicken, 158
probiotic-rich spritzer recipe, 235
probiotics, 16
prolactin, 234
protein
  adding to meals, 51, 56
  increased need for during pregnancy, 3, 6
  overview, 17–18
  for postpartum recovery, 9, 14t, 36–37t
  role in lactation, 11
  in various types of milk, 57
protein add options, 56
  breads and muffins, 88–89, 92–93, 97–99
  breakfast, 100–101, 104, 106–107
  broth, 64–66
  pantry meals, 182–183, 187–189
  salad, 190
  sandwiches and wraps, 123, 128–129, 136–137

soup, 146–147, 160–161, 191
protein-rich recipes
  breakfast, 84–87, 94–96, 108–115
  casserole, 62–63, 68–69
  drinks and smoothies, 216–217, 219–221
  meat-based, 60, 70–71, 76–79, 82–83, 142, 152–153, 156–158
  plant-based, 61, 72–73, 80–81, 148–150, 154–155, 172–173, 184–185
  salad, 118–122
  sandwiches and wraps, 124–126, 130–131, 171
  snacks and desserts, 198, 206–210
  soup, 72–73, 176–177, 180–181
  spaghetti sauce, 60–61
  stew, 74–75
Pudding, Creamy Chia Seed, 105
Pulled BBQ Pork Sandwich, 171
Pumpkin Chocolate Chip Muffins, 98–99
Pumpkin Smoothie, My Little, 216–217

Q
Quesadillas, Oven Black Bean, 184–185

R
Rainbow Hummus Sub, 128–129
Ramen Noodle Soup, 176–177
recovery stages, 8–10
respiratory system, 4–5
rice, recipes using, 114–115, 159, 182–183
Rice Krispies Treats, Pop's, 196–197

S
salad recipes
  Caesar, 123
  chicken, 122, 127, 132–133
  chickpea, 118–119, 190
  egg, 127
  salmon, 134–135
  taco, 120–121
  tuna, 118–119
Salmon and Veggies, Teriyaki, 186
sample weeklong menu, 49t
sandwich recipes
  BTLT: BBQ Tempeh, Lettuce, and Tomato, 130–131
  Elevated PB&J Sandwich, 124–125
  Grilled Cheese, 174–175
  Pulled BBQ Pork Sandwich, 171
  Rainbow Hummus Sub, 128–129
Sassy Spritzer, 235

Savory Baked French Toast, 112
Savory Congee Bowl, 114–115
seafood recipes, 108–109, 118–119, 134–135, 140–141, 176–177, 186
Seaweed Stew (Miyeok Guk), 164–165
Sheet-Pan Fish and Chips, 140–141
Sheet-Pan Steak Fajitas, 156–157
Shredded Beef Tacos, 170
Shredded Meat (3 Ways), 79
Shrimp Boil, One-Pan, 144–145
sleep disruption, 8–9
Smoked Salmon Spread, 108–109
smoothies
   Cherry Antioxidant Smoothie, 222–223
   Daycare Defender Smoothie, 214–215
   Green Goddess Smoothie, 216–217
   Iron Infuser, 218
   It's a Girl! Smoothie, 220–221
   Midwife Mix-Up Smoothie, 220
   Mocha Mama Smoothie, 219
   My Little Pumpkin Smoothie, 216–217
   Tata's Morir Soñando, 222–223
   Smooth Move Mocktail, 238–239
snacks, 194–195, 198, 206–207, 210
soup recipes
   Butter Bean French Onion Soup, 180–181
   Butternut Squash Soup, 160–161
   Grandma's Tomato Soup, 174–175
   Life-Giving Lentil Soup, 72–73
   Mateo's Minestrone, 146–147
   Ramen Noodle Soup, 176–177
   Sopa de Nopalitos, 191
Spaghetti Sauce, Lentil, 61
Spaghetti Sauce, Mom's, 60
Spinach Artichoke Pasta, 168–169
staple ingredients, 42–43
Steak Fajitas, Sheet-Pan, 156–157
stew recipes
   Chicken Barley Stew, 151
   Ironclad Beef Stew, 74–75
   Seaweed Stew (Miyeok Guk), 164–165
Strawberry-Lime Mock-a-Rita, Frozen, 232–233
Sugar, Spice, and Everything Nice Cream (4 Ways), 204–205
Summer Shandy, 235
supplements
   biotin, 21
   calcium, 25
   choline, 25
   collagen, 18
   docosahexaenoic acid (DHA), 19–20
   iron, 27
   prenatal vitamins, 13
   probiotic, 16
   vitamin B12, 22
   vitamin D, 24
   zinc, 29
Sweet Potato Hash, Baked, 113

T
Tata's Morir Soñando, 222–223
Tea, Brewed Fennel, 234
Tea, Nana's Aynar Spiced, 242–243
Teriyaki Salmon and Veggies, 186
Thai Peanut Chicken Salad, 132–133
Three Bean (3-Bean) Chili, 150
thyroid, 26–27
Titi Rita's Horchata, 230–231
tofu, recipes using, 86–87, 96, 126, 136–137, 154–155, 172–173, 176–177, 179, 199
Trail Mix, Midnight, 194–195
triglycerides, 11, 33
Tuna and Chickpea Salad, 118–119
Turkey Burgers, Mediterranean, 82–83

U
Upgraded Boxed Mac and Cheese, 178
uterus, 7, 9

V
Vegan Breakfast Burritos, 86–87
Vegetable Broth, Homemade, 66
vegetarian. See plant-based option; plant-based recipes
Veggie Fried Rice, 182–183
Virgin Piña Colada, (She Ain't a), 226–227. See also mocktail recipes
vitamin A, 14t, 20–21, 36–37t
vitamin A-rich recipes, 67–68, 113, 154–155, 160–161
vitamin B complex, 21–22, 36–37t
vitamin B complex-rich recipes, 67–68, 82–83, 140–141, 150, 171, 200–201
vitamin C
   degradation during cooking, 47–48
   and iron, 29
   overview, 22–23
   for postpartum recovery, 9, 14t, 36–37t
   recipes requiring a boost of (See freezer meals)

vitamin C-rich recipes
  drinks and smoothies, *214–215*, 218, *222–223*,
    228–229, *232–233*
  meals, *154–155*, *172–173*, *182–183*, 191
vitamin D, 9, 23–24, 36–37t
vitamin E, 23, 36–37t
vitamin E-rich recipes, *194–195*, *206–207*

W

water, 30–31. *See also* hydrating recipes
Watermelon Lime Cooler, 228
White Bean Chicken Chili, *70–71*
wrap recipes
  Baby Caesar Salad Wrap, 123
  Buffalo Tofu Wrap, *136–137*
  Customizable Tofu Wrap, 126

Z

zinc
  overview, 29
  for postpartum recovery, 8–9, 14t, 36–37t
  role in collagen production, 17–18, 22
zinc-rich recipes, *80–81*, *100–101*, *148–149*, 171

Acknowledgments

Writing a cookbook is a deliciously challenging project. We are grateful to everyone who has contributed to making this book a reality.

First and foremost, we want to thank our husbands, Andrew and Eric, for their unwavering support during this process. From watching the boys during hours of early morning Zoom calls to endless recipe testing, we could not have accomplished this without you.

To our families, we owe you so much. Your encouragement and confidence in us has allowed us to dream big and pursue our goals. Our love of food started in your homes and will now be shared with many more.

A heartfelt thanks to Blue Star Press and the entire publishing team, whose guidance helped us turn this book from an idea into a comprehensive resource. We appreciate your hard work and everything you did to support this project.

Last but not least, to the postpartum women who will use these recipes to help their incredible bodies recover. You deserve to prioritize your health, too. We hope you enjoy these recipes and that they bring joy to your families' tables.

With love,
DIANA AND ASHLEY

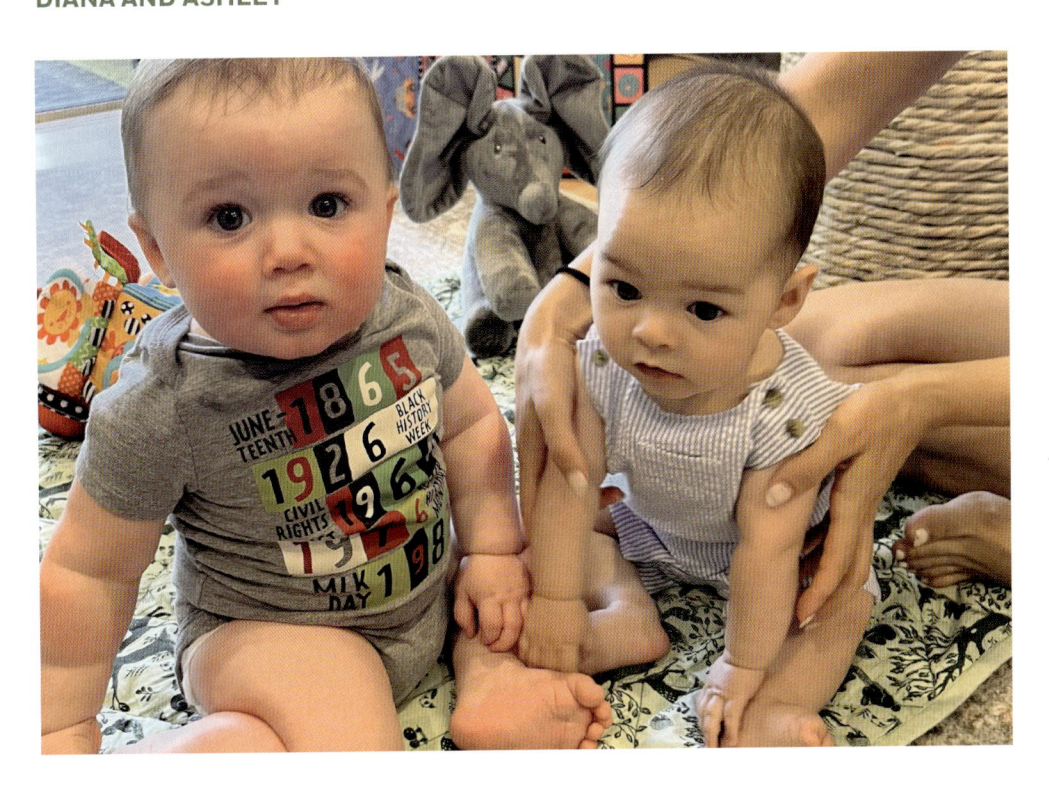

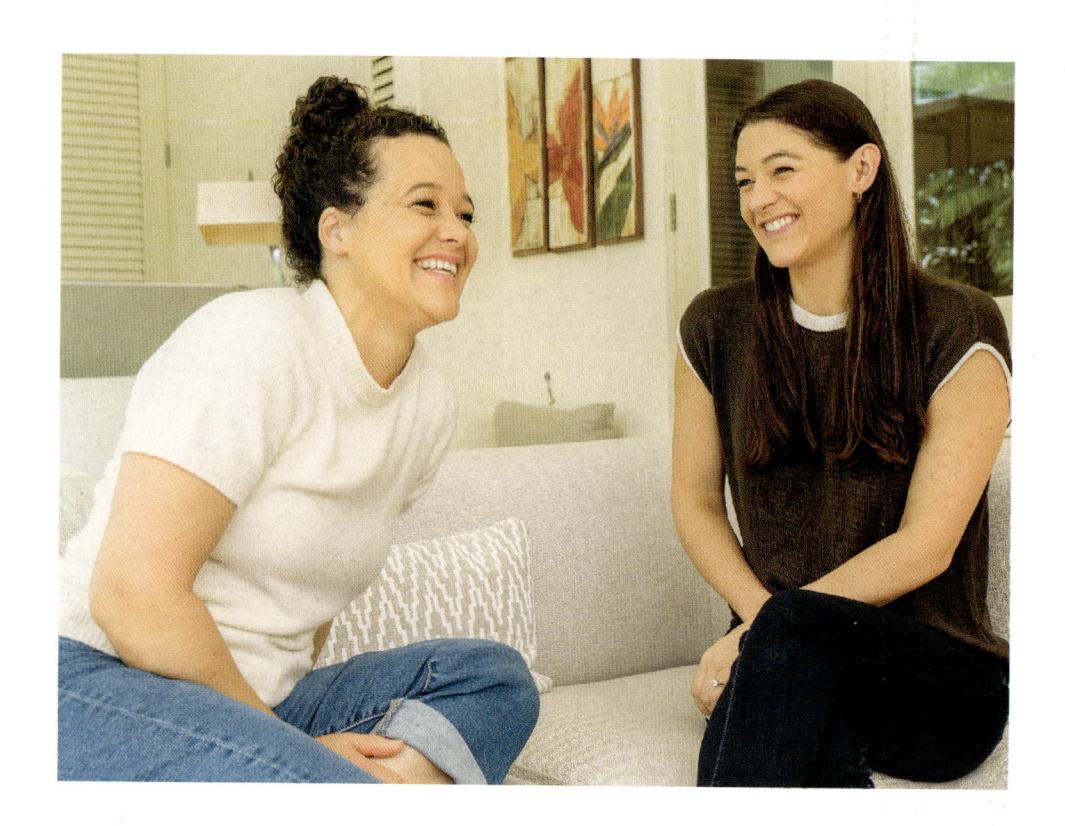

About the Authors

Diana Licalzi is a registered dietitian and cookbook author originally from Guaynabo, Puerto Rico. She currently resides in London, England, with her husband, Andrew, and son, Mateo. She received her education and dietetics training from Villanova University, Tufts University, and UC San Diego Health. In addition to postpartum nutrition, Diana specializes in diabetes management. She runs the Type 2 Diabetes Revolution, an online platform that counsels individuals on how to adopt nutrition and lifestyle modifications to treat prediabetes and type 2 diabetes. Diana has authored several cookbooks, including *Drinking for Two*, *Mocktail Party*, and *The Type 2 Diabetes Revolution*.

Ashley Reaver is a registered dietitian and cookbook author. Originally from Emmitsburg, Maryland, she currently resides in Los Gatos, California, with her husband, Eric, and son, Miles. She received her education and dietetics training from Cornell University, Tufts University, and California State Polytechnic University, Pomona. Ashley combines her expertise in nutrition and dietetics as a lecturer at the University of California, Berkeley, where she educates future dietitians and shares her passion for cooking. Ashley also owns a private nutrition counseling practice, guiding clients toward balanced lifestyles that help them reach their health and performance goals. In addition to postpartum nutrition, she specializes in cholesterol management.